M000206747

We are committed to the notion that our most vulnerable population should have access to the best and most current evidence-based care. From the moment we took on this project, this book has been a labor of love. The entire process has been punctuated with extreme highs and lows. Throughout it all, we enjoyed incredible support from our families, friends, and colleagues. Sadly, in 2013, we lost two of our most faithful and constant supporters: Kimberly Holmes (Linda's daughter) and Estelle Drozdz (Sandi's mother). Our book is dedicated to their memory. These two amazing women never met, but both demonstrated remarkable strength in their lives. We are forever in their debt.

Contents

Acknowledgments

No project this big can be accomplished alone. We are fortunate to have had the support of those closest to us as we worked to bring this book to completion. Deepest gratitude goes to our families for allowing us the time to work on this project. We'd also like to acknowledge the many professional colleagues whose work continues to inspire us and our elderly patients who have motivated us. Finally, we wish to thank Victor Van Beuren, the acquisitions editor from the American Diabetes Association for planting the seed for this book. Without his kind and gentle support over the past few years, this project would not have been possible.

List of Contributors

VOLUME EDITORS

Sandra Drozdz Burke, PhD, ANP-BC, CDE, FAADE
Clinical Associate Professor
UIC College of Nursing at Urbana
Urbana, IL

Linda B. Haas, PhC, RN, CDE
Diabetes Consultant
Burien, WA
Clinical Assistant Professor
University of Washington, Seattle, WA

CONTRIBUTORS

Charlene S. Aaron, PhD, RN
Assistant Professor
Illinois State University
Normal, IL

Debbie Hinnen, APN, BC-ADM, CDE, FAAN, FAADE
Director of Education Services
Mid-America Diabetes Associates
Wichita, KS

Naushira Pandya, MD, CMD, FACP
Professor and Chair
Department of Geriatrics
Director Geriatrics Education Center
Nova Southeastern University College of Osteopathic Medicine
Davie, FL

Meenakshi Patel, MD, FACP, MMM, CMD
Associate Professor
Wright State University
Director of Geriatrics
Miami Valley Hospital
Dayton, OH

Laurie Quinn, PhD, RN, APN, CDE, FAAN
Clinical Associate Professor
Department of Biobehavioral Health Science
College of Nursing
University of Illinois at Chicago
Chicago, IL

Elizabeth Quintana, EdD, RD, LD, CDE
Clinical Associate
West Virginia University
School of Medicine
Section of Endocrinology
Morgantown, WV

Jeffrey M. Robbins, DPM
Director, Podiatry Service VACO
Louis Stokes Cleveland, VAMC
Cleveland, OH

Professor, Podiatric Medicine
Kent State University College of Podiatric Medicine
Independence, OH

Clinical Assistant Professor
Case Western University School of Medicine
Department of Surgery
Cleveland, OH

Katie Sikma, BSN, RN
Staff Nurse
Riverside Medical Center
Cardiac Intensive Care Unit
Kankakee, IL

Carrie Swift, MS, RD, BC-ADM, CDE
Certified Diabetes Educator and
    Registered Dietitian
Kadlec Regional Medical Center
Richland, WA

Ann Wagle, PhD, RN, NEA-BC
Green House Project Educator
Education and Research
Department of Veterans Affairs
Danville, IL

Meghan Warren, PT, MPH, PhD
Associate Professor
Department of Physical Therapy and
    Athletic Training
Northern Arizona University
Flagstaff, AZ

Ann S. Williams, PhD, RN
Research Associate Professor
Case Western Reserve University
Frances Payne Bolton School of Nursing
Cleveland, OH

Donald K. Zettervall, RPH, CDE
National Director, Diabetes Management
    Strategies
Sanofi, US
Bridgewater, NJ

1

Introduction

Linda B. Haas, PhC, RN, CDE, and Sandra Drozdz Burke, PhD, APN, CDE, FAADE

INTRODUCTION

The older adult population is growing rapidly in the U.S.[1] In fact, 10,000 baby boomers are turning 65 years old every day. At the same time, the prevalence of diabetes, particularly type 2 diabetes (T2D), is surging. An estimated number of ~26 million Americans now have this chronic, often-debilitating disease and an additional 79 million have a condition known as "prediabetes," which predisposes them to develop T2D.[2] The dual epidemics of diabetes and aging in the U.S. are coming together and are about to strike a blow in tsunami-like fashion. Certainly, most of the baby-boom population will not be admitted to long-term care (LTC) facilities on their 65th birthday, but clinicians already are seeing the impact of diabetes in LTC facilities. The prevalence of diabetes in skilled nursing facilities (SNFs) has been reported to range from 22 to 33%,[3,4] with the prevalence being highest in non-Caucasians.[5] Put another way, SNFs now have 1,462,000 occupied beds.[6] If current estimates of diabetes in this population are accurate, then one in every three or four beds is occupied by someone with diabetes. Overall, caring for residents in LTC facilities, particularly in the SNF, is becoming increasingly complex, and residents with diabetes account for one of the most complex populations in these facilities.

Undoubtedly, this high prevalence of diabetes and its complexity already represents a major problem for clinicians, and the issues related to care of the resident with diabetes will continue to take center stage for some time to come. Experts estimate there will be a 4.5-fold increase in the number of people with diabetes ≥65 years old by 2050.[7] Three trends are thought to contribute to the increased prevalence of diabetes in the elderly. First is the aging of the general population. Diabetes often is called a disease of aging, and it is clear that the age-group with the highest prevalence of diabetes is elders ≥65 years old.[2] Second is the increasing incidence of diabetes in all age-groups, but particularly in the 54- to 64-year-old age-group. This population most likely will be residents of LTC in the not too distant future. Finally, people with diabetes are living longer after being diagnosed and even after developing long-term complications of diabetes,[8] as well as other diseases and conditions associated with aging, including geriatric syndromes.[9]

As clinicians prepare to deal with diabetes in the older adult population, it is important to consider various aspects of aging as well as the health care environment. Living arrangements for the older adult population range from living independently to long-term residence in an institutional care facility. Older adults can utilize LTC in their homes, in senior centers, at community centers,

DOI: 10.2337/9781580404730.01

at adult day care centers, or in special retirement or assisted-living facilities. According to the Health Insurance Association of America, nearly 1.4 million individuals receive home health services and ~745,000 older adults live in continuing care retirement communities. More than 1.1 million seniors live in some type of senior housing community in the United States. More than 150,000 individuals receive care and services at an adult day center and nearly a million more live in assisted-living residences. In 2012, the majority of the older adult population continued to live independently; only ~3% of the population >65 years old resided in SNFs.[1]

As the U.S. population ages, the younger old initially will make up the vast majority of older adults. This population may need nursing care assistance following hospitalization, but for the most part, even those with diabetes will continue to live independently. Conversely, the oldest old are much more likely to be living in the LTC environment. The oldest old represent the fastest growing, and the most frail, segment of the older adult population.[1] For this reason, this book focuses on care in the nursing home or SNF. The SNF resident with diabetes is likely to be very old, frail, vulnerable, and require complex care.

COMPLEXITY OF CARE

Diabetes care is complex for many reasons. Over the past two decades, many changes have been made in the number and types of medications available for diabetes management; the nutritional recommendations for people with diabetes have undergone several revisions; and guidelines for management of diabetes, particularly in the elderly, have been inconsistent and confusing.[10-14] Other, less obvious reasons for the complexity of care are that residents with long-term diabetes are more likely to have visual impairments and have higher rates of both kidney failure and cardiovascular disease[15] than residents without diabetes. Residents with known diabetes also have higher rates of depression, falls,[16] functional impairment, dependency, and dementia[17,18] than residents without diabetes.

Residents with diabetes in SNF have more:

- depression
- falls
- functional impairment
- dependency
- dementia

As a result of these complexities, residents with diabetes consume more resources, including time, than do other residents. In 2012, for example, nursing home costs for residents with diabetes were estimated at $12 billion, with 80% of those costs going to residents who were ≥65 years of age.[19] Overall, the cost of care for residents with diabetes was twice that of residents without diabetes.

Adding to the complexity of diabetes management in the older adult is the diversity of the disease in this population. Some residents will have diabetes on admission and others will develop diabetes during their stay in a SNF. LTC clinicians and staff need to be alert to the possibility of diabetes in all SNF residents as there is a high rate of newly diagnosed diabetes in this population.[20] In fact, to identify new onset disease, some experts recommend that all residents be screened at admission and yearly thereafter. Residents with known or long-standing diabetes already may have chronic complications, such as neuropathy, diabetic kidney disease, or visual impairment. Furthermore, diabetes in the older adult often is accompanied by other comorbidities, as well as geriatric syndromes, each of which requires attention.

CONFUSING TIMES

It seems that considerable variation in care coordination and delivery exists within the LTC setting. The primary intent of this book was to present evidence in each chapter so that administrators, providers, and all staff would have a single resource to use when developing policies, procedures, and plans for the care of residents with diabetes. To the extent possible, that has been done. Unfortunately, there is a need for considerably more research. To date, the elderly with diabetes, particularly those >75 years of age and those with multiple comorbidities are seldom included in large randomized controlled trials.[3,21,22] In recent publications that address diabetes management in older adults, however, the experts have attempted to generalize existing evidence to older adults in LTC.[3,22–24] In many of the areas addressed in this book, expert opinion has been the source of guidelines presented. Where applicable, these guidelines have been included in chapters. Each clinician remains responsible for interpreting these expert guidelines relative to the clinical setting and the individual resident with diabetes. Numerous studies specific to LTC have been descriptive in nature. Several authors have included these studies in their chapters, and thus readers can compare their own settings and evaluate whether the authors' recommendations are applicable to the readers' setting. Unfortunately, few studies linked the descriptions or processes to outcomes.[4] Administrators and clinicians, however, may be able to translate the guidelines into practice and link these to outcomes. The International Diabetes Federation (IDF) Guideline may be particularly helpful in this endeavor, as it identifies outcomes that can be used in quality improvement projects.[22] The book also may be a reference to diabetes specialists to assist staff in LTC facilities to monitor processes, implement indicated changes, monitor progress of these changes, evaluate the changes, and revise if indicated.

Each chapter in this book addresses a specific topic or issue important in the management of diabetes. Each chapter stands alone as a resource or reference. The book can be used as a tool to help health care workers engaged in practice at the SNF level to evaluate their settings, determine whether changes are needed, and identify methods to make changes. This book also is a resource for diabetes experts who need to expand their understanding of the older adult in SNF settings. Greater knowledge in this area can enable consultants to assist SNF staff to make any changes they deem necessary to improve the quality of diabetes care provided. The editors have attempted to emphasize or summarize salient points and identify resources to facilitate use of the book.

In developing plans of care for residents with diabetes, the heterogeneity of this population should be kept in mind and care should be individualized, considering life expectancy, comorbidities and geriatric syndromes, unique nutrition issues, activity needs, and functional and cognitive status. Although setting glycemic targets is flexible, premeal hyperglycemia (glucose levels >200 mg/dl) and hypoglycemia (glucose levels <70 mg/dl) at any time, should be avoided. Residents and families, where appropriate, should be included in the development, implementation, and revisions of care plans.[3,18,21] Although each setting is unique and each resident is an individual, some principles are applicable to all settings and all individual residents with diabetes. Ultimately, although caring for residents with diabetes can be challenging, it is our hope that this book will facilitate LTC staff to develop processes of care that will enable appropriate, safe, and cost-effective care for LTC residents with diabetes and provide a rewarding environment for LTC staff.

REFERENCES

1. Administration on Aging (AoA). *A Profile of Older Americans: 2012.* Washington, DC, U.S. Department of Health and Human Services, 2012, p. 1–16. Available from http://www.aoa.gov/AoARoot/Aging_Statistics/Profile/2012/docs/2012profile.pdf. Accessed 12 February 2014.
2. Centers for Disease Control and Prevention. *National Diabetes Fact Sheet: National estimates and general information on diabetes and pre-diabetes in the United States, 2011.* Atlanta, GA, Centers for Disease Control and Prevention, 2011, p. 1–12. Available from http://www.cdc.gov/diabetes/pubs/pdf/ndfs_2011.pdf. Accessed 12 February 2014.
3. Kirkman MS, Briscoe VJ, Clark N, et al. Diabetes in older adults. *Diabetes Care* 2012;35:1–15.
4. Garcia TJ, Brown SA. Diabetes management in the nursing home: A systematic review of the literature. *The Diabetes Educator* 2011;37(2):167–187.
5. Resnick HE, Heineman J, Stone R, Shorr RI. Diabetes in U.S. nursing homes, 2004. *Diabetes Care* 2008;31:287–288.
6. Jones AL, Dwyer LL, Bercovitz AR, Strahan GW. The National Nursing Home Survey: 2004 overview. National Center for Health Statistics. Vital Health Stat 13(167). 2009. Available from http://www.cdc.gov/nchs/data/series/sr_13/sr13_167.pdf. Accessed 12 February 2014.
7. Narayan KM, Boyle JP, Geiss LS, Saaddine JB, Thompson TJ. Impact of recent increase in incidence on future diabetes burden: U.S., 2005–2050. *Diabetes Care* 2006;29:2114–2116.
8. Hayes AJ, Leal J, Gray AM, Holman RR, Clark PM. UKPDS Outcomes Model 2: a new version of a model to simulate lifetimes outcomes of patients with type 2 diabetes mellitus using data from the 30 year United Kingdom Prospective Diabetes Study: UKPDS 82. *Diabetologia* 2013;56:1925–1933.
9. Cigolle CT, Langa KM, Kabeto MU, Tian Z, Blaum CS. Geriatric conditions and disability: The Health and Retirement Study. *Annals of Internal Medicine* 2007;147:156–164.

10. American Diabetes Association. Standards of medical care in diabetes—2013. *Diabetes Care* 2013;36(Suppl1):S11–S66.
11. American Geriatrics Society Expert Panel on the Care of Older Adults with Multimorbidity. (2012). Guiding Principles for the Care of Older Adults with Multimorbidity: An Approach for Clinicians. *Journal of the American Geriatrics Society, 60*(10), E1-E25. doi: 10.1111/j.1532-5415.2012.04188.x
12. American Medical Directors Association. *Guidelines for diabetes management in the long-term care setting.* Columbia, MD, Author, 2010.
13. Brown AF, Mangione CM, Saliba D, Sarkisian CA, California Healthcare Foundation/American Geriatrics Society Panel on Improving Care for Older Persons with Diabetes. Guidelines for improving the care of the older person with diabetes mellitus. *Journal of the American Geriatric Society* 2003;51(5):S265–S280.
14. Sinclair AJ, Paolisso G, Castro M, Bourdel-Marchasson I, Gadsby R, Rodriguez Mañas L. European diabetes working party for older people 2011 clinical guidelines for type 2 diabetes mellitus. Executive summary. *Diabetes and metabolism* 2011;37(Suppl3)(0):S27–S38.
15. Zhang X, Decker FH, Luo H, et al. Trends in the prevalence and comorbidities of diabetes mellitus among nursing home residents in the United States: 1995-2004. *Journal of the American Geriatrics Society* 2010;58(4):724–730.
16. Maurer MS, Burcham J, Cheng H. Diabetes mellitus is associated with an increased risk of falls in elderly residents of a long-term care facility. *Journals of Gerontology Series A: Biological Sciences and Medical Sciences* 2005;60(9):1157–1162.
17. Morley JE. Diabetes and aging: Epidemiologic overview. *Clinics in Geriatric Medicine* 2008;24:395–405.
18. Gadsby R, Barker P, Sinclair AJ. People living with diabetes resident in nursing homes—assessing levels of disability and nursing needs. *Diabetic Medicine* 2011;28:778–780.
19. American Diabetes Association. Economic costs of diabetes in the U.S. in 2012. *Diabetes Care* 2013;36(4):1033–1046.
20. Sinclair AJ, Paolisso G, Castro M, Bourdel-Marchasson I, Gadsby R, Manas L, R. European diabetes working party for older people 2011 clinical guidelines for type 2 diabetes mellitus. Executive summary. *Diabetes and Metabolism* 2011;37:S27–S38.
21. Abdelhafiz AH, Sinclair AJ. Hypoglycaemia in residential care homes. *British Journal of General Practice* 2009;59:49–50.
22. Sinclair AJ, Dunning T, Colagiuri S, IDF Working Group. *International Diabetes Federation—managing older people with type 2 diabetes: Global guideline.* 1st ed. Brussels, Belgium, International Diabetes Federation, 2013.
23. American Diabetes Association. Standards of medical care diabetes—2014. *Diabetes Care* 2014;37(Suppl1):S14–S80.
24. Moreno G, Mangione CM, Kimbro L, Vaisberg E, American Geriatrics Society Expert Panel on the Care of Older Adults with Diabetes Mellitus. *Guidelines for improving the care of older adults with diabetes mellitus.* 2nd ed. New York, American Geriatrics Society, 2013. Available at www.GeriatricsCareOnline.org. Accessed 14 January 2014.

2

The Medical Director's Viewpoint

Naushira Pandya, MD, CMD, FACP and Meenakshi Patel, MD, FACP, MMM, CMD

INTRODUCTION

Patients with diabetes constitute some of the most medically complex patients in nursing facilities. They usually have existing macro- and microvascular complications and are prone to frequent infections, cardiovascular events, injurious falls, electrolyte disturbances, cognitive impairment, weight fluctuations, and hypoglycemia. They have a greater degree of functional impairment and dependence and constitute some of the "heaviest care" patients in the facility.[1]

The challenges of managing diabetes in long-term care (LTC) may be characterized as attributable to resident and disease, institution, staff and practitioner, and medication management factors.[2] These factors are displayed in Table 2.1. To address some of these challenges or to minimize their impact requires engagement of the medical director as well as his or her clinical, administrative, communication, and interpersonal skills. In addition, a working knowledge of the regulations regarding processes of care and monitoring is valuable.

Institutional Factors

Nurse managers or facility champions who are engaged in improving diabetes care, implementing any protocols, or training first-line caregivers are crucial individuals for the success of any care process in the LTC setting.[3] Staff turnover is a major issue because the benefits of staff development for registered nurses (RNs), licensed practical nurses (LPNs), and certified nursing assistants (CNAs) will be diminished as staff members leave the facility. According to the 2004 National Nursing Home Survey, the annualized staff turnover rate was highest among CNAs at 74.5%, followed by RNs at 56.1%, and LPN/LVNs at 51%.[3] The tenure of the director of nursing (usually the lead clinician in the facility), the RN hours per patient day, and the CNA hours per patient day were associated with lower turnover and higher staff retention rates.[4] High staff turnover and frequent changes to patient–resident assignments become problematic because they result in a lack of familiarity with residents as well as in a failure to recognize unmet needs and atypical symptoms of hypoglycemia, especially in those with dementia or delirium.

Many nursing facilities continue to offer restricted diets, such as "no concentrated sweets," and the "1,800 calorie ADA diet," to residents with diabetes despite recommendations from the American Diabetes Association,[5] the American Medical Director's Association,[6] and the Academy of Nutrition and

DOI: 10.2337/9781580404730.02

Table 2.1 Sources of Challenges in Managing Diabetes in LTC

Resident and disease	Institution	Staff and practitioner	Medication management
Altered pharmacokinetics and pharmacodynamics	Staff turnover and lack of familiarity with residents	Knowledge deficits (disease, complications, selection and modification of therapies)	Multiple and changing treatment approaches
Increased risk of hypoglycemia	Restricted dietary practices	Lack of team communication (hyperglycemia, glucose excursions)	Reliance on potentially dangerous sliding-scale insulin protocols
Irregular meal consumption	Inadequate review of glucose logs	Therapeutic pessimism	Inappropriate dosing or timing of insulin
Cognitive dysfunction and depression	Lack of facility–specific diabetes treatment algorithms	Failure to individualize care (A1C, BP, lipids)	Hypoglycemia management (delayed recognition or overcorrection)
Psychological insulin resistance (individual opposition to starting or taking insulin)	Lack of established blood glucose parameters for physician/provider notification	Failure of timely and stepwise rational advances in therapy	Lack of comfort with newer insulins and injectable agents, and delivery systems
Impaired vision and manual dexterity			
Greater potential for age related adverse effects and drug interactions			

Source: Adapted from Prandya N. Common clinical conditions in long-term care. In *A pocket guide to long-term care medicine.* Fenstemacher PA, Winn P, Eds. New York, NY,

Dietetics[7] that older adults with diabetes should consume a regular diet. The medical director, in collaboration with a staff or consulting dietitian, can have a significant influence in formulating facility policies regarding special diets and the specific clinical situations in which they should be offered. Chapter 7 provides more specific details on the nutritional recommendations for LTC residents with diabetes.

Unlike in the outpatient setting in which diabetes patients are seen every 3–4 months, and blood glucose logs or glucose meters may not be available to the clinician, practitioners in LTC are positioned uniquely to manage diabetes well. Except possibly in rural settings, practitioners often visit their LTC facilities on a weekly or biweekly basis. Residents in these settings get regular (often too many!) blood glucose checks and these are documented on a flow chart. Consequently, nursing staff are able to notify practitioners in a timely manner if hypoglycemic episodes occur, glucose levels show increased fluctuations, or the patient experiences a change of condition. Clinicians then are able to examine glucose logs (flow charts), clinically assess the resident, and make targeted changes to the therapeutic regimen instead of having to rely on inadequate information for empiric changes.

Pertinent Point

Practitioners in SNF have an opportunity to manage diabetes well if they have:

- Regular and documented glucose monitoring
- Readable glucose logs that can facilitate glycemic management

---

Unfortunately, in the current environment, practitioners do not always examine glucose logs to assess trends and often give excessive importance to A1C levels or blood glucose values from serum chemistry profiles. Moreover, the manner in which capillary blood glucose values commonly are documented makes an analytical review of glucose trends prohibitive. Currently, practice standards require documentation of blood glucose levels, along with the insulin dose, injection site, and the nurse's initials on the Medication Administration Record (MAR). This information is documented in tiny cells on a single page for an entire month. Identifying the resident's blood glucose trends from such a form is not practical. The medical director could work with the director of nursing to create and implement a more functional glucose log that includes blood glucose parameters for notifying the resident's provider. Such care processes have been described in detail in the American Medical Director's Association Clinical Practice Guideline on the Management of Diabetes in the Long-Term Setting, last revised in 2010.[6] Figure 2.1 illustrates an example of a glucose log that could be adopted by a facility. Many facilities, however, now are adopting electronic health record systems, which do display blood glucose values in a clear manner and also allow these values to be trended and analyzed.

Assessment of Facility Management of Diabetes

Successful implementation of facility-wide diabetes evaluation, treatment, and monitoring protocols is possible if there is support from the administration and if there is effective education of, and communication with, practitioners, nursing staff, and medical assistants in the LTC facility. The role of each discipline should be defined and a "diabetes nurse" or champion could ensure the implementation of any protocols that are created.

One way to determine the need for a comprehensive diabetes protocol is to conduct a facility-wide quality improvement program. The medical director and director of nursing could select one or more outcome or process indicators (Table 2.2) and review all patients with diabetes in the facility with regard to

Patient Name: _____   **Month:**_____

Residence/Room #:_____   **Physician:**_____

Notify clinician if—

-Blood glucose is <70 and unresponsive

-Blood glucose is <70 on two occasions

-Blood glucose is >250 with new medical symptoms

-Blood glucose is >300 during all or part of 2 days

Date	Fasting/prebreakfast			Prelunch			Predinner			Prebedtime		
	Blood glucose	Insulin type & dose	Initial	Blood glucose	Insulin type & dose	Initial	Blood glucose	Insulin type & dose	Initial	Blood glucose	Insulin type & dose	Initial
1												
2												
3												
4												
5												
6												
7												
8												
9												
10												
11												
12												
13												
14												
15												

Figure 2.1 Sample Diabetes Management/Glucose Log.

Table 2.2 Examples of Process and Outcome Measures

Process indicators	Outcome indicators
Appropriate decision-making and care planning based on individual patient goals	Average A1C levels
Appropriate diet orders	Prevalence of hypoglycemia and symptomatic hyperglycemia
Limited prevalence of sliding-scale insulin use	Rate of hospitalizations and emergency-room visits for complications related to poor glucose control
Consistency of basal, bolus, and correction insulin use	Rate of lower extremity amputations, infections, and ulcers
Appropriate monitoring (e.g., A1C, lipid profile, and albumin–creatinine ratio, if clinically appropriate)	
Appropriate number of evaluations for eye, nutritional, and foot problems	

Source: Adapted from American Medical Directors Association. *Clinical practice guideline; Management of diabetes in the long-term setting.* Columbia, MD:AMDA, 2008, revised 2010. p. 38. Reprinted with permission from the publisher.

performance in the selected criteria. These data then would be shared with all department heads and relevant staff at a quality assurance–improvement meeting. Examining such data, brainstorming collectively, and following trends on a regular basis can be a powerful driving force to improve the care of residents with diabetes and achieve mutually defined goals.[6]

KNOWLEDGE BARRIERS AND ATTITUDES

The knowledge base of diabetes and its complications, therapeutic options, and drug delivery systems is growing constantly. This presents a challenge for all health care providers involved in the LTC setting. In particular, the LPNs and RNs who are the primary clinicians may have received their professional training many years prior and therefore may be unaware of current guidelines, protocols, and treatment recommendations for diabetes management. Although staff development is required in all nursing facilities, scheduling of in-service training programs often conflicts with patient care responsibilities, making it difficult to reach staff on all shifts on any given subject. In-service programs tend to be brief and competency based. In practice, therefore, it is not unusual to see confusion related to insulin types and brands, which also is not surprising given that product names are so similar. Confusion about insulin, however, can result in a rapid-acting insulin analog being administered 30 minutes before a meal (too early) or a long-acting basal analog being inappropriately withheld when a morning blood glucose level is lower than desired.

Most facilities have an open-staff model, which has its merits, but also has the inherent problem that each practitioner has different attitudes and beliefs about managing diabetes. This variability among providers makes diabetes management confusing for the caregiving staff. In practice, inconsistent protocols will affect the resident's glycemic control and A1C goals, affect the facility thresholds for reporting very high or very low glucose levels, and may result in therapeutic inertia with regard to timely use of insulin, the frequency of glucose monitoring, and willingness to address staff concerns and questions. These factors cannot all be regulated by policies and procedures, but the medical director can facilitate the development and implementation of basic policies and procedures that ensure a level of caregiver competence that results in enhanced patient safety. Examples of such policies and procedures might include the following:

■ Hypoglycemia management
■ Practitioner notification parameters for hypoglycemia or hyperglycemia
■ Practitioner notification criteria for other related acute changes of condition
■ Policies to minimize the use of sliding-scale insulin (SSI)

Communication

According to U.S. federal regulations, the medical director of the nursing home is responsible for implementing medical care policies and coordinating medical care in the facility.[8] It therefore is clear that effective communication is of paramount importance to overcome the challenges associated with diabetes management in the long-term care facility. Changes in practice often are difficult. When, however, the director of nursing, the administrator, and the medical director have a mutual agreement on the priorities and the issues that need to be addressed, it is easier for nurses and direct care staff as well as other professionals to implement changes and comply with new policies. Systems rarely are perfect. When new policies and procedures are implemented, a process must be in place for direct caregivers to provide feedback to the administrators. As well, the administrators should devise a process for evaluating the effectiveness of the practice changes. In effect, successful implementation of any new policy requires the surveillance needed for quality control. Additionally, given the challenges of the open staff model, the relationship between the medical director and other practitioners, as well as open noncumbersome modes of communication, will make it easier to communicate new priorities and implement change.

Critical Point

Collaboration of Medical Directors, Directors of Nursing, and a Diabetes Champion (with administration support) can bring about change to improve diabetes management.

Collaboration with the Pharmacist

In the LTC setting, one of the most important relationships is the one developed between the consultant pharmacist and the medical director. Together they can effect change in several disease processes. In diabetes, specifically, the consultant pharmacist can play an important role in assisting the resident's primary care provider achieve established metabolic goals. Although the resident's primary provider will determine the goals of treatment for the individual resident, a discussion and mutual understanding of factors determining the "tightness" of control and evidence pertaining to frail elders would be helpful to both professionals.

Consultant pharmacists can review charts and glucose logs to monitor glucose excursions, and monitor blood pressure (BP) readings to see whether the BP is controlled adequately. Laboratory values such as A1C, urine microalbumin, and serum lipid profile results can be reviewed and recommendations to obtain a needed lab test can be made. When lab results are outside of the target range, the consultant pharmacist can recommend (to the provider) appropriate changes in the treatment plan. The pharmacist also can review the medication list for potential drug–drug and drug–disease interactions—for example, recommending an alternative to a thiazolidinedione in a resident with New York Heart Association Class III or IV heart failure, or a substitution for metformin in someone with Stage 4 chronic kidney disease. The pharmacist would also review whether appropriate medications have been prescribed for other conditions. For example, residents with renal insufficiency or albuminuria may need an angiotensin-converting enzyme inhibitor or an angiotensin receptor blocker to protect renal function, and someone with uncontrolled BP may need an additional antihypertensive.

Importantly, the pharmacists can review the use of SSI in the facility. They can assist the medical director in effecting change in the management practices of the attending provider by making recommendations to change from SSI to scheduled insulin and by educating nursing staff. In facilities with an in-house pharmacist, the pharmacist can even become the diabetes champion for the facility.

Sliding-Scale Insulin

The high prevalence and persistent use of SSI is inconsistent with the American Medical Director's Association guideline as well as current recommendations from the American Diabetes Association. Additional studies are needed to evaluate outcomes associated with prolonged SSI use in LTC facilities.[9] The following practices, although outdated, continue to be used in many LTC facilities and include the persistence of now-discredited SSI protocols without scheduled mealtime insulin or rational adjustment to regimens; the tendency to use one-size-fits-all regimens; and the continued reliance on human insulin, delivered using vial and syringe, despite compelling data supporting the advantages of insulin analogs. Data from a retrospective study reveals that ~70% of the blood glucose results done by finger-stick have no action taken in individuals on SSI.[10] The same SSI regimen may be in effect for several months regardless of blood glucose levels, giving nurses a false sense of security that there is "coverage" for any glucose level and therefore no need to notify the practitioner.

The use of SSI generally depends on frequent blood glucose monitoring. The cost of monitoring blood glucose four times a day includes test strip, lancet, and machine cost and the time involved for the individual performing these tests. There is an additional cost on the resident side with an effect on quality of life in terms of increased pain related to frequent finger-sticks. When SSI is changed to scheduled insulin dosing, blood glucose control improves and the number of finger-sticks done per day can be reduced significantly. Scheduled insulin dosing results in fewer incidences of hypoglycemia and hyperglycemia, and the disease is managed proactively rather than reactively. In short, blood glucose control improves, and the resident enjoys improved quality of life.

FEDERAL REGULATIONS FOR NURSING HOMES

Federal regulations for nursing homes are commonly known as F-tags.[11] Citations for failure to follow regulations can be given at an annual state licensing survey or during a complaint survey, which could occur at any time of the year. Diabetes is linked to several F-tags. Some of the more common regulations are discussed in this section.

F-Tag 309

F-Tag 309[10] pertains to the facility's provision of quality care. It states, "Each resident must receive and the facility must provide the necessary care and services to attain or maintain the highest practicable physical, mental, and psychosocial well-being, in accordance with the comprehensive assessment and plan of care." Residents whose diabetes is not well controlled may have symptoms of hypoglycemia with or without neurological sequelae and hyperglycemia leading to a feeling of malaise, worsening neuropathic pain, worsening wounds, incontinence secondary to polyuria, falls and fractures related to urgency, and frequency of urination secondary to uncontrolled hyperglycemia. Sometimes severe hyperglycemia also can lead to dehydration. In essence, failure to prevent blood glucose extremes represents noncompliance with this regulation.

F-Tag 314

The intent of F-Tag 314[10] is that the facility provides care and services to promote the prevention of all types of wounds, promotes the healing of all types of wounds (including infection), and prevents additional wounds from occurring. Uncontrolled hyperglycemia can delay wound healing.

F-Tag 315

F-Tag 315[10] deals with urinary incontinence. Residents with diabetes are at risk for urinary incontinence, which may be caused by or worsened by the polyuria associated with uncontrolled hyperglycemia.

F-Tag 323

F-Tag 323[10] addresses the prevention of falls. In residents with diabetes, falls may increase secondary to rushing to the bathroom due to the urgency and polyuria, with worsening neuropathy or during periods of hypoglycemia.

F-Tag 329

F-Tag 329[10] pertains to the use of unnecessary medications or inappropriate medication management. With respect to diabetes, this would include prolonged, nonemergency use of the SSI. Use of SSI is a clear violation of F-Tag 329 when it is the only treatment for diabetes for months, with no interventions to start scheduled medication.

F-Tag 501

F-Tag 501,[10] specifying the functions of a medical director, were codified in Title 42 483.75(i)(2). The functions are to implement resident care policies and coordinate medical care in the facility. This includes developing policies for appropriate SSI use and procedures to get residents on scheduled medications and insulin regimens to help to manage their diabetes.

IMPROVED CARE TRANSITIONS

Residents with diabetes often are hospitalized for acute medical problems, including infections, renal failure, and cardiovascular compromise. It is vital that the current medication record accompanies the patient to the acute care setting along with the transfer sheet and other pertinent information, such as the history and physical, the problem list, recent laboratory data, and relevant nursing and practitioner progress notes leading up to the hospital transfer. In the hospital, not uncommonly, an oral regimen is changed to SSI only, or previously scheduled insulin regimens may be changed to SSI and basal insulin. Diligent medication reconciliation is important on readmission to the facility, and most facilities now implement this process to ensure that important medications have not been missed, duplications in therapy are corrected, and medications that are no longer clinically appropriate are discontinued rather than resumed automatically. Medical directors can lead this process by ensuring that appropriate information is sent to and received from referring institutions (discharge summaries, consultations, key test results) and that diabetes treatment regimens are optimized once patients are eating normally and improving clinically.

Avoiding Errors

Critical Point: Exquisite attention to medication reconciliation prevents errors during transitions to and from acute care facilities.

CONCLUSION

The management of diabetes in LTC residents is complex. It is affected by the duration of disease and complications related to diabetes in each resident, institutional culture, practices and protocols, staff and practitioner knowledge, attitudes, and competency, as well constantly changing options for medical management. The medical director has a challenging role in guiding diabetes management in the facility, providing education, and monitoring care processes and outcomes, all the while ensuring that diabetes management is individualized, especially in residents with limited life expectancy. Collaboration with the director of nursing and the support and buy-in of the facility administrator is central to the success of this endeavor.

REFERENCES

1. Travis SS, Buchanan RJ, Wang S, et al. Analyses of nursing home residents with diabetes at admission. *Journal of the American Medical Directors Association* 2004;5:320–327.
2. Pandya N. Common clinical conditions in long-term care. In *A pocket guide to long-term care medicine*. Fenstemacher PA, Winn P, Eds. New York, NY, Humana Press, 2011, p. 75–122.
3. Jones AL, Dwyer LL, Bercovitz AR, Strahan GW. The national nursing home survey: 2004 overview. *Vital Health Stat* 2009;13(167):1–155.
4. Donoghue C. Nursing home staff turnover and retention. An analysis of national level data. *Journal of Applied Gerontology* 2010;29(1):89–106.
5. American Diabetes Association. Standards of medical care in diabetes—2012. *Diabetes Care* 2012;35:S11–S63.
6. American Medical Directors Association. *Clinical practice guideline on the management of diabetes in the long-term setting*. Columbia, MD, AMDA, 2008, revised 2010.
7. Dorner B, Freidrich EK, Posthauer ME. Position paper: The nutritional approach for older adults in health care communities. *Journal of the American Dietetic Association* 2010;110:1549–1553.
8. Levine, JM, Savino F, Siegel F. Introduction to the revised federal guidelines for nursing home medical directors: F-Tag 501. *Annals of Long Term Care* 2008. Available at http://annalsoflongtermcare.com/article/6528. Accessed on 4 March 2012.
9. Pandya N, Thompson S, Sambamoorthi U. The prevalence and persistence of sliding scale insulin use among newly admitted elderly nursing home residents with diabetes mellitus. *Journal of the American Medical Directors Association* 9(9) 663–669, 2008.
10. Pandya N, Wei W, Kilpatrick BS, et al. Burden of sliding scale insulin use in elderly long-term care residents with type 2 diabetes. *J Am Geriatr Soc* 2013;61:2103–2110.
11. Centers for Medicare and Medicaid. Appendix PP. Guidance to surveyors for long term care facilities; Section 483.29. In *State operations manual*. Available from http://www.cms.gov/Regulations-and-Guidance/Guidance/Manuals/Internet-Only-Manuals-IOMs-Items/CMS1201984.html. Accessed 12 February 2014.

3

Diabetes Management in Long-Term Care Settings: Nursing Perspective

Charlene S. Aaron, PhD, RN

INTRODUCTION

Interdisciplinary health care professionals should follow the most current protocols to maintain glycemic control, as well as respond appropriately to glycemic changes. Management of diabetes in the nursing home environment can be challenging for many reasons. The increasing numbers of older adults in nursing homes with diabetes calls for the development of a reference that includes the latest protocols, strategies, and treatment algorithms to guide medical and nursing directors as they set policies for professional staff who care for residents with this complex disease. In the U.S., the American Diabetes Association (ADA), American Geriatric Society (AGS), and American Medical Directors Association (AMDA) all have established guidelines for the treatment of diabetes in older adults, but only the AMDA guidelines are specific to the long-term care setting.[1-5] Two other key resources for the management of diabetes in this vulnerable group are the European-based clinical guideline for type 2 diabetes (T2D) in older people and the recently published global guideline for the management of diabetes in older adults.[6,7]

INDIVIDUALIZING TARGETS

The AMDA Clinical Practice Guideline for Diabetes specifically mentions the need to individualize therapy in nursing home patients. Factors to consider when determining interventions to manage blood glucose levels of nursing home residents include the resident's quality of life, number of comorbidities, duration and severity of diabetes, life expectancy, and, importantly, the resident's preferences.[2] The AGS Clinical Practice Guidelines (CPG) support the notion that clinicians caring for older adults with diabetes must consider individual heterogeneity when determining and prioritizing treatment goals.[8]

Diabetes control commonly is measured with the A1C test. The results indicate glucose control over the previous 2- to 3-month time period.[9] A1C is measured easily using a venous blood sample, but it also can be measured at the point of care with a capillary blood sample. The optimal frequency of A1C measurement in T2D continues to be debated. To identify those with undiagnosed diabetes, the ADA[1] recommends that A1C, oral glucose tolerance, or fasting plasma glucose be tested every 1–3 years in overweight adults or at ≥45 years of age.

DOI: 10.2337/9781580404730.03

Complications are found in persons newly diagnosed with diabetes, according to ADA.[1] Fortunately, complications from T2D can be prevented or delayed in middle-aged clients with lifestyle interventions, and careful monitoring of their labs determines effectiveness of the interventions.[1]

Once diagnosed, glucose control targets are likely to vary according to a number of factors. According to the U.S. Department of Veterans Affairs and the U.S. Department of Defense,[10] elderly people with diabetes who are well-functioning and free of multiple morbidities are best controlled with A1C levels <7 %. Although the ADA recommends a target A1C level of ≤7% for most adults, this target level may be higher or lower depending on the individual.[1] Current evidence from the U.K. Prospective Diabetes Study (UKPDS), which enrolled participants 65 years of age, found microvascular benefits from glycemic control behaviors resulting in decreased mortality and myocardial infarctions framed as "the legacy effect" of glycemic control.[11] Three randomized controlled trials followed the UKPDS, the Action to Control Cardiovascular Risk in Diabetes (ACCORD) trial, the Action in Diabetes and Vascular Disease: Preterax and Diamicron MR Controlled Evaluation (ADVANCE) trial, and the Veterans Affairs Diabetes Trial (VADT). These trials studied the effects of glycemic control in middle-age and older adults with a goal of reducing glucose levels to near-normal levels (A1C 6.0 or 6.5%). In the ACCORD trial, older participants experienced more hypoglycemia and other adverse effects. In the ADVANCE trial, nephropathy was reduced in all participants, regardless of age.[12] In addition, Gao et al.[13] studied community-dwelling older adults and found that those with A1C levels of ≥7% had a high risk of cardiovascular mortality and dementia compared with older adults who had A1C levels <7%. These studies all seem to confirm the uncertainty surrounding the risks and benefits of glycemic control in older adults, especially those with a long history of diabetes or severe hypoglycemia. As a result of an ADA consensus conference to address diabetes management in older adults, which was convened in 2012, an A1C target based on individual characteristics is now recommended (see Chapter 5, Table 5.1).[14]

Overall, the evidence supports the need for individualized targets in the management of diabetes for older adults. Healthy elders in the community may be able to meet the usual adult targets, but identifying the best A1C value for older adults in nursing home environments is likely to be more challenging. Expert opinion supports the need for nursing home residents with diabetes to have variable, but generally higher A1C levels based on their comorbidities,[15] the duration of their diabetes, and their functional status.[14] The recent consensus document by the ADA as well as the European Association for the Study of Diabetes[16] and the AMDA[2] all recommend a target A1C of 7–7.5% or lower for healthy elders, and support an individualized holistic approach in treating hyperglycemia for nursing home residents with diabetes. The AGS[8] also targets an A1C of 7% in healthy elders with good functional ability, but it recommends an A1C of 8% for frail elderly with a life expectancy of <5 years. The 2013 AGS guidelines continue these recommendations.[5] More recently, the European Diabetes Working Party for Older People recommended a target A1C range of 7.6–8.5% for frail patients who are at high risk for glucose extremes.[4] These patients include nursing home residents with multiple comorbidities and those with diminished functional or cognitive capacity. Zarowitz et al.[17] supported the application of evidenced-based principles in managing glucose control in elders in nursing homes by using the ADA-AMDA-AGS treatment goals. A recent consensus panel concluded, however, that the evidence for diabetes management of older adults in long-term care settings is alarmingly thin.[14] At present, all three associations support using a conservative A1C target of 8–8.5% with the rationale of avoiding hypoglycemia in frail elders in the nursing home. To assist the interdisciplinary health care team in meeting the goal of glucose control while avoiding the complication of hypoglycemia, it is important to understand how health care professionals weigh the risks and benefits of applying evidenced-based principles to the development of individualized interventions for institutionalized elderly.

Geriatric Syndromes and Diabetes

Diabetes is associated with an increased prevalence of geriatric syndromes, specifically, functional disabilities, depression, falls, urinary incontinence, malnutrition, and cognitive impairment.[18] Geriatric syndromes not only contribute to loss of independence and decreased quality of life but also complicate the treatment and care of patients with diabetes.[18] Contributing factors to geriatric syndromes include vascular complications, comorbid conditions, and aging in general.[2] It is imperative for interdisciplinary health care professionals to use current and evidence-based guidelines for comprehensive geriatric assessment of geriatric syndromes.[16] The multifactorial nature of diabetes requires a variety of interventions to achieve and maintain glucose control. At a minimum, interventions are directed toward meal planning, activity, medication management, and social and psychological support.[1] To meet the goal of glucose control in the long-term care setting, administrators must ensure that all interdisciplinary team members are competent to meet the needs of elders with diabetes.[19]

Because the presence of geriatric syndromes complicates the management of diabetes, assessment of geriatric syndromes must occur regularly and from a multidisciplinary perspective.[8,18] Older adults with geriatric syndromes and multiple comorbid conditions should have individualized treatment goals to manage their blood glucose.[2,8,17,20] Individualized management of blood glucose in older adults with diabetes requires a holistic approach that addresses age, life expectancy, patient preference, pain, falls, incontinence, polypharmacy, and cognitive impairment.

Certified nursing assistants (CNAs), nurses, activities directors, social workers, and consultants can all be involved in assessing the resident's activities of daily living, instrumental activities of daily living, gait and balance, visual acuity, risk and history of falls, continence status, pain level, and support systems. Cognition and mental state can be assessed periodically using instruments such as the Mini Mental Status Exam and the Beck Depression Inventory. Orthostatic hypotension can be identified by measuring supine and standing blood pressure while the functional ability of the older adult's urinary bladder can be assessed with residual volume measurements.[18] The latter information is useful in planning for individualized ambulation and toileting needs and assisting to identify the root cause of falls in some residents. Because hypoglycemia also can place the resident at risk for falls, knowledge of risk factors such as the ones secondary to geriatric syndromes will help the care team individualize glucose targets and thus provide for a safer clinical environment.

Glucose Control

Elevated blood glucose (hyperglycemia) may be directly responsible for many forms of the geriatric syndrome, including functional disability resulting from general malaise, malnutrition associated with increased protein catabolism, urinary incontinence linked to polyuria, and the cognitive impairment that occurs secondary to significant hyperglycemia. Typical symptoms of hyperglycemia include excessive urination, thirst, fatigue, and dehydration.[1] Importantly, the symptoms of hyperglycemia may be masked in older adults as a result of the normal aging processes or symptoms from other comorbidities. For example, older adults commonly have a decreased sensation of thirst and many will urinate frequently if they are taking diuretics for the management of blood pressure or heart failure. Hyperglycemia contributes to poor health outcomes in older adults in long-term care. Hyperglycemia is the technical term for elevated blood glucose, clinically defined as a blood glucose level higher than the person's target range set by their physician,[1] and a consistent glucose >200 mg/dl.[21] Long-term poor glucose control affects cognitive function[22-26] and puts older adults with diabetes at risk for infection.[18]

Hypoglycemia, the most common metabolic complication in older adults with diabetes, leads to substantial morbidity and mortality.[27] Hypoglycemia is the technical term for low blood glucose, clinically defined as a blood glucose level <70 mg/dl. Common symptoms of hypoglycemia include sweating, tremors, headache, palpitations, blurred vision, confusion, or anger. Hypoglycemia has been attributed to an increased incidence of falls in the elderly.[28] and it has been attributed to increased incidences of falls in the elderly.[29] In the Health, Aging and Body Composition Study of well older adults using insulin, an A1C level of <6% was associated with an increased risk of falls.[24] Examining a community-dwelling population, Nelson et al.[29] found that adults >75 years are at increased risk for falls when their A1C is ≤6%, regardless of frailty status. Insulin secretagogues continue to be commonly prescribed for older adults with T2D. Those individuals with A1C levels <6% who are taking insulin or insulin secretagogues may be experiencing hypoglycemia. Translating this finding to the nursing home, where residents with diabetes tend to be very frail, it is reasonable to conclude that hypoglycemia will lead to more frequent falls. Quality indicators for falls in frail elderly that require monitoring include medication review, gait and balance, blood pressure, vision changes, nutrition and cognitive status, and keeping glycemic control between 8 and 9%.[8]

Medical directors tend to set different diabetes treatment limits for the resident who is cognitively impaired.[30] This is due, in part, to the difficulties preventing hypoglycemia in this group. Cognitively impaired residents with diabetes not only have altered eating patterns but also have difficulty recognizing the symptoms of hypoglycemia.

Hypoglycemia can be treated easily and reversed when the symptoms are felt. Like hyperglycemia, however, typical symptoms may not be clear or obvious in the older adult. In the nursing home setting, because the ratio of residents to caregivers is high, recognition and treatment of hypoglycemia may be delayed. In a recent study involving residents with diabetes who participate in scheduled activities, nearly one-third of the participants experienced hypoglycemia, yet no treatment protocols were available.[31]

Importantly, protocols for treating hypoglycemia need to be in place. Knowing the resident well and becoming aware of their usual behavior, allows members of the health care team to create an individualized plan of care that addresses A1C goals and avoids acute complications arising from poor glycemic control.

Self-Care

In the same way as anyone else with T2D, older adults need to practice good self-management behaviors to maintain their physical and mental health. Understanding the daily routines and self-management behaviors of older adults with T2D is important as they might be highly motivated for diabetes management. In the long-term care setting, residents will have less functional ability and less personal control to adhere to self-management protocols.[32] Older adults with diabetes living in nursing homes can contribute to the plan for diabetes care, and receive coaching from the interdisciplinary team. It is important for the care team to show respect for the elder's independence regarding their diabetes care.[19] In the nursing home setting, the interdisciplinary team of physician, nurse, pharmacist, and dietitian can assist the resident and their family in coordinating appropriate diabetes self-care and screenings.[1,33] More detailed information about self-care can be found in Chapter 6.

MANAGEMENT MODALITIES

Nutrition

According to some authors, a diet that promotes good glucose control and appropriate weight management is the cornerstone of diabetes treatment for each resident. Many care home staff members, however, do not understand diabetes and feel uncertain about how to manage the condition.[19] In the nursing home, a common challenge is working with frail residents to maintain a safe weight. Residents with swallowing problems and those who need to be fed by staff have the best chances for maintaining their weight when staff receive appropriate training on dietary management of diabetes. Hydration status is also important in the elder with diabetes. Important measures to include in the plan of care for residents with diabetes are monitoring of food consumption, fluid intake, and weight status.

In the recent past, nursing facilities have embraced a more liberalized nutritional approach for elders with diabetes. In fact, it may be best to serve residents in long-term care facilities a regular diet to avoid malnutrition. Many residents with T2D have poor nutritional intake, dysphasia, weight loss, wounds, and other comorbidities.[28] Food management should be tailored to the individual to address their nutritional needs and should be culturally appropriate.[8] This, and more detailed information about meal planning can be found in Chapter 7.

Physical Activity and Glycemic Control

Interventions for elderly residents with diabetes include exercise as well as diet therapy. In a 16-week exercise resistance training program muscle strength and glycemic control was improved in older adults with diabetes.[34] Tai chi has been found to be effective in preventing falls in elderly residents with diabetes.[35] In nursing home residents with diabetes, those who participated in more activity hours were more likely to achieve A1C goals.[31] Additional benefits from participating in activities have been found in the oldest old with diabetes who are suffering from depression, and who may need psychological interventions such as social support, cognitive behavioral therapy, and exercise training.[31] Chapter 8 addresses physical activity in greater detail.

Depression, Glycemic Control, and Older Adults

Diabetes is considered to be the most psychologically and behaviorally demanding chronic illness.[22] The American Diabetes Association[36] and AGS[8] recommends completing a psychosocial assessment on people with diabetes, and changes should prompt further screening for depression. Although this recommendation is not directed to the older adult population, it turns out that elderly adults with diabetes are twice as likely as younger adults to be depressed.[37] Participation in psychosocial and behavioral activities has been shown to improve symptoms of depression in older adults.[31,38] Socialization through activities has a positive effect on emotional health for residents with T2D.[31] Today's nursing homes are filled with scheduled social activities, including games, crafts, shopping trips, and happy hour. Social activities like these provide opportunities for sharing fun, fellowship, and the always-available snacks. Interestingly, residents who participate in more activities seemed to be more likely to attain better A1C levels and have relatively few hypoglycemic episodes.[31] It seems clear that social activities are beneficial for all residents, including those with diabetes.

Medications

T2D is a progressive disease. In addition to diet and exercise, most people often require an oral antihyperglycemic medication and generally will progress to insulin for effective treatment of the disease. Because of the heterogeneity of the population and the absence of clear guidelines, treatment decisions rest on individual cases of diabetes severity, resident needs, and practitioner preferences. All members of the health care team need a good understanding of how medications for diabetes management work and the risk of hypoglycemia that comes with many of these drugs.

Blood glucose levels reflect the interaction between medications, food intake, and activity. It takes a balanced approach and concerted effort from all caregivers to help residents stay on a schedule with mealtimes and snacks. Diabetes medications used in nursing homes include the sulfonylurea family of drugs, including glyburide, glipizide, and glimepiride; the biguanide class (metformin); and insulin. Other classes of drugs are available and may be gaining popularity in the older adult. Medication administration, particularly with prandial insulin and some oral hypoglycemic drugs, needs to be coordinated around meals and activities to maintain a safe glucose level. Chapters 5, 9, and 10 provide detailed information about drugs and medication management.

Monitoring

Organizational factors can affect diabetes care in nursing homes. Diabetes management in long-term care facilities requires an interdisciplinary approach with resident input.[39] Findings from the Yarnall study[39] demonstrated that only 45% of nursing home residents were asked to contribute to their care plans. Allowing the residents to contribute to their plan of care will aid in compliance.[1,33] Monitoring residents who have both diabetes and functional and cognitive impairment was approached less aggressively.[30] A change in organizational systems with an interdisciplinary approach to monitoring diabetes in all elderly residents could decrease episodes of hypoglycemia.[30]

Skin and Foot Care

Nursing home residents >70 years of age are susceptible to developing pressure ulcers.[40] Older males in long-term care facilities are more likely to develop pressure ulcers than females.[41] In fact, according to Horn et al.[42] and Capon et al.,[43] severe illness, severe disability, cognitive impairment, confusion, and poor mental status are predictors of pressure ulcers in long-term care facilities. Diabetes, Alzheimer's disease, chronic obstructive pulmonary disease, stroke, heart failure, Parkinson's disease, and rheumatoid arthritis also have effects on pressure ulcer development.[44]

Assessment of the skin in nursing homes is to be completed on admission, quarterly and annually and when conditions change.[45] One factor that influences the performance of skin assessments in long-term care facilities is the staffing levels. Capon et al.[43] recommended that nursing and ancillary staff provide at least five staff members per 10 beds to result in a decreased likelihood of pressure ulcer development. More direct care time by registered nurses, licensed practical nurses, and CNAs per resident per day have been significantly related to lower incidences of pressure ulcer development in long-term care facilities.[42]

Foot care is important to older adults with diabetes as they can acquire ulcers that can become infected and spread systemically.[19] When diabetes is poorly controlled, nerve damage (neuropathy) can result. Subsequently, foot ulcers may occur and, if unnoticed, these can lead to infections on the feet. Diabetic wounds present differently than other chronic wounds. If the wounds are not adequately assessed and treated, consequences for the patient can be devastating, leading to major amputation or death.[46] When neuropathy is accompanied by poor circulation, these infections can lead to lower extremity amputations. Good nursing care for people with diabetes who live in long-term care facilities should include a focus on skin and foot care. See Chapter 12 for a more detailed discussion of foot care.

Skin Assessment

The Braden Scale[47] is a popular tool for skin assessment in long-term care and includes six risk factors: mobility, activity, sensory perception, skin moisture, nutritional status, and friction or shear. Previous studies have shown that poor mobility,[48,49] long periods of being confined to bed,[41] impaired self-positioning in bed,[51] difficulty turning in bed,[52] decreased pain perception,[53] friction or shear, dry skin, urinary, and fecal incontinence,[48-50,52] moisture,[50] eating problems,[42] poor appetite,[48] poor nutritional status,[54] a low ankle-brachial index value,[41] and low albumin levels[51,54] are all risk factors for skin breakdown in residents of long-term care facilities. When older adults have diabetes and any of these risk factors, nursing home personnel should be extra vigilant in reaching the patient goal of maintaining skin integrity.

Clinical Notes

Risk factors for skin breakdown:

- Poor mobility
- Confined to bed for long periods
- Impaired self-positioning in bed
- Friction or shear
- Dry skin
- Urinary and fecal incontinence
- Moisture
- Eating problems
- Poor appetite
- Poor nutritional status
- Low serum albumin levels
- Low ankle-brachial index
- Decreased pain perception

Transitions in Diabetes Care

Transitions include considering the structured environment of the nursing home and how nursing care provision is aligned with evidenced-based prevention, practice, and monitoring procedures.[55] Previous research comparing monitoring of older adults with diabetes in the community and those who live in the nursing home showed that types of monitoring differed between settings. For example, A1C testing occurred more often in the nursing home[56,57] than in the community setting.[58-60] Conversely, dilated eye examinations and lipid profile testing occurred more often in community settings than in nursing homes.[61] Overall, physicians reported being less likely to order special diets and order routine lipids panels for patients with impaired functional and cognitive status.[30]

Eighty-six percent of nursing home admissions are short-term rehabilitation stays, which currently are covered by Medicare. One-tenth of all nursing home stays are attributable to diabetes.[1] A number of challenges are associated with managing diabetes during short-term stays, not the least of which is the difficulty in teaching, modifying, and monitoring self-management of diabetes behavior before discharge. A systems approach to the care of people with diabetes in the nursing home is critical in monitoring symptoms and preventing complications of diabetes.[55] Transitions in diabetes care are the focus of Chapter 15.

Staff Education on Diabetes Nursing Care

Some research indicates that the structured environment of long-term care allows for more consistent application of guidelines driven care for residents with diabetes.[55] For this to occur, however, the guidelines need to be clear and the caregivers must be well-versed in application of the guidelines. Currently, there are multiple approaches to the management of diabetes in nursing homes and all recognize the lack of a comprehensive evidence base.[1,2,4,8] In the absence of consistent guidelines, nursing home staff are faced with the challenges associated with wide variations of clinical care. A better understanding of diabetes in general and diabetes in the elderly, in particular, will assist staff in the day-to-day application of diabetes care.

The structure of nursing home care for older adults with diabetes is critical to meet the competencies necessary to monitor and prevent complications. Meeting this challenge begins with education on evidenced-based practice, with educational tools appropriate for nurses at varying experience levels. In an interesting study examining the frequency of staff in-service training on diabetes in 13 long-term care facilities across six states, 46% of the respondents were unsure whether they had ever received diabetes content.[20]

There are significant barriers to staff education. The first barrier is the variability in the training and preparation of the health care team members. Nurses are part of the care team; often serving as directors of nursing, charge nurses, and advance practice nurses (as primary care givers). The Hartford Foundation promotes certification in gerontological nursing care. Yet only 2% of nurses are certified in gerontological nursing. Perhaps nursing facilities should offer financial support for the preparation and examination fees for certification for current and prospective nurses, but requiring certification may negatively affect recruitment of nurses into long-term care.

Licensed nurses are essential to the care team, but the direct care providers in long-term care typically are nursing assistants, orderlies, and attendants. The mean age of these workers is 46 years old. Although ~20% of CNAs and home health aides have not graduated from high school, >30% have attended some college. Thus, a barrier for many of these health care workers is education. A third major barrier to a well-educated staff is attrition. Approximately 50% of direct care workers are employed full time, and the average national turnover rate for CNAs is 71%. Ultimately, to be effective, any educational materials developed must be accessible so that new staff can be trained efficiently and the materials must meet the needs of multiple care providers who come from various backgrounds.

CONCLUSION

Generally, there is minimal current evidence to drive translation of diabetes care in nursing homes into practice.[30] The prevalence of diabetes in older adults in U.S. nursing homes is at 26%, according to the Minimum Data Set.[62] The problem is that adequate screening for diabetes is not initiated on admission. Undiagnosed diabetes is a serious problem as evidence has linked diabetes to cognitive impairment,[22-27] and therefore, screening elders with dementia may reveal undiagnosed diabetes.[63] Knowledge of diabetic conditions can lead to formulation of effective interventions to improve A1C levels. This, in turn, may lead to improved physical and cognitive function and may limit the occurrence of acute diabetes complications.

Many questions remain unanswered in the management of diabetes in long-term care facilities. Should the resident with diabetes be allowed or even encouraged to take advantage of the snacking opportunities during social activities? Is a liberalized diet more likely to contribute to reduced psychosocial distress and improved quality of life? What is the best way to educate staff on resident-centered care, resident choice, and resident well-being in the maintenance of glycemic control in the nursing home setting? What measures should be taken to address elevated evening blood glucose resulting from excessive overeating at activity gatherings? Perhaps greater supervision by professional staff is required at psychosocial activity gatherings to encourage the residents with diabetes to make better snack choices.

Research Questions

- Should residents with diabetes be allowed/encouraged to have snacking opportunities at social events?
- Does a liberalized meal plan improve quality of life?
- What is/are the best way(s) to educate staff regarding diabetes management?
- How should elevated bedtime glucose readings after evening social events be handled?

Numerous gaps in the literature concerning diabetes in nursing home systems remain. A study by Feldman, Rosen, and DeStasio,[20] examined the systems for diabetes management in 13 nursing homes across six states. Interviews with directors of nursing and medical directors, as well as chart reviews, revealed that only 1 of the 13 facilities had a quality improvement tool to evaluate compliance with current policies. Recommendations from this study for diabetes management in the nursing home included individualizing treatment goals and developing a strategic quality improvement program to allow facilities to track utilization of the diabetes management plan to identify what worked well and what needed further improvement.[20] Overall, management of diabetes in long-term care facilities has been understudied. Existing research demonstrates a need for more staff education in diabetes management, system changes in admission processes, assessment, staffing, care coordination, and discharge teaching. The recent AGS guidelines[8] and the consensus report on managing diabetes in older adults[14] are person centered and can be incorporated into plans of care for elders living in nursing homes. The influx of baby boomers reaching older adulthood and the increasing prevalence of diabetes in the U.S. warrants further exploration of this important topic. The relationship between poor diabetes management and cognitive decline is startling, particularly given the increasing numbers of people in the nursing home with diabetes. The culture in the nursing home setting needs transformation. Imagine what could be realized if the entire interdisciplinary team selected, followed, and evaluated the results of implementation of just one set of recommended guidelines.

REFERENCES

1. American Diabetes Association. Standards of medical care diabetes—2014. *Diabetes Care* 2014;37(Suppl1):S14–S80.
2. American Medical Directors Association. *Diabetes management in the long-term care setting: Clinical practice guideline.* Columbia, MD, American Medical Directors Association, 2008.
3. Brown AF, Mangione CM, Saliba D, et al. Guidelines for improving the care of the older person with diabetes mellitus. *Journal of the American Geriatric Society* 2003;51:S265–S280.
4. Sinclair AJ, Paolisso G, Castro M, Bourdel-Marchasson I, Gadsby R, Manas LR. European Diabetes Working Party for Older People 2011: Clinical guidelines for type 2 diabetes. Executive summary. *Diabetes and Metabolism* 2011;37:S27–S38.
5. Moreno G, Mangione CM, Kimbro L, Vaisberg E, Mellitus A. Guidelines abstracted from the American Geriatrics Society guidelines for improving the care of older adults with diabetes mellitus: 2013 update. *Journal of the American Geriatrics Society* 2013;61:2020–2026.
6. International Diabetes Federation. Managing older people with type 2 diabetes: A global guideline. In *IDF working group on older adults.* 1st ed. Brussels, Belgium, International Diabetes Federation, 2013.
7. Sinclair A, Morley JE, Rodriguez-Manas L, Paolisso G, Bayer T, Zeyfang A. Lorig K. Diabetes mellitus in older people: Position statement on behalf of the International Association of Gerontology and Geriatrics (IAGG), the European Diabetes Working Party for Older People (EDWPOP), and the International Task Force of Experts in Diabetes. *Journal of the American Medical Directors Association* 2012;13(6):497–502.
8. American Geriatrics Society. Guidelines abstracted from the American Geriatrics Society guidelines for improving the care of older adults with diabetes mellitus: 2013 update. *Journal of the American Geriatrics Society* 2013;61:2020–2026.
9. Lindau ST, McDade TW. Minimally invasive and innovative methods for biomeasure collection in population-based research. In *National Research Council (US) Committee on Advances in Collecting and Utilizing Biological Indicators and Genetic Information in Social Science Surveys.* Weinstein M, Vaupel JW, Wachter KW (Eds.). Biosocial Surveys. Washington, DC, National Academies Press, 2008. Available from http://www.ncbi.nlm.nih.gov/books/NBK62423. Accessed 14 February 2014.
10. Department of Veterans Affairs. *Executive summary: Health services research and development service. Evidenced-based synthesis program self-monitoring of*

blood glucose in patients with type 2 diabetes mellitus: Meta-analysis of effective-ness. Washington, DC, 2007

11. Holman RR, Paul SK, Bethel MA, et al. 10 year follow-up of intensive glucose control in type 2 diabetes. *New England Journal of Medicine* 2008;359:1577–1589.
12. Patel A, MacMahon S, Chalmers J, Neal B, Billot L, et al. Intensive blood glucose control and vascular outcomes in patients with type 2 diabetes. *New England Journal of Medicine* 2008;358(24):2560–2572.
13. Gao L, Matthews FE, Sargeant LA, Brayne C. An investigation of the popu-lation impact of variation in HbA1c levels in older people in England and Wales: From a population based multi-centre longitudinal study. *British Medical Community Public Health* 2008;8:54.
14. Kirkman MS, Jones Briscoe V, Clark N, Florez H, Haas LB, et al. Diabetes in older adults. *Diabetes Care* 2012;35:2342–2356.
15. Meyers RM, Broton JC, Woo-Rippe KW, et al. Variability in glycosolated hemoglobin values in diabetic patients living in long-term care facilities. *Journal of the American Medical Directors Association* 2007;8:511–514.
16. Inzucchi SE, Bergenstal RM, Buse JB, et al. Management of hyperglycemia in type 2 diabetes: A patient-centered approach. Position Statement of the American Diabetes Association (ADA) and the European Association for the Study of Diabetes (EASD). *Diabetes Care* 2012;35:1364–1379.
17. Zarowtz BJ, Tangalos EG, Hollenack K, O'Shea T. The application of evi-dence-based principles of care in older persons: management of diabetes mel-litus. *Journal of the American Medical Directors Association* 2006;3(3):234-240.
18. Araki A, Ito H. Diabetes mellitus and geriatric syndromes. *Geriatric Geron-tological Society International* 2009;9:105–114.
19. Heeley-Creed D, Brown K. Comprehensive management of diabetes in care homes. *Nursing and Residential Care* 2009;11(9):458–461.
20. Feldman SM, Rosen R, DeStasio J. Status of diabetes management in the nursing home setting in 2008: A retrospective chart review and epidemiol-ogy study of diabetic nursing home residents and nursing home initiatives in diabetes management. *Journal of the American Medical Directors Association* 2009;10:354–360.
21. Smelzer S, Bare B. Chronic illness and disability. In *Textbook of Medical-Surgical Nursing.* 13th ed. Hinkle J, Cheever K (Eds.). Philadelphia, PA, Wolters Kluwer Health/Lippincott Williams & Wilkins, 2010, p. 131–148.
22. Ciechanowski PS, Katon WJ, Russo JE. Depression and diabetes: Impact of depressive symptoms on adherence, function, and costs. *Archives of Internal Medicine* 2000;160:3278–3285.
23. Hagemann R, Sartory G, Hader C, Kobberling J. Mood and cognitive func-tion in elderly diabetic patients living in care facilities. *Dementia Geriatric Cognitive Disorders* 2005;19:369–375.
24. Maraldi C, Volpato S, Penninx BW, et al. Diabetes mellitus, glycemic con-trol, and incident depressive symptoms among 70-79 year old persons: The health, aging, and body composition study. *Archives of Internal Medicine* 2007;167:1137–1144.

25. Perlmuter LC, Hakami MK, Hodgson-Harrington C, et al. Decreased cognitive function in aging non-insulin dependent diabetic patients. *American Journal of Medicine* 1984;77:1043–1048.
26. Reaven GM, Thompson LW, Nahun D, Haskins E. Relationship between hyperglycemia and cognitive function in older NIDDM patients. *Diabetes Care* 1990;13(1):16–21.
27. Kagansky N, Levy S, Rimon E, Cojocaru L, Fridman A, Ozer Z, et al. Hypoglycemia as a predictor of mortality in hospitalized elderly patients. *Archives of Internal Medicine* 2003;163:1825–1829.
28. Dorner B. A liberalized approach to diets for diabetes in long-term care. *The Director* 2002;10(4):132–136.
29. Nelson JM, Durfraux K, Cook PF. The relationship between glycemic control and falls in older adults. *Journal of American Geriatrics Society* 2007;55:2041–2044.
30. McNabney MK, Pandya N, Iwuagwu C, et al. Differences in diabetes management of nursing home patients based on functional and cognitive status. *Journal of American Medical Directors Association* 2005;6:375–382.
31. Bellissimo JL, Holt RM, Maus SM, Marx TL, Schwartz FL, Shubrook DO. Impact of activity participation and depression on glycemic control I older adults with diabetes: Glycemic control in nursing homes. *Clinical Diabetes* 2011;29(4):139–144.
32. Chelbowy D, Hood S, LaJoie A. Facilitators and barriers to self-management of type 2 diabetes among urban African American adults. *Diabetes Educator* 2010;36(6):897–905.
33. Inzucchi SE, Bergenstal RM, Buse JB, et al. Management of hyperglycemia in type 2 diabetes: A patient-centered approach. Position Statement of the American Diabetes Association (ADA) and the European Association for the Study of Diabetes (EASD). *Diabetes Care* 2012;35:1364–1379.
34. Castaneda C, Layne JE, Munoz-Orians L, et al. A randomized controlled trial of resistance exercise training to improve glycemic control in older adults with type 2 diabetes. *Diabetes Care* 2002;25:2335–2341.
35. Gillespie LD, Gillespie WJ, Robertson MC, Lamb SE, Cumming RG, Rowe BH. Interventions for preventing falls in elderly people. *Cochrane Database of Systematic Reviews* 2003;4:CD000340.
36. American Diabetes Association. Standards of medical care in diabetes. *Diabetes Care* 2012;35(Suppl1):S11–S63.
37. Munshi M. Managing the geriatric syndrome in patients with type 2 diabetes. Consultant Pharmacology 2008;(Suppl. B):12–16.
38. Meeks S, Young CM, Looney SW. Activity participation and affect among nursing home residents: support for a behavioral model of depression. *Aging and Mental Health* 2007;11:751–760.
39. Yarnall AJ, Hayes L, Hawthorne GC, Candish CA, Aspray TJ. Short report: Care delivery, diabetes in care homes: Current care standards and resident's experience. *Diabetic Medicine* 2011;29:132–135.
40. Dellefield ME. Prevalence rate of pressure ulcers in California nursing homes. *Journal of Gerontological Nursing* 2004;30(11):13–31.

41. Okuwa B, Sanada, Sugama, J, Inagaki M, Konya C, Kitagawa A, Tabata K. A prospective cohort study of lower extremity pressure ulcer risk among bedfast older adults. *Advances in Skin and Wound Care* 2006;19(7):391–397.
42. Horn S, Bender S, Ferguson M, Smout R, Bergstrom N, Taler G, Cook A, Sharkey S, Voss AC. The national pressure ulcer long-term care study: Pressure ulcer development in long-term care residents. *Journal of the American Geriatrics Society* 2004;52(3):359–367.
43. Capon A, Pavoni N, Mastromattei A, DiLallo D. Pressure ulcer risk in long-term units: Prevalence and associated factors. *Journal of Advanced Nursing* 2007;58(3):263–272.
44. Margolis DJ, Allen-Taylor L, Hoffstad O, Berlin JA. Diabetic neuropathic foot ulcers: Predicting which ones will not heal. *American Journal of Medicine* 2003;115:627–631.
45. Centers for Medicare and Medicaid (CMS). Centers for Medicare/Medicaid and Quality Care for the Elderly. Improving the care of dual eligible: What's ahead? *Annals of Long-Term Care and Aging* 2011;19(9):26–30.
46. Bently J, Foster A. Management of the diabetic foot ulcer: Exercising control. *British Journal of Community Nursing* 2008;13(3):S16–S20.
47. Bergstrom N, Braden B, Laguzza A, Hulman V. A clinical trial of the Braden scale for predicting pressure sore risk. *Nursing Clinics of North America* 1987;22:417–428.
48. Papanikolaou Y, Palmer H, Binns MA, Jenkins DJA, Greenwood CE. Better cognitive performance following a low glycaemic-index compared with a high glycaemic-index carbohydrate meal in adults with type 2 diabetes. *Diabetologia* 2006;49(5):855–862.
49. Berquist S. Pressure ulcer prediction in older adults receiving home health care: Implications for use with the OASIS. *Advances in Skin and Wound Care* 2003;16(3):132–139.
50. Berquist B, Frantz R. Braden scale: Validity in community based-older adults receiving home health care. *Journal of Applied Nursing Research* 2001;14:26–43.
51. Mino-Leon D, Figueras A, Amato D, et al. Treatment of type 2 diabetes in primary health care: A drug utilization study. *Annals of Pharmacotherapy* 2005;39:441–445.
52. Baumgarten M, Margolis D, van Doorn C, Gruber-Baldini AL, Hebel JR, Zimmerman S, Magaziner J. Black/White differences in pressure ulcer incidence in nursing home residents. *Journal of the American Geriatrics Society* 2004;52(8):1293–1298.
53. Ash D. An exploration of the occurrence of pressure ulcers in a British spinal injuries unit. *Journal of Clinical Nursing* 2002;11(4):470–478.
54. Reed RL, Hepburn K, Adelson R, Center B, McKnight P. Low serum albumin levels, confusion, and fecal incontinence: are these risk factors for pressure ulcers in mobility-impaired hospitalized adults? *Gerontology* 2003;49(4):255–259.
55. Quinn CC, Gruber-Baldini AL, Port CL, May C, Stuart B, Hebel JR, Zimmerman, Magaziner J. The role of nursing homes: Admission and dementia

status on care for diabetes mellitus. *Journal of American Geriatrics Society* 2009;57:1628–1633.

56. Holt RM, Schwartz FL, Shubrook JH. Diabetes care in extended-care facilities; Appropriate intensity of care? *Diabetes Care* 2007;30:1454–1458.
57. Meyers RM, Broton JC, Woo-Rippe KW, et al. Variability in glycosolated hemoglobin values in diabetic patients living in long-term care facilities. *Journal of the American Medical Directors Association* 2007;8:511–514.
58. Arday DR, Flemming BB, Keller DK, et al. Variation in diabetes care among states: Do patient characteristics matter? *Diabetes Care* 2002;25:2230–2237.
59. Ellerbeck EF, Engelman KK, Williams NJ, et al. Variations in diabetes care and the influence of office systems. *American Journal of Medical Quality* 2004;19:12–18.
60. Jenks SF, Huff ED, Cuerdon T. Change in the quality of care delivered to Medicare beneficiaries: 1998-1999 to 2000-2001. *Journal of the American Medical Association* 2003;289:305–312.
61. White BA, Jablonski RA, Falkerstern SK. Diabetes in the nursing home. *Annals of Long-Term Care* 2009;17(8):42–46.
62. Travis SS, Buchanon RJ, Wang S, Kim M. Analysis of nursing home residents with diabetes at admission. *Journal of American Medical Directors Association* 2004;5:320–327.
63. Aspray TJ, Nesbit K, Cassidy TP, et al. Diabetes in British nursing and residential homes: A pragmatic screening study. *Diabetes Care* 2006;29(3):707–708.

4

Geriatric Syndromes and Diabetes

Sandra Drozdz Burke, PhD, ANP-BC, CDE, FAADE, and Katie Sikma, BSN, RN

INTRODUCTION

Diabetes is a chronic condition characterized by variable levels of blood glucose. Normally, fasting blood glucose levels range from 70 to 99 mg/dl. Impaired glucose tolerance or impaired fasting glucose is now known as prediabetes; it is associated with blood glucose levels between 100 and 125 mg/dl. Diabetes, which occurs when fasting blood glucose levels are consistently at 126 mg/dl or higher, occurs frequently in the aging population. Because blood glucose levels rise insidiously, many people fail to experience symptoms of hyperglycemia until the blood glucose level is consistently well above 300 mg/dl. For this and other reasons, diabetes often goes undiagnosed for many years. With uncontrolled hyperglycemia, clinicians often expect to see classic signs and symptoms of polyuria, polydipsia, and extreme fatigue. Given the expected physiologic changes associated with aging, these signs and symptoms may not be present in the older adult. Instead, urinary incontinence (UI) and confusion are symptoms that should lead to the suspicion of diabetes in the older adult.[1] Moreover, older adults with new onset diabetes may present with hyperosmolar, hyperglycemic state, an acute form of extreme hyperglycemia.

Although type 1 diabetes (T1D) can occur at any point during the lifetime, type 2 diabetes (T2D) is, by far, the most common form of the disease in older adults. Current Centers for Disease Control and Prevention (CDC) data suggest that at least 27% of people age ≥65 years have diabetes and an additional 50% have prediabetes. Among the oldest old-age group, the prevalence of diabetes remains relatively high, and it has been speculated that the prevalence is even greater than reported.[2–5] Diabetes is common in the long-term care (LTC) environment. More than a decade ago, researchers reported that nearly 58% of nursing home patients in the U.K. already had or were at risk for T2D.[6]

Diabetes is at now at epidemic proportions throughout the world. Uncontrolled diabetes is commonly known to increase the risk of heart attack and stroke and lead to kidney failure, blindness, and loss of limb.[7,8] Overall, the individual with diabetes has more than twice the amount of medical expenses and double the risk of death as someone at the same age without diabetes.[7,9,10] Diabetes is becoming more prevalent, especially in older adults, and is the seventh leading cause of death in the U.S.[7] All diabetes complications can occur in older adults, and typically they occur more frequently compared with younger populations.[1]

DOI: 10.2337/9781580404730.04

33

For most individuals with diabetes, management includes a balance between meal planning, physical activity, and medications. Commonly, treatment is guided by blood glucose monitoring and periodic measurement of hemoglobin A1C values. In addition to these metabolic measures, management decisions also are influenced by quality-of-life issues.[11]

Diabetes can be difficult to control in any population, but it may be particularly problematic for the older adult in LTC. This is true partly because the LTC resident with diabetes will have different needs depending on the type of diabetes, the duration of diabetes, and the type or number of diabetes complications. Each of these situations is unique because it will affect both the level of diabetes control needed and the expected response to treatment. Management also is complicated when "self-management" is replaced by "shared" or "collective" management. In the LTC environment, multiple caregivers who have markedly different levels of professional training are involved in the day-to-day management of a resident's diabetes.

The complexity of diabetes management in older adults also is associated with the number of coexisting chronic illnesses and the expected physiologic changes that go along with the aging process.[1] Normal aging typically results in changes in functional status. The older adult who has difficulty with activities of daily living (ADLs) often will be unable to follow complex diabetes self-management plans without assistance. This is especially noticeable in the cognitively impaired individual.[1] Older adults are expected to have multiple chronic illnesses. In the Health and Retirement Study, researchers found that while ~65% of Medicare patients have two or more chronic conditions, 43% have three or more.[12,13] In general, multiple comorbidities are associated with higher levels of functional dependencies. In other words, when older adults have many chronic conditions, they are less likely to be able to remain independent.

Diabetes management in LTC can be affected by:

- Physiologic changes of aging
- Comorbidities
- Geriatric syndromes

Physiologic changes of aging also affect glucose regulation. The normal renal glucose threshold is 180 mg/dl, but aging kidneys do not filter blood as efficiently as younger kidneys, so the renal threshold increases.[1,14] Blood glucose levels may go well >200 mg/dl before excess glucose spills over into the urine. Essentially, it takes longer for the body to respond to an abnormally high glucose level. Typically, high levels of glucose are expected to cause osmotic diuresis. This results in polyuria, one of the classic signs of uncontrolled hyperglycemia. Polyuria should lead to activation of the thirst mechanism and subsequent polydipsia. Because aging alters the body's normal thirst mechanism, however, an older adult may not feel thirsty and will not replace lost fluids. Dehydration can occur very quickly in these residents.

Diabetes management is complicated by the presence of multiple comorbid conditions and a number of the geriatric syndromes. Although chronic conditions typically are associated with practice guidelines developed by clinical experts, when multiple chronic illnesses coexist, it is important to focus holistically on the individual rather than on the various disease states.

GERIATRIC SYNDROMES

Experts in gerontology often refer to the "geriatric syndromes." These so-called syndromes are actually individual conditions, characteristics, or features that tend to cluster together and they increase the older adult's risk for poor health outcomes.[13,15,16] Many common conditions found in older adults, including delirium, falls, frailty, dizziness, syncope, and UI, are classified as geriatric syndromes. When the literature is reviewed, however, it becomes difficult to identify which specific conditions constitute the geriatric syndromes.

Sixteen geriatric syndromes are listed in the table of contents of the *American Geriatric Society Core Curriculum*, 8th ed. These include frailty, visual impairment, hearing impairment, dizziness, syncope, malnutrition, eating or feeding difficulty, UI, gait impairment, falls, osteoporosis, pressure ulcers and wound care, dementia, behavior problems in dementia, delirium, and sleep problems.[17] Inouye et al.[16] identified delirium, falls, UI, frailty, and functional decline as the geriatric syndromes. A publication of the American Geriatric Society's Foundation for Health in Aging lists "vision and hearing problems, bladder problems, dizziness, falls, delirium, and dementia as conditions that can interfere with activities of daily living, limit independence and impair quality of life."[18] In a report from the Agency for Healthcare Research and Quality, Kane et al.[19] identified eight of the most common geriatric syndromes, including cognitive impairment, frailty, disability, sarcopenia, malnutrition, homeostenosis, chronic inflammation, and polypharmacy. More recently, Rosso et al.[20] defined the geriatric syndromes as depression, dizziness, falls, hearing or vision impairment, osteoporosis, polypharmacy, syncope, sleep disturbances, and UI. Although a number of conditions are common among authors, it would appear that a great deal of inconsistency and confusion surrounds what does or does not constitute the geriatric syndromes. It is clear that geriatric syndrome is a term used to capture clinical conditions in older people that do not fit into discrete disease categories. An underlying notion is that when geriatric syndromes are clustered together, they commonly are associated with functional dependency.

As individuals age, they are more likely to develop chronic illnesses. Although the term "geriatric syndrome" is not interchangeable with the term "chronic illness," the geriatric syndromes certainly are more common in patients with chronic illnesses.[13,21] Individuals with multiple chronic illnesses (i.e., multimorbidities) are more likely to experience functional dependencies.

Geriatric Syndromes

- Conditions, characteristics or features that cluster together and can lead to poor outcomes

- Geriatric syndromes include:

  ❏ frailty

  ❏ visual or hearing impairment

  ❏ dizziness or syncope

  ❏ eating/feeding difficulty, sarcopenia, malnutrition

  ❏ urinary incontinence

  ❏ gait impairment

  ❏ osteoporosis

  ❏ pressure ulcers/wound care

  ❏ dementia/behavior problems, delirium

  ❏ sleep problems

  ❏ functional decline

  ❏ cognitive impairment

  ❏ depression

  ❏ polypharmacy

Several geriatric syndromes used to describe the health complications associated with diabetes have been shown to decrease the functional ability and quality of life in older adults.[22-24] In diabetes, these typically include depression, UI, falls, functional disabilities, cognitive impairment, polypharmacy, and malnutrition. Each geriatric syndrome can lead to frailty, loss of independence, an overall decrease in daily functioning, and complications in the treatment and management of diabetes.[23] Each of these syndromes will be discussed briefly in the following sections.

Depression

Depression, with or without diabetes, has a negative impact on quality of life.[25-27] Depression is twice as common among individuals with diabetes as it is in the general population and it can adversely affect diabetes management.[25,26,28,29] Overall, depression can be expected to occur in more than one-third of all LTC residents.[30] In the community-dwelling elder, unrecognized or untreated depression interferes with self-management choices which can lead to poor diabetes control, subsequent chronic complications, and reduced quality of life.[27] Screening for depression in LTC is an essential requirement for all residents, but it is particularly important in those with known diabetes.[23,30] Simple screening tools are available.[31] In the LTC setting, older adults with diabetes who become permanent residents tend to be at high risk for depression.[22,32] Moreover, individuals with depression tend to be at high risk for diabetes.[26]

Urinary Incontinence

UI is a common problem among women. As many as 40% of women <60 years of age and half of all older women experience UI.[33] Urology specialists define seven categories of UI: stress, urge, overactive bladder, functional, overflow, mixed, and transient.[34] Table 4.1 defines the various types of incontinence. Urge, functional, mixed, and overflow incontinence are common to LTC residents. The relationships between UI, functional dependence, quality of life, and use of resources have been clearly established.[35-38] Moreover, although the number varies considerably, up to 65% of all nursing home residents experience some degree of bowel or bladder incontinence.[39]

Risk factors for UI include race and ethnicity, BMI, number of pregnancies, various medications, and a history of diabetes, vascular disease, and gynecologic surgery.[33] Specifically, white women are more likely than non-Hispanic black women to develop UI. It is more common in women who are overweight or obese. Muliparity also is implicated in UI. Women who have had three or more children are at a higher risk, as are women who have had hysterectomies. Hormone replacement therapy, diuretics, calcium channel blockers, and angiotensin-converting-enzyme inhibitors all seem to increase the likelihood of UI. Diabetes and vascular disease also put women at higher risk to experience UI. In and of

Table 4.1 The Types of Urinary Incontinence

Stress	Leakage of small amounts of urine during physical movement (coughing, sneezing, exercising).
Urge	Leakage of large amounts of urine at unexpected times, including during sleep.
Overactive bladder	Urinary frequency and urgency, with or without urge incontinence.
Functional	Untimely urination because of physical disability, external obstacles, or problems in thinking or communicating that prevent a person from reaching a toilet.
Overflow	Unexpected leakage of small amounts of urine because of a full bladder.
Mixed	Usually the occurrence of stress and urge incontinence together.
Transient	Leakage that occurs temporarily because of a situation that will pass (infection, taking a new medication, colds with coughing).

Source: Adapted from National Institutes of Health.[34]

itself, UI does not predict a decline in ADLs, nursing home admission, or death, but UI is a marker of frailty.[34] Incontinence can lead to depression, falls, fractures, and social isolation. A number of pharmacological or behavioral interventions are available to treat UI.[15]

Clinical Note

Urinary Incontinence

- More common in females
- A marker of frailty
- Can lead to falls
- Associated with mobility impairment, decreased cognition, ADL impairment, UTIs, pressure ulcers, hospitalizations

---

Falls

Falls constitute another geriatric syndrome associated with diabetes, and they are common in LTC settings. Falls are said to be the eighth-leading cause of unintentional injury for older adults.[40] Moreover, 50–75% of all LTC residents fall at least once a year.[40,41] Risk factors can be personal or environmental.[41,42] Using Minimum Data Set (MDS) data, Leland et al.[43] found that 40% of all newly admitted residents reported a history of falling and ~20% fall within the first 30 days of admission. In addition to advanced age, personal risk factors for falling might include impaired vision, gait, balance, or cognition. Of note, 92% of newly admitted residents in 2006 reported impaired balance during their admission assessment.[43] High-risk medications also put a resident at risk for falls. A number of medications commonly are cited, but those that affect the central nervous system (e.g., antianxiety agents, antipsychotics, and hypnotics) seem to be most worrisome.[42,43] Examples of risk factors in the environment include such things as poor lighting, slippery or uneven surfaces, and improper footwear.

Chronic diseases have been shown to increase the odds of falling. Conditions whose pathophysiology or treatment tend to affect gait or balance, limit

---

Clinical Note

Falls

- 50–75% of LTC residents fall at least annually
- 20% of newly admitted residents fall within first 30 days
- Central nervous system medications increase risk
- Falls can start a downward spiral of functional disability

---

mobility, impair cognition or functional status, and reduce visual acuity can lead to falling or a fear of falling. Common conditions include arthritis, coronary heart disease (CHD), depression, diabetes, hypertension, Parkinson's disease, and heart failure.

Falls tend to be more common in older women than in men, are more likely to cause injury, and are closely associated with frailty.[42] Falls can lead to fractures, a decline in glycemic control, and a decrease in quality of life. Even if a fall does not cause serious harm, falling can cause anxiety and reduce participation in physical and social activities.[23] Indeed, falling creates a downward spiral of functional ability as most elders who fall report being fearful of falling again. According to Cayea and Durso,[15] exercise programs are strongly associated with a decrease in the incidence of falls; however, the Panel on Prevention of Falls in Older Adults[41] suggested that exercise may increase the risk of falling in some older adults and found limited research supporting widespread adoption of exercise programs in high-risk residents.

Experts agree that fall risk assessment is an essential element of good care. In an online resource from the Hartford Institute for Geriatric Nursing, Gray-Micelli and Quigley[44] outlined a nursing standard of practice for fall prevention that includes comprehensive assessment and follow-up.

Functional Disability

Restriction of ability ranges in severity and can be measured on a continuum that ranges from independent living to complete dependence on caregivers.[45] Functional disability is considered one of the most serious and debilitating of the geriatric syndromes. A person with a functional disability has trouble performing even the most simple ADLs, such as bathing or getting dressed, as well as experiencing difficulty with instrumental activities of daily living (IADLs), such as banking, shopping for necessities, and cooking.[23] In the LTC environment, this translates to a need for assistance with ADLs. People with diabetes ≥60 years old have mobility difficulties.[8] They are three times more likely to have problems climbing stairs, walking a minimum of a quarter of a mile, and doing normal household duties.[7] When a person has difficulty doing daily tasks and tires easily, physical activity becomes a struggle and that struggle could lead to a two to four times higher chance of a heart-disease related death.[7]

It is important to distinguish functional disability from frailty. Functional disability is associated with a reduction in ability to perform ADLs.[23] Frailty occurs when individuals are not only more vulnerable but are also less able to compensate for physiologic stressors.[46] As many as 50% of all elders >85 years old may be frail.[47] Weight loss, self-reported exhaustion, weakness, slowed walk speed, and reduced activity levels are clinical characteristics of the frail elder.[48] Clegg et al.[47] also suggested that frail elders are more likely to exhibit delirium and what they call "fluctuating disability," which is more commonly known as "good days" and "bad days" (p. 753). Frail elders are more likely to experience functional decline, especially when diabetes is an underlying condition.[8] Moreover, frail elders are nearly four times more likely to fall than nonfrail elders.[49] At the end of the day, it is the lack of functional ability that leads to institutionalization, but it is the frailty that results in poor outcomes, including death.[8,45,48]

Frailty

- Increased vulnerability
- Can't compensate for physiologic stressors
- Common in "oldest old" (>85 years of age)

Cognitive Impairment

Mild cognitive impairment (MCI) is associated with changes in cognitive functioning that are more pronounced than what normally is expected during the aging process.[50] The two types of MCI are amnesic and nonamnesic. Clinical characteristics of amnesic MCI tend to be limited to increasing levels of forgetfulness. The evidence linking diabetes to cognitive impairment identifies specific deficits that relate to memory, suggesting that individuals with diabetes are likely to have the amnesic form of MCI.[15,23] Various factors, including duration of diabetes, hyperglycemia, severe hypoglycemia, and cerebrovascular disease, have been linked with cognitive decline in diabetes.[23,51,52] Some evidence suggests that improving glucose control will improve cognitive function.[23] A delicate balance exists here. Tight glycemic control is associated with frequent and possibly severe hypoglycemia and severe hypoglycemia is also a risk factor for impaired cognition. In the LTC environment, it is essential to evaluate residents for changes in cognition. A variety of instruments are available. Two of the more common tools are the Mini-Mental State Examination and the Mini-Cog.[53] Useful instructional videos on assessing cognition in the older adult are available on the Hartford Geriatric Institute website.[54]

Polypharmacy

The geriatric syndrome known as polypharmacy affects the majority of individuals who are ≥65 years old. Although there is no clear definition of the number of prescription medications needed to establish polypharmacy, the term represents a situation that occurs when unnecessary or clinically inappropriate medications are added to an individual's drug regimen.[55] Authors often refer to polypharmacy when an individual is taking five to six or more prescription medications.[55-57] Polypharmacy can increase the chances of having adverse drug side effects and drug-to-drug interactions and also can worsen other geriatric syndromes. In the community and assisted-living environments, it also can lead to a diminished quality of life, needless drug expense, and difficulty following recommended medication therapies.[23] Polypharmacy can increase the risk for adverse drug events as well as lead to drug-related emergency room visits or to hospitalizations. In some cases, polypharmacy can be directly responsible for drug-related deaths. Upon admission to the LTC facility and during all transitions of care (from nursing home to hospital or home and back again), the resident's list of medications should be reconciled. Ongoing communication about any medication-related issues should be part of routine care conferences. Ideally, the resident or a family caregiver can participate in these conferences to provide their perspective. Detailed information related to the pharmacologic needs of residents with diabetes can be found in Chapter 9.

Malnutrition

The simplest definition of malnutrition is that it is a condition resulting from inadequate nutritional intake or poor absorption of nutrients.[58] Unhappily, malnutrition is common in older adults. It is noted to occur in as many as 80% of nursing home residents.[59,60] In the older adult population, malnutrition can be considered a geriatric syndrome associated with disability, increased rates of mortality, and potentially life-threatening complications.[23] The multifactorial causes of malnutrition include physiologic changes of aging, restricted diets, depression, cognitive or swallowing disorders, drug-related anorexia, vitamin and mineral deficiencies, and conditions that cause difficulty with self-feeding, as well as numerous institutional factors, such as high staff turnover, inadequate training, and lack of personal assistance during feeding.[59] Individually or collectively, these changes result in diminished hunger, decreased interest in food, early satiety, poor absorption of nutrients, and reduced intake.[61] Most authors agree that although malnutrition is a serious problem, it typically remains underrecognized in the LTC setting.

A related problem, sarcopenia, refers to an age-related and progressive loss of muscle mass. Sarcopenia can be a significant problem in up to half of all older adults.[46] The sarcopenic individual is underweight with little fat mass, reduced skeletal muscle mass, low BMI, and reduced waist circumference.[62] This is the resident who is clearly emaciated; certainly not the picture of the typical person with T2D.

There tends to be a cycle of disability that accompanies malnutrition. Sarcopenia increases the risk of health care–acquired infections in institutionalized elders. Malnourished and sarcopenic older adults are more likely to be frail and to develop pressure ulcers.[59] Frailty, another geriatric syndrome, increases the risk of falling and perpetuates multiple other geriatric syndromes, including depression, persistent malnutrition, altered cognition, and even UI.

BLENDING DIABETES WITH THE GERIATRIC SYNDROMES

Conventional wisdom as well as more than two decades of research tells us that control of hyperglycemia is important. For many years the American Diabetes Association (ADA) defined well-controlled diabetes with a hemoglobin A1C <7%. The American Association of Clinical Endocrinologists promoted a more stringent A1C goal of ≤6.5%. To better understand hemoglobin A1C values, think about the percentage as it relates to the average level of glucose in the bloodstream. The ADA now has an estimated average glucose (eAG) calculator available on its website.[63] Table 4.2 provides an excerpt that illustrates target blood glucose levels with their respective eAG values. Well-controlled diabetes reduces the risk of complications, and hypoglycemia was the only limitation to tight control. Whichever set of guidelines clinicians followed, they applied the recommendations to all adults, including the elderly. Early research rarely included older adults, however, and more current recommendations now recognize the need for individualized blood glucose target values.

Table 4.2 Comparison of Recommended Hemoglobin A1C Targets to Estimated Average Glucose Levels

Targets	A1C value	Estimated average glucose (eAG)
American Association of Clinical Endocrinologists	6.5%	140 mg/dl
American Diabetes Association	7%*	154 mg/dl
American Geriatrics Society	8%	183 mg/dl
Frail elders (multiple recommendations)	8.5%	197 mg/dl

Note: Formula to calculate eAG: 28.7 × A1C − 46.7 = eAG.
*For healthy, functional adults.
Source: Adapted from the American Diabetes Association.[63]

Glucose control is still important, but the ideal level of control in the older adult is not yet known. This is particularly true for the *frail* older adult who may be dealing with many simultaneous geriatric syndromes.[64] Research evidence now suggests that focusing on management of cardiovascular risk factors instead of concentrating on tight glycemic control is more likely to decrease morbidity and mortality rates in the older adult.[65,66] As indicated in Chapter 14, strong evidence from clinical trials supports the notion that the treatment of hypertension in the older adult improves quality of life in a relative short time frame. The time frame to realize benefit is important. It takes ~8 years to benefit from well-controlled diabetes compared with only 2–3 years of blood pressure and lipid control.[65,67–71] Clinicians would be well advised to take time to benefit into account when setting glycemic goals for residents.

In the LTC setting, individualizing diabetes control is complicated. Considering the impact of diabetes on each of the more common geriatric syndromes may make it easier for the LTC clinician to determine the resident's level of frailty and then set reasonable glycemic goals based on their individual risks.

Depression and Diabetes

Depression is an issue in the LTC population because it interferes with successful diabetes management. As a result of depressed mood, the resident may exhibit poor appetite and reluctance to participate in physical activity. In fact, depression is the most common reason for weight loss in the older adult population.[48] Normal diabetes medications are based on eating and activity habits. Changes in these patterns will have a direct impact on blood glucose levels. Reduced carbohydrate intake typically lowers blood glucose values. This puts the resident who is taking insulin or insulin secretagogues at risk for hypoglycemia. On the other hand, blood glucose levels may rise when a physically active resident reduces the amount of physical activity. A reduction in nutritional intake combined with a reduction in physical activity in an LTC resident creates an unpredictable situation. When a resident is at high risk for hypoglycemia, it is important to add periodic monitoring of finger-stick blood glucose levels whenever the routine changes. Regular communication with the resident's primary care provider during periods of change is important. Diabetes medication dosages may need to be altered or even discontinued. The team pharmacist may be able to provide recommendations for change. Keep in mind that sliding-scale insulin dosing is no longer recommended because it is associated with inconsistent blood glucose levels and overall poor glycemic control. More information about this can be found in Chapter 2. If the resident is not eating well, consult with a dietitian to determine the type and time frame for nutritional supplementation.

Beyond blood glucose values, the resident with depression is likely to need additional help with basic ADLs. Interference with ADLs, UI, poor perceived health status, visual impairment, and a higher number of hospitalizations are all directly related to the severity of depression.[7,23] During acute depression, there is little desire to perform even the most basic self-care functions much less participate in normal or usual activities. Failure to participate in social activities can further isolate the resident and potentially even worsen the depression.

Urinary Incontinence and Diabetes

Women with diabetes are at a higher risk for UI than women in the general population.[15,23,72,73] It is reasonable to conclude that this also applies to women in LTC environments. Importantly, because geriatric syndromes, including UI, tend to occur at younger ages in women with diabetes, monitoring for UI in residents with diabetes should begin earlier.[72] Urge, stress, and mixed UI are most common in women with diabetes.[23,33] Because these data were collected from community-dwelling women, however, it is reasonable for caregivers to also focus on functional and overflow incontinence as these tend to be fairly common in residents of LTC. Overall, UI has been associated with impairments in mobility, cognitive ability, and ADLs, as well as increased numbers of urinary tract infection, pressure ulcers, and hospitalizations.[73]

According to Lawhorne et al.,[38] of all the most common geriatric syndromes, UI is the most neglected. They found that incontinence pads and briefs were used as the default intervention, and although considered to be very helpful, toileting schedules are not applied consistently in LTC. Because depression is so common to both diabetes and UI, it makes sense to focus intervention on evaluation and management of UI to improve quality of life and reduce the risk for depression.

On admission and periodically thereafter, the resident needs to be screened for the risk factors of UI, and those who are cognitively intact should participate in developing a toileting schedule; this often is called "prompted voiding." One form of assessment recommended by the Hartford Institute for Geriatric Nursing is the Urogenital Distress Inventory Short Form.[75] This simple assessment tool can easily be incorporated into admission and periodic assessments. Continence charts and records can be used to document the frequency and severity of involuntary urine loss.

Caregivers need to understand that continence status can change over time. Urinary tract infections commonly cause frequent urination and, in the older adult, short-term or more pronounced UI. Residents with significant hyperglycemia (e.g., blood glucose values consistently >250 mg/dl), may experience osmotic diuresis and develop UI as a result of this hyperglycemia.

Treatment for UI can include both pharmacological and nonpharmacological therapy. It is important to minimize the impact of known risk factors. For example, clinicians should review the resident's drug regimen and discontinue (if possible) known offenders. If they must be used, diuretics should be given during the early part of the day and a toileting plan should take into account the time frame the drug was given. Similarly, foods and fluids that contain caffeine should be minimized. Limiting overall fluid intake is not beneficial, but decreasing intake after dinner may be helpful in reducing nighttime incontinence. Although it is not effective in preventing nighttime incontinence, prompted voiding can reduce UI up to 40% in nursing home residents.[74] Daily routines should include bathroom breaks before all meals to allow for incontinence pads and briefs as well as soiled clothing to be changed. Failure to do so can result in a resident that refuses to participate in communal meals, and then becomes isolated and subsequently depressed. Importantly, changing soiled briefs guards against the development of urinary tract infection, a condition that actually worsens UI. Finally, attempts should be made to keep diabetes control relatively stable and in the target range, keeping in mind that each resident's blood glucose target values will differ according to the type and duration of diabetes and their level of frailty. Chapter 11 provides more detailed information on monitoring.

Falls and Diabetes

All LTC residents are at risk of falling. The resident with long-standing diabetes may also have a number of diabetes complications that predisposes him or her to falls.[76] One form of diabetic nerve disease, for example, is diabetic peripheral neuropathy (DPN). Symptoms of DPN can range from tingling in the extremities to complete numbness or loss of feeling in the feet and legs. It is easy to slip, trip, or fall if both feet are numb. When normal gait is impaired, the individual may need to transition to an assistive device, such as a cane or walker. Caregivers need to spend extra time with the resident as she or he adjusts to this change in mobility. Remind the resident that extra time will be needed to complete ADLs and to get to and from activities. A toileting schedule or routine not only will prevent problems related to UI but also may reduce the likelihood of a fall from rushing to get to the bathroom.

Autonomic neuropathy (AN) is another form of diabetic nerve disease. Some people with AN develop orthostatic hypotension and can fall if they try to get up and move quickly before their blood pressure can accommodate changes in posture. To routinely evaluate for orthostatic changes, residents with diabetes should have blood pressure checked in both sitting and standing or lying and sitting positions. Orthostasis is defined as fall in systolic pressure of ≥20 mmHg and fall in diastolic pressure of ≥10 mmHg.[42] To prevent orthostatic-related falls, residents should be reminded to dangle their feet at the bedside for several minutes to allow the blood pressure to stabilize. Failure to wait for the blood pressure to stabilize may result in a fall.

Clinical Note

Fall risk related to diabetic neuropathy

- Sensory—decreased feeling, proprioception
- Motor—foot deformities, gait impairment
- Autonomic—orthostatic hypotension

Visual complications of diabetes include retinopathy, glaucoma, macular degeneration, and cataracts. The resident with decreased vision will be at high risk for falls. Retinopathy ranges in severity. Residents with visual alterations may have reduced peripheral vision or complete blindness. As with other complications, to prevent falls, caregivers must allow increased time for ADLs and other activities. A few universal recommendations will help the visually impaired resident avoid falling. Keep the floor of the resident's room free from clutter, avoid moving furniture around, ensure that grab-bars and rails are present and in good working order, and have assistive devices (including patient call devices) accessible to the resident. Much more comprehensive information on this topic is available in Chapter 13.

The two acute complications of diabetes are hypoglycemia and hyperglycemia. Both can lead to falls. An early warning symptom of hypoglycemia is hunger. If the resident develops hypoglycemia, she or he will want to treat it immediately, call for help, or do both. Glucose tablets, gel, or some form of simple carbohydrate must be accessible to the resident. Keep simple carbohydrates in a bedside table and in other locations that are readily available. Be sure to let the resident know where to find this "treatment" and remind him or her to call for help when hypoglycemia occurs. Extreme hyperglycemia can result in daytime polyuria or nocturia, which in and of itself places the resident at risk for falling. As a result of polyuria, the resident's normal toileting routine will be compromised. Additionally, polyuria will lead to volume depletion with subsequent orthostatic changes to blood pressure, which presents another risk for falling. Caregivers will need to frequently check the resident to assist him or her with the frequent urination caused by elevated blood glucose levels and to make every attempt to keep the resident well hydrated.

Polypharmacy is common in older adults, particularly in residents of LTC. Complex drug regimens not only are associated with increased risks for medication errors and adverse drug reactions, but in diabetes, polypharmacy also is linked to higher rates of hypoglycemia.[31] High or low blood glucose levels can cause falls as the resident is rushing to treat hypoglycemia or rushing to the bathroom to urinate during periods of extreme hyperglycemia. Combine this "rushing" with visual impairment or diabetic nerve disease and you now have a resident who is at extremely high risk for falling.

Functional Disability, Frailty, and Diabetes

Diabetes is a risk factor for nursing home placement, and individuals with diabetes are typically younger on admission than other residents.[8,31,77] Following hospitalization, frail elders with diabetes are more likely to be admitted to LTC facilities. Because frailty is associated with reductions in physiologic reserve, it can result in functional disability, further decline, and, in some cases, death. Frailty makes care of the institutionalized elder with diabetes complex and time-consuming. Frail elderly residents with diabetes are likely to experience falls, rehospitalization, and sustained disability.[46] An important aspect of assessment for residents upon admission is assessment of frailty. According to Clegg et al.,[47] the Canadian Study of Health and Aging (CSHA) clinical frailty scale is the gold standard for assessment. The CSHA is time-consuming, however, and must be conducted by a geriatrics specialist. Reasonable alternatives include the Fried Frailty Phenotype and the Edmonton Frail Scale.[47,78,79]

A goal of care for these residents is to improve functional capacity, strength, and physiologic reserve. Weight maintenance, muscle strengthening, and fall prevention are all important goals in restoring functional ability to the frail elder.[80] Sarcopenia and muscle weakness are common in the older adult with diabetes; however, those individuals who were more independent before institutionalization will experience functional decline to a lesser degree.[47,81] Involving physical and occupational therapists, consultant dietitians, and family caregivers with the LTC staff will optimize the resident's potential for recovery. Barriers to success include chronic complications of diabetes, such as CHD, stroke, diabetic kidney disease (nephropathy), and diabetic nerve disease (neuropathy). Residents with chronic complications may have the capacity to regain limited functional abilities, but they should work to achieve their highest possible level of functioning. Impaired cognitive ability presents another barrier to regaining independence in functional ability. When residents are not given the opportunity to participate in their care, improvement in functional capacity is unlikely. The plan of care should encourage resident engagement that is continual and progressive. Fall risk assessments can be conducted routinely. Body weight should be recorded weekly and changes brought to the attention of the charge nurse and medical director. It might be useful to assess grip strength regularly and document changes. The key to success with this resident population is modest but continued improvement in functional ADLs.

Polypharmacy and Diabetes

Older adults with diabetes are particularly prone to polypharmacy. These residents are just as likely as anyone else to have degenerative arthritis and other common diseases of aging. Having diabetes tends to increase the individual's risk for cataracts, glaucoma, and Alzheimer's disease. Each of these conditions requires an array of medications. Diabetes typically coexists with several other chronic conditions, including depression, hypertension, elevated cholesterol, and possibly heart disease. Each of these conditions needs specific medications. Finally, medication management just for diabetes can be incredibly complex. To control T2D, an individual may take oral medications, insulin, other injectable diabetes drugs, or some combination of all three.

All of the issues with polypharmacy listed earlier can occur in the resident with diabetes. Add to the list of drug-to-drug interactions, increased frequency of adverse reactions, and hospitalization, the potential for diabetes specific problems. First and foremost among these problems is hypoglycemia. It is the most common complication of diabetes drug therapy. Multiple medications may increase the resident's risk for this complication. Clinicians need to consider the risk of hypoglycemia when setting blood glucose target levels because the older adult may not have clear symptoms when blood glucose levels drop.[54] Front-line primary caregivers often know the residents best. They often are the ones who will recognize when a resident's behavior is different and may indicate a need for finger-stick glucose testing. These caregivers should be familiar with hypoglycemia treatment protocols and have easy access to simple carbohydrates for rapid treatment.

Orthostasis presents a dual risk for the resident with diabetes. In diabetes complicated by autonomic neuropathy, orthostatic hypotension is not uncommon. Polypharmacy, however, is another possible cause of orthostasis in the resident with uncomplicated diabetes. Because hypertension is so common in people with diabetes, caregivers in nursing homes should expect that residents with diabetes will be taking at least one and possibly two or three different antihypertensive medications for blood pressure control. Multiple medications for hypertension may increase the risk for orthostatic hypotension. The combined risks for hypoglycemia and orthostatic changes increase the resident's risk of falling.

Care conferences should address medication management. It is likely that multiple medications will be needed to control the various clinical conditions existing in the resident with diabetes. The consultant pharmacist should be involved in frequent review of the resident's medication lists and feel comfortable making recommendations for change. Much more detailed information can be found in Chapter 9, which deals with pharmacologic management of diabetes.

Malnutrition and Diabetes

There is an interesting paradox in thinking about malnutrition in the resident with diabetes. Current CDC data reveal that 90% of all people with T2D are overweight or obese. How can malnutrition be possible in an obese individual? In actuality, even obese individuals can be undernourished. Perhaps this is part of the reason that malnutrition is underrecognized and underdiagnosed in LTC.

Excess body fat combined with reduced lean body mass is known as sarcopenic obesity; it has been shown to alter muscle strength and insulin sensitivity resulting in poor glycemic control.[82] Considering the complexity of diabetes management in the frail elder, weight loss may not be appropriate for LTC residents with diabetes who are at such high risk for malnutrition.[23] Living on their own, older adults are more likely to be undernourished than frail elders in LTC settings who ingest a variety of fruits and vegetables.[83] When undernourished, residents who take insulin or insulin secretagogues are more likely to experience hypoglycemia and suffer falls.

The main issue becomes one of finding the best, most appropriate diet for the individual with diabetes. Many caregivers continue to believe that a strict "diabetic" or sugar-restricted diet is needed for proper glucose control. Individualized care actually makes more sense. The most current guidelines for diabetes management in LTC suggest a regular diet that includes a variety of foods and consistency in carbohydrate and dietary fiber intake.[22] The recommended guidelines certainly will require more coordination for residents taking antihyperglycemic medications, but the outcome should be safer management and better quality of life for the resident. Chapter 7 provides more detailed information about this aspect of care.

CONCLUSION

T2D develops slowly and, fundamentally, it is a disease of aging. We are all more likely to develop diabetes as we grow older. In the older adult, the silent nature and slow development of diabetes can be particularly problematic because as many as 50% of these patients are unaware they have the disease.[84] Years of poorly controlled diabetes is what leads to chronic complications, such as heart disease, kidney failure, and blindness. In the LTC setting, residents may have diabetes (complicated or uncomplicated) at admission, or they may develop diabetes during the course of their stay. The frail elder with diabetes is at high risk for a number of geriatric syndromes, and the combination of these syndromes with diabetes increases the complexity of care. The acute complications, hypoglycemia and extreme hyperglycemia, put the resident at an even higher risk. Testing for diabetes upon admission is one way to identify the individuals who have not yet been diagnosed. By being aware of diabetes in a resident, the staff can design and implement a plan care that reduces the risk of injury from extremely high or low blood glucose values.

REFERENCES

1. Chau D, Edelman SV. Clinical management of diabetes in the elderly. *Clinical Diabetes* 2001;19(4):172–175.
2. Davey A, Lele U, Elias MF, Dore GA, Siegler IC, Johnson MA, for the Georgia Centenarian Study. Diabetes mellitus in centenarians. *Journal of the American Geriatrics Society* 2012;60(3):468–473.
3. Ferrer A, Padrós G, Formiga F, Rojas-Farreras S, Perez J, Pujol R. Diabetes mellitus: Prevalence and effect of morbidities in the oldest old. The Octabaix Study. *Journal of the American Geriatrics Society* 2012;60(3):462–467.
4. Hermans MP, Pepersack TM, Godeaux LH, Beyer I, Turc AP. Prevalence and determinants of impaired glucose metabolism in frail elderly patients: The Belgian Elderly Diabetes Survey (BEDS). *Journal of Gerontology* 2005;60A(2):241–247.

5. Zhang X, Decker FH, Luo H, Geiss LS, Pearson WS, Saaddine JB, Albright A. Trends in the prevalence and comorbidities of diabetes mellitus in nursing home residents in the United States: 1995–2004. *Journal of the American Geriatrics Society* 2010;58(4):724–730.

6. Sinclair AJ, Gadsby R, Penfold S, Croxson SCM, Bayer AJ. Prevalence of diabetes in care home residents. *Diabetes Care* 2001;24(6):1066–1068.

7. Centers for Disease Control and Prevention. *National diabetes fact sheet: National estimates and general information on diabetes and pre-diabetes in the United States, 2011.* Atlanta, GA, Centers for Disease Control and Prevention, 2011.

8. Clement M, Leung F. Diabetes and the frail elderly in long-term care. *Canadian Journal of Diabetes* 2009;33(2):114–121.

9. American Diabetes Association. Economic costs of diabetes in the U.S. in 2007. Diabetes Care 2008;31(3):596–615.

10. Boyle JP, Thompson TJ, Gregg EW, Barker LE, Williamson DF. Projection of the year 2050 burden of diabetes in the US adult population: dynamic modeling of incidence, mortality, and prediabetes prevalence *Population Health Metrics* 2010;8(29):1–12.

11. Landman GWD, van Hatteren KJJ, Kleefstra N, Groenier KH, Gans ROB, Bilo HJG. Health-related quality of life and mortality in a general elderly population of patients with type 2 diabetes (Zodiac-18). *Diabetes Care* 2010;33(11):2378–2382.

12. American Geriatrics Society, Expert Panel on the Care of Older Adults with, Multimorbidity. Guiding principles for the care of older adults with multimorbidity: An approach for clinicians. *Journal of the American Geriatrics Society* 2012;60(10):E1–E25.

13. Lee PG, Cigolle C, Blaum C. The co-occurrence of chronic diseases and geriatric syndromes: The Health and Retirement Study. *Journal of the American Geriatrics Society* 2009;57(3):511–516.

14. Migdal A, Yarandi SS, Smiley D, Umpierrez GE. Update on diabetes in the elderly and in nursing home residents. *Journal of the American Medical Directors Association* 2011;12(9):627–632.e622

15. Cayea D, Durso SC. Management of diabetes mellitus in the nursing home. *Annals of Long Term Care* 2007;15(5):27–33.

16. Inouye SK, Studenski S, Tinetti ME, Kuchel GA. Geriatric syndromes: Clinical research and policy implications of a core geriatric concept. *Journal of the American Geriatric Society* 2007;55(5):780–791.

17. Durso SC, Sullivan GM, Eds. Geriatrics Review Syllabus. 8th ed. New York, American Geriatrics Society, 2013.

18. AGS Foundation for Health in Aging. Guide to "geriatric syndromes"—part I, n.d. Available at http://www.clinicalgeriatrics.com/images/cg1108Guide.pdf. Accessed 20 March 2013.

19. Kane RL, Talley KM, Shamliyan T, Pacala JT. Common syndromes in older adults related to primary and secondary prevention. (AHRQ Pub No. 11-05157-EF-1). Rockville, MD, AHRQ, 2011.

20. Rosso AL, Eaton CB, Wallace R, Gold R, Stefanick ML, Ockene JK, Michael YL. Geriatric syndromes and incident disability in older women:

Results from the women's health initiative observational study. *Journal of the American Geriatrics Society*, 2013;61(3):371–379.

21. Cigolle CT, Langa KM, Kabeto MU, Tian Z, Blaum CS. Geriatric conditions and disability: the Health and Retirement Study. *Annals of Internal Medicine* 2007;147(3):156–164.

22. American Medical Directors Association. *Guidelines for Diabetes Management in the Long-Term Care Setting.* Columbia, MD, American Medical Directors Association, 2010.

23. Araki A, Ito H. Diabetes mellitus and geriatric syndromes. *Geriatrics and Gerontology International* 2009;9(2):105–114.

24. Garcia TJ, Brown SA. Diabetes management in the nursing home: A systematic review of the literature. *The Diabetes Educator* 2011;37(2):167–187.

25. de Groot M, Anderson R, Freedland KE, Clouse RE, Lustman PJ. Association of depression and diabetes complications: A meta-analysis. *Psychosomatic Medicine* 2001;63:619–630.

26. Kan C, Silva N, Golden SH, Rajala U, Timonen M, Stahl D, Ismail K. A systematic review and meta-analysis of the association between depression and insulin resistance. *Diabetes Care* 2013;36(2):480–489.

27. Maraldi C, Volpato S, Penninx BW, et al. Diabetes mellitus, glycemic control, and incident depressive symptoms among 70- to 79-year-old persons: The health, aging, and body composition study. *Archives of Internal Medicine* 2007;167(11):1137–1144.

28. Anderson RJ, Freedland KE, Clouse RE, Lustman PJ. The prevalence of comorbid depression in adults with diabetes: A meta-analysis. *Diabetes Care* 2001;24:1069–1078.

29. Lustman PJ, Clouse RE. Depression in diabetic patients: The relationship between mood and glycemic control. *Journal of Diabetes Complications* 2005;19:113–122.

30. Thakur M, Blazer DG. Depression in long-term care. *Journal of the American Medical Directors Association* 2008;9(2):82–87.

31. Pinkstaff SM. Aging with diabetes—An underappreciated cause of progressive disability and reduced quality of life. *Clinical Geriatrics* 2004;12(9):45–56.

32. Travis SS, Buchanan RJ, Wang S, Kim M. Analyses of nursing home residents with diabetes at admission. [11/23/12]. *Journal of the American Medical Directors Association* 2004;5:320–327.

33. Danforth KN, Townsend MK, Curhan GC, Resnick NM, Grodstein F. Type 2 diabetes mellitus and risk of stress, urge and mixed urinary incontinence. *The Journal of Urology* 2009;181(1):193–197.

34. National Institutes of Health. Urinary incontinence in women. U.S. Department of Health and Human Services, NIH Publ. No. 08–4132. October 2007. Available from http://kidney.niddk.nih.gov/KUDiseases/pubs/uiwomen/UI-Women_508.pdf. Accessed 4 March 2013.

35. Devore EE, Townsend MK, Resnick NM, Grodstein F. The epidemiology of urinary incontinence in women with Type 2 Diabetes. *The Journal of Urology* 2012;188(5):1816–1821.

36. DuBeau CE, Simon SE, Morris JN. The effect of urinary incontinence on quality of life in older nursing home residents. *Journal of the American Geriatrics Society* 2006;54(9):1325–1333.

37. Holroyd-Leduc JM, Mehta KM, Covinsky KE. Urinary incontinence and its association with death, nursing home admission and functional decline. *Journal of the American Geriatrics Society* 2004;52(5):712–718.
38. Lawhorne LW, Ouslander JG, Parmelee PA, Resnick B, Calabrese B. Urinary incontinence: a neglected geriatric syndrome in nursing facilities. *Journal of the American Medical Directors Association* 2008;9(1):29–35.
39. Leung FW, Schnelle JF. Urinary and fecal incontinence in nursing home residents. *Gastroenterology Clinics of North America* 2008;37(3):697–707.
40. Oliver D, Healy F, Haines TP. Preventing falls and fall-related injuries in hospitals. *Clinic Geriatric Medicine* 2010;26(4):645–692.
41. Panel on Prevention of Falls in Older Persons. Summary of the updated American Geriatrics Society/British Geriatrics Society clinical practice guideline for prevention of falls in older persons. *Journal of the American Geriatrics Society* 2011;59(1):148–157.
42. Martin FC. Falls risk factors: Assessment and management to prevent falls and fractures. *Canadian Journal on Aging* 2011;30(1):33–44.
43. Leland NE, Gozalo P, Teno J, Mor V. Falls in newly admitted nursing home residents: A national study. *Journal of the American Geriatrics Society* 2012;60(5):939–945.
44. Gray-Micelli D, Quigley PA. Falls. Nursing standard of practice protocol: Fall prevention, 2012. Hartford Institute for Geriatric Nursing. Available at http://consultgerirn.org/topics/falls/want_to_know_more#Wrap. Accessed 1 June 2013.
45. Bourdel-Marchasson I, Berrut G. Caring the elderly diabetic patient with respect to concepts of successful aging and frailty. *Diabetes and Metabolism* 2005;31(Spec No 2):5S13–5S19.
46. Atiénzar P, Abizanda P, Guppy A, Sinclair AJ. Diabetes and frailty: An emerging issue. Part 1: Sarcopaenia and factors affecting lower limb function. *British Journal of Diabetes and Vascular Disease* 2012;12(3):110–116.
47. Clegg A, Young J, Iliffe S, Rikkert MO, Rockwood K. Frailty in elderly people. *Lancet* 2013;381(9868):752–762.
48. Morley JE, Haren MT, Rolland Y, Kim MJ. Frailty. *Medical Clinics of North America* 2006;90(5):837–847.
49. Nelson JM, Dufraux K, Cook PF. The relationship between glycemic control and falls in older adults. *Journal of the American Geriatrics Society* 2007;55(12):2041–2044.
50. Petersen RC. Mild cognitive impairment. *New England Journal of Medicine* 2011;364(23):2227–2234.
51. Morley JE. Diabetes, sarcopenia, and frailty. *Clinics in Geriatric Medicine* 2008;24(3):455–469.
52. Bruce DG, Davis WA, Casey GP, Starkstein SE, Clarnette RM, Almeida OP, Davis TME. Predictors of cognitive decline in older individuals with diabetes. *Diabetes Care* 2008;31(11):2103–2107.
53. Braes T, Milisen K, Foreman MD. Assessing cognitive function, 2012. Hartford Institute for Geriatric Nursing. Available at http://consultgerirn.org/topics/assessing_cognitive_function/want_to_know_more. Accessed 1 June 2013.
54. Hartford Geriatric Institute. Assessing cognitive function. Available at http://consultgerirn.org/topics/assessing_cognitive_function/want_to_know_more. Accessed 1 March 2013.

55. Good CB. Polypharmacy in elderly patients with diabetes. *Diabetes Spectrum* 2002;15(4):240–248.

56. Hajjar ER, Cafiero AC, Hanlon JT. Polypharmacy in elderly patients. *The American Journal of Geriatric Pharmacotherapy* 2007;5(4):345–351.

57. Abdelhafiz AH, Sinclair AJ. Hypoglycaemia in residential care homes. *British Journal of General Practice* 2009;59(558):49–50.

58. Merriam Webster. http://www.merriam-webster.com/dictionary/malnutrition. Accessed 1 March 2013.

59. Cowan DT, Roberts JD, Fitzpatrick JM, While AE, Baldwin J. Nutritional status of older people in long term care settings: current status and future directions. *International Journal of Nursing Studies* 2004;41(3):225–237.

60. Guigoz Y, Lauque S, Vellas BJ. Identifying the elderly at risk for malnutrition. The mini nutritional assessment. *Clinics in Geriatric Medicine* 2002;18(4):737–757.

61. Labossiere R, Bernard MA. Nutritional considerations in institutionalized elders. *Current Opinion in Clinical Nutrition and Metabolic Care* 2008;11(1):1–6.

62. Waters DL, Baumgartner RN. Sarcopenia and obesity. *Clinics in Geriatric Medicine* 2011;27(3):401–421.

63. American Diabetes Association. Estimated average glucose (eAG) calculator. Available at http://professional.diabetes.org/GlucoseCalculator.aspx. Accessed 4 March 2013.

64. Sinclair AJ, Paolisso G, Castro M, Bourdel-Marchasson I, Gadsby R, Rodriguez Mañas L. European Diabetes Working Party for Older People 2011. Clinical guidelines for type 2 diabetes mellitus. Executive summary. *Diabetes and Metabolism* 2011;37(Suppl3):S27–S38.

65. Stratton IM, Adler AI, Neil HA, et al. Association of glycaemia with macrovascular and microvascular complications of type 2 diabetes (UKPDS 35): Prospective observational study. *British Medical Journal* 2000;321:405–412.

66. Kirkman MS, Briscoe VJ, Clark N, Florez H, Haas LB, Halter JB, Swift C.S. Diabetes in older adults. *Diabetes Care* 2012;35(12):2650–2664.

67. American Diabetes Association. Standards of medical care in diabetes—2012. *Diabetes Care* 2013;35(Suppl1):S11–S63.

68. Brown AF, Mangione CM, Saliba D, Sarkisian CA, California Healthcare Foundation/American Geriatrics Society Panel on Improving Care for Older Persons with Diabetes. Guidelines for improving the care of the-older person with diabetes mellitus. *Journal of the American Geriatric Society* 2003;51(5):S265–S280.

69. Holman RR, Paul SK, Bethel MA, Matthews DR, Neil HA. 10-year follow-up of intensive glucose control in type 2 diabetes. *New England Journal of Medicine* 2008;359:1577–1589.

70. Sinclair A, Morley JE, Rodriguez-Manas L, Paolisso G, Bayer T, Zeyfang A, Lorig K. Diabetes mellitus in older people: position statement on behalf of the International Association of Gerontology and Geriatrics (IAGG), the European Diabetes Working Party for Older People (EDWPOP), and the International Task Force of Experts in Diabetes. *Journal of the American Medical Directors Association* 2012;13(6):497–502.

71. UK Progressive Diabetes Study (UKPDS) Group. Intensive blood glucose control with sulfonylureas or insulin compared with conventional treatment

and risk of complications in patients with type 2 diabetes (UKPDS 33). *Lancet* 1998;352(9131):837–853.

72. Cigolle CT, Lee PG, Langa KM, Lee Y, Tian Z, Blaum CS. Geriatric conditions develop in middle-aged adults with diabetes. *Journal of General Internal Medicine* 2011;26(3):272–279.

73. Phelan S, Kanaya AM, Subak LL, Hogan PE, Espeland MA, Wing RR, et al. Prevalence and risk factors for urinary incontinence in overweight and obese diabetic women: Action for Health in Diabetes (Look AHEAD) study. *Diabetes Care* 2012;32(8):1391–1397.

74. Zarowitz BJ, Tangalos EG, Hollenack K, O'Shea T. The application of evidence-based principles of care in older persons (Issue 3): management of diabetes mellitus. *Journal of the American Medical Directors Association* 2006;7(4):234–240.

75. Hartford Institute for Geriatric Nursing. Urogenital distress inventory short form. Available at http://consultgerirn.org/topics/urinary_incontinence/want_to_know_more. Accessed 5 March 2013.

76. Maurer MS, Burcham J, Cheng H. Diabetes mellitus is associated with an increased risk of falls in elderly residents of a long-term care facility. *The Journals of Gerontology Series A: Biological Sciences and Medical Sciences* 2005;60(9):1157–1162.

77. Resnick HE, Heineman J, Stone R, Shorr RI. Diabetes in U.S. nursing homes, 2004. *Diabetes Care* 2008;31(2):287–288.

78. Rockwood K, Song X, MacKnight C, Bergman H, Hogan DB, McDowell I, Mitnitski A. A global clinical measure of fitness and frailty in elderly people. *Canadian Medical Association Journal* 2005;173(5):489–495.

79. Poltawski L, Goodman C, Iliffe S, Manthorpe J, Gage H, Shah D, Drennan V. Frailty scales—their potential in interprofessional working with older people: A discussion paper. *Journal of Interprofessional Care* 2011;25(4):280–286.

80. Benefield LE, Higbee RL. Frailty and its implications for care, 2007. Hartford Institute for Geriatric Nursing. Available at http://consultgerirn.org/topics/frailty_and_its_implications_for_care_new/want_to_know_more. Accessed on 1 June 2013.

81. Atiénzar P, Abizanda P, Guppy A, Sinclair AJ. Diabetes and frailty: an emerging issue. Part 2: Linking factors. *British Journal of Diabetes and Vascular Disease* 2012;12(3):119–122.

82. Prado CM, Wells JC, Smith SR, Stephan BC, Siervo M. Sarcopenic obesity: A Critical appraisal of the current evidence. *Clinical Nutrition* 2012;31(5):583–601.

83. Haas L. Functional decline in older adults with diabetes. *American Journal of Nursing* 2007;107(6):50–54.

84. Meneilly GS, Tessier D. Diabetes in elderly adults. *Journal of Gerontology* 2001;56A(1):M5–M13.

RECOMMENDED READING

Bourdel Marchasson I, Doucet J, Bauduceau B, Berrut G, Blickle JF, Brocker P, et al. Key priorities in managing glucose control in older people with diabetes. *Journal of Nutrition, Health and Aging* 2009;13(8):685–691.

Fitzner KA, Dietz DA, Moy E. How innovative treatment models and data use are improving diabetes care among older African American adults. *Population Health Management* 2011;14(3):143–155.

He XZ. Diabetes care for older patients in America. *International Journal of Clinical Practice* 2012;66(3):299–304.

5

Glycemic Management in Long-Term Care

Debbie Hinnen, APN, BC-ADM, CDE, FAAN, FAADE

INTRODUCTION

The epidemic of type 2 diabetes (T2D) is escalating and has far-reaching effects in long-term care (LTC). In the 2008 national nursing home survey, it was identified that nearly 25% of residents in LTC have diabetes.[1] More than two-thirds (69%) of the residents with diabetes in LTC have two or more chronic diseases—most often hypertension (56%) and various cardiovascular problems (80%). These complicated comorbidities require multiple medications, contributing to polypharmacy in these residents.

In diabetes, glycemic control is measured in multiple ways. The A1C is the gold standard for biochemical measurement. This test measures the overall average blood glucose for the previous 2- to 3-month period. Fasting plasma glucose (FPG) is another commonly used test. It provides a simple snapshot of the individual's current glucose level. Although it may be helpful in some situations, the FPG is not particularly useful in determining glycemic control. Capillary (finger-stick) blood glucose (CBG) testing is another commonly used procedure. Although not as precise as plasma glucose obtained by venipuncture, the CBG provides a rapid and reasonably accurate picture of current blood glucose values. The A1C test is reported as a percent. FPG and CBG results are both reported in milligrams per deciliter (mg/dl) of plasma. Over the years, many people with diabetes have had trouble understanding how the percent value of the A1C related to their finger-stick blood glucose values. Now, there is a simplified conversion chart called the estimated average glucose (eAG) that patients and care providers can use to make the A1C results more meaningful. An eAG calculator can be found on the American Diabetes Association website (see Table 4.2).[2] Throughout this chapter, the A1C will be used as the primary reference point for glycemic control.

Determining evidenced-based glycemic goals in the elderly with T2D is challenging, as there are no randomized controlled trials targeting this population. Glycemic control and complications have been evaluated in retrospective studies. One study of older persons with T2D showed a U-shaped association between A1C and mortality. In this study, those older persons with the lowest risk for death had an A1C of ~7.5%. High and low mean A1C values were associated with increased all-cause mortality and cardiac events.[3] The Kaiser aging study demonstrated similar results. In this retrospective cohort study of >70,000 people with T2D, there was also a U-shaped relationship between mortality and A1C in those who were ≥60 years of age. Mortality risk was lower for A1C between 6.0 and 9.0%. These mortality patterns generally were seen across older age-groups: the young old (60–69), the middle old (70–79), and the oldest old (>80 years).[4]

DOI: 10.2337/9781580404730.05

CLINICAL PRACTICE GUIDELINES AND
GLYCEMIC MANAGEMENT

Several sources have suggested glycemic goals. The goal of diabetes treatment as recommended by the American Medical Directors Association (AMDA), the national professional organization representing attending physicians and medical directors who care for residents in the LTC setting, is to "improve blood glucose control, optimize cardiovascular risk factors and minimize complications while taking into account individual preferences, life expectancy, and quality of life as defined by the patient."[5] The AMDA recommendation is to achieve an A1C <7%. The European Diabetes Working Party for Older People guidelines for treating people with diabetes >70 years old, recommends an A1C range of 7 to 7.5% for older adults without major comorbidities, but adds that a level of 7.6 to 8.5% is more appropriate for frail residents.[6] The Working Party for Older People defined frailty as dependent, having multisystem disease, or as care home residency, including those with dementia, where hypoglycemia risk may be high and the benefit relatively low. Another group providing guidelines for glycemic control is the U.S. Department of Veterans Affairs and Department of Defense (VA/DOD).[7] The VA/DOD 2010 Diabetes Guidelines for Primary Care focus on patient status rather than age.[7] These guidelines are meant for primary care; however, they may be considered in the LTC setting if residents meet the stated criteria:[7]

- The patient with no or very mild microvascular complications, free of major concurrent illnesses, and a life expectancy of at least 10–15 years, should have an A1C target of <7%, if this target can be achieved without risk.
- The patient with longer duration diabetes (>10 years) or with comorbid conditions, and who requires a combination medication regimen including insulin, should have an A1C target of <8%.
- The patient with advanced microvascular complications or major comorbid illnesses, or a life expectancy of <5 years is unlikely to benefit from aggressive glucose-lowering management and should have an A1C target of 8–9%. Although lower targets (<8%) can be established on an individual basis.

In its annual clinical practice guidelines document, the American Diabetes Association (ADA) recommended that goals for older adults should be individualized based on duration of diabetes, age and life expectancy, comorbid conditions, known cardiovascular disease (CVD) or advanced microvascular complications, hypoglycemia unawareness, and individual resident considerations. In addition, the ADA suggests that the clinician consider issues such as cognition and polypharmacy when setting goals for glycemic management The ADA recommendation for the general diabetes population is an A1C <7%.[8,9] Depending on these factors, more stringent or less stringent glycemic goals may be appropriate for individual LTC residents. AMDA goals are consistent with ADA based on prospective randomized clinical trials, such as the U.K. Prospective Diabetes Study (UKPDS). There is little evidence to suggest that goals established in adults with diabetes are not appropriate for healthy, active elderly patients. Many LTC residents, however, may not be considered healthy, active older adults.

Adding the American Geriatrics Society (AGS) similar guidelines of an A1C <7% for relatively healthy older adults with good functional status, there is good consistency among the major organizations.[10] A more conservative target, such as A1C ≤8% should be considered for elderly residents who are frail, have a life expectancy of <5 years, or in whom the risks of intensive glycemic control appear to outweigh the benefits.[10] ADA and AMDA also agree with this premise.

A 2012 consensus statement from an ADA conference on the diabetes care in older adults reviewed evidence from many studies and systematic reviews and concluded that glycemic targets for older people must be individualized.[11] The information in Table 5.1 was suggested for clinicians to organize their thinking about this issue. This table has been included in the ADA's *Standards of Medical Care in Diabetes—2014.*[9] Even if life expectancy is relatively short, maintaining reasonable glucose control will reduce symptoms of hyperglycemia, such as frequent urination and incontinence, which usually occur when the blood glucose levels are >200 mg/dl (A1C >8.5–9%).[11]

Table 5.1 Framework for Considering Treatment Goals for Glycemia in Older Adults with Diabetes

Patient characteristics and health status	Rationale	Reasonable A1C goal (%)	Fasting or preprandial glucose (mg/dl)	Bedtime glucose (mg/dl)
Healthy (few coexisting chronic illnesses, intact cognitive and functional status)	Longer life expectancy	<7.5	90–130	90–150
Complex/intermediate (multiple coexisting chronic illnesses, or 2+ instrumental activities of daily living impairments, or mild-moderate cognitive impairment	Intermediate life expectancy, high treatment burden, hypoglycemia vulnerability, fall risk	<8	90–150	100–180
Very complex/poor health (long-term care or end-stage chronic illness, or moderate-severe cognitive impairment, or 2+ activities of daily living dependencies	Limited life expectancy makes benefit uncertain	<8.5	100–180	110–200

Source: Adapted from Kirkman, et al. Consensus report: Diabetes in older adults. *Diabetes Care* 2012;35:1–15, epub ahead of print: 25 October 2012.

Factors Affecting Glucose Control

Managing glycemia in LTC is complicated by many factors, not all of which are resident related. Direct care staff may not have a broad understanding of the diabetes disease state, causes of complications and current medication actions and side effects. In the LTC setting, direct care typically is entrusted to the certified nursing assistant and the medication aide and overseen by a licensed nurse, often a licensed practical nurse or a licensed vocational nurse. Although these care providers often are knowledgeable about the residents under their care, they may not be comfortable with the most current diabetes guidelines. Staffing issues, such as frequent turnover, complicates the issue further and can contribute to less-than-optimal care. Registered nurses serve a coordinating and supervising role in care, but they may not be accessible to direct care providers. Consultant pharmacists, dietitians, and advanced practice nurses and physicians are even less available to assess and intervene in residents' care.

Residents with diabetes have many confounding issues related to diabetes management. It is common to find physical limitations, various prescription medications, other medical diagnoses, or diabetes complications, as well as changes in cognition, mobility, and communication. Impaired renal clearance affecting drug excretion, poor or inconsistent nutritional intake, altered counterregulatory hormones, and slowed intestinal absorption all may increase the risk of hypoglycemia. In the aging system, because a change in the counterregulatory response is seen, the common signs and symptoms of hypoglycemia may not be present. Instead, the more insidious neuroglycopenic symptoms of confusion, lack of motor skills, and tiredness, may be the only outward warning of low blood glucose. Those symptoms often are misinterpreted as something other than hypoglycemia and are not promptly and appropriately treated.

Helpful Hint: Counterregulatory hormones are stimulated by hypoglycemia and work to raise blood glucose levels

Hormone	Secreted by	Action
Glucagon	Pancreas (alpha cells)	Increases glucose production in the liver
Epinephrine	Adrenal glands	Inhibits insulin secretion Stimulates glucagon

---

Recognizing Glucose Extremes

Hyperglycemia in the elderly may be difficult to recognize. One- to two-hour glucose levels consistently >180 mg are considered hyperglycemia.[8] Higher levels may be acceptable, however, in frail elderly residents, with limited life expectancy and high risk for hypoglycemia.[6,10,11] Possible signs and symptoms of hyperglycemia in the elderly might include new or worsening confusion, lethargy, weight loss, blurred vision, fruity breath (if the resident has type 1 diabetes), worsening incontinence, polydipsia, and polyphagia.[5]

Uncontrolled hyperglycemia leads to multiple complications. Infections and vascular changes may exacerbate the risk of pressure sores. The highly regulated nursing home industry addresses several problems frequently occurring in diabetes. With regard to uncontrolled diabetes, the Medicare State Operations manual addresses pressure sores in F-Tag 314: "Institutions must ensure that a resident who enters the facility without pressure sores does not develop pressure sores unless the individual's clinical condition demonstrates they were unavoidable."[12]

Clinical Note

Hyperosmolar, Hyperglycemic State Potentially fatal condition associated with hyperglycemia and dehydration Risk factors include:

- Undiagnosed diabetes
- "Diabetogenic medications," e.g., high-dose corticosteroids
- Omission of diabetes medication(s)
- Infection/stress

Physiologic cascade

Hyperglycemia
↓
Dehydration
↓
Kidneys shutdown to preserve fluids
↓
Oliguria
↓
Extreme hyperglycemia as kidneys can't excrete glucose

Prevention

- Ensure adequate hydration
- Monitor intake and output and urine specific gravity
- Increase glucose monitoring frequency if "diabetogenic" medications started
- Don't stop basal insulin

Hypoglycemia may be equally challenging to identify in the elderly. The following may indicate hypoglycemia: altered behavior or mental function; poor concentration and coordination, leading to falls; hallucinations; irritability; altered level of consciousness; drowsiness; lethargy; pallor; sweating; seizure, or stroke.[5] With a long duration of diabetes, diminished counterregulatory function may cause hypoglycemia to occur without symptoms, making it doubly important to regularly monitor blood glucose levels. The AMDA guidelines for diabetes in LTC identify hypoglycemia as particularly problematic in residents who may not perceive or communicate the symptoms. As with other people with diabetes, glycemic management in the older adult includes the tools of medical nutrition therapy, physical activity, and diabetes medication management. See Chapters 7–10 for more comprehensive information on these topics.

Diabetes Medications and Glycemic Management

To achieve target glucose levels, the geriatric resident with diabetes may be managed with oral agents (Tables 5.2 and 5.3) or insulin or other injectables. Comorbid conditions such as congestive heart failure (CHF), extreme age, gastrointestinal disorders, liver disease, lower-extremity edema, and renal insufficiency, must be considered when individualizing therapy. Adverse drug reactions and drug–drug or drug–food interactions are likely even greater considerations in the resident with diabetes.[5,13] A number of new medications for treating T2D have emerged since 2005 and even more are in development. Although these drugs are more expensive initially, they may be a better consideration for the elderly in the long run. Reducing the potential for adverse drug reactions or interactions and giving medications with lower dose or lower frequency may reduce nursing time and ultimately be a more cost-effective consideration. As a general rule, the lowest possible dosage should be initiated, with gradual increases until glycemic targets are reached.

According to standard algorithms, metformin is generally the preferred initial starting medication in T2D.[8,9,14] Before initiating metformin, however, the older adult will need to be evaluated carefully for chronic kidney disease or CHF. Because age- or disease-related declines in renal function may be common in this population, the starting metformin dose should be reduced if the resident's estimated glomerular filtration rate (eGFR) is between 30 and 60 and, importantly, metformin should not be used if a resident's eGFR is <30.[11] Upset stomach, gas, diarrhea, and other common gastrointestinal side effects may be mitigated by using the extended-release metformin. Metformin ER (XR) 500 mg is a common dosage on preferred formulary and pharmacy benefit plans. Poor oxygenation, hypoxia, CHF, or infection may increase the risk of lactic acidosis, which is a rare complication. It is not uncommon for metformin to be discontinued during hospitalization. Whether or not it can or should be resumed upon discharge will vary with the individual. Metformin's action primarily targets nocturnal glucose release via reducing glycogenolysis and gluconeogenesis. When initiating this medication, a modest dose with the evening meal potentially will result in reduced morning fasting blood glucose levels. Taking the medication after the meal and increasing the dose weekly may reduce side effects. Hypoglycemia is rare with metformin. The maximum clinically therapeutic dose is 2000 mg/d usually in divided doses.[5,13,15–17] Morning fasting blood glucose readings are the primary "report card" on the effectiveness of metformin. If the resident has attained near-normal fasting blood glucose levels, and postmeal blood glucose levels are elevated, the next medication to consider is from a category that will "nudge" the β-cells of the pancreas, which make insulin. Additional information about metformin can be found in Chapter 9.

Table 5.2 Oral Medications for Diabetes and Their Pharmacokinetics

Medication class	Primary mode of action	Agent	Trade name	Expected decrease in A1C	Onset of action	Typical dose
Second-generation sulfonylureas	Stimulate increased insulin production by pancreatic islet β-cells	Glyburide	Micronase		2 hours	Initially, 2.5 mg once daily with breakfast or first main meal. Dose range 1.25–20 mg/d in single or divided doses.
			DiaBeta		2 hours	Elderly start at 1.25 mg with gradual increases. Max dose 10 mg/d. *Note:* The Beers Criteria recommend not using glyburide in the elderly (Fick et al., 2012).
		Glyburide (micronized)	Glynase PresTab		2 hours	Initially, 1.5–3 mg once daily with breakfast or first main meal. Dose range usually 0.75–12 mg/d; increases of 1.5 mg/d weekly. Elderly start at 0.75 mg. Max dose 12 mg/d.
		Glipizide	Glucotrol	1.5%	90 minutes	Initially, 5 mg once daily before breakfast. Adjust at 2.5 mg to 5 mg intervals. Dose range 2.5–20 mg/d. Max dose 20 mg/d. Elderly start at 2.5 mg once daily.
		Glipizide (extended release)	Glucotrol XL		90 minutes	Initially, 5 mg once daily with breakfast. If needed, increase to 10 mg/d. Max dose 20 mg/d. (Max dose may not increase benefit.) Hypoglycemia is more common with long-acting formulations.
		Glimepiride	Amaryl		1 hour	Initially, 1–2 mg once daily with breakfast or first main meal. After 2 mg/d, wait 1–2 weeks between increases. Dose range 1–4 mg once daily. Max dose 8 mg/d. Elderly start at 1 mg/d.

(Continued)

Table 5.2 Oral Medications for Diabetes and Their Pharmacokinetics (Continued)

Medication class	Primary mode of action	Agent	Trade name	Expected decrease in A1C	Onset of action	Typical dose
Meglitinides	Increase insulin release from the pancreas	Repaglinide	Prandin	1–1.5%	<1 hour	For recently diagnosed patients or those with A1C <8%, 1–2 mg up to 30 minutes before meals. Monitor fasting (or postprandial) blood glucose. Increase weekly to 4 mg after meals until results obtained. Take up to 4 times daily. Max dose 16 mg/d.
		Nateglinide	Starlix		20 minutes	Starting and maintenance dose alone or in combination therapy, 120 mg 3 times daily before meals. Max dose 360 mg/d. If close to A1C target when starting, initiate at 60 mg 3 times daily.
α-Glucosidase inhibitors	Reduce postprandial glucose absorption	Acarbose	Precose	0.5–0.8%	<15 minutes	Initially, 25 mg 3 times daily at start of meal (may decrease GI side effects). Max dose 300 mg/d if >60 kg. If <60 kg or elderly, max dose 150 mg/d.
		Miglitol	Glyset		<15 minutes	Initially, 25 mg 3 times daily with first bite of each meal. (Starting at 25 mg once daily for 1 week may decrease GI side effects.) After 4–8 weeks, titrate to 50 mg 3 times daily. Max dose 100 mg 3 times daily. All doses at first bite of each meal.
Biguanides	Decrease insulin resistance, primarily by decreasing hepatic glucose output; minor increase in muscle glucose uptake	Metformin	Glucophage	1.5%	Maximum level 4–8 hours	500 mg daily. Increase by 500 mg intervals every 1–3 weeks, 2–3 times daily. Max dose 2550 mg/d. Often limited to 2,000 mg/d as most effective dose.
		Metformin extended release	Glucophage XR		Maximum level 4–8 hours	Initially, 500 mg once daily with evening meal. Increase by 500 mg weekly as needed up to max dose 2000 mg/d with evening meal. Consider splitting dose for greater control.

Drug class	Action	Generic name	Brand name	A1C	Onset/Peak	Dosing
Thiazolidinediones	Decrease hepatic output and increase insulin-dependent muscle glucose uptake (decreases insulin resistance)	Rosiglitazone	*Avandia	0.5–1.4%	Peak 1 h	Initially, 4 mg daily, single or divided dose. Increase to 8 mg at 12 weeks if needed. Max dose 8 mg/d, taken with or without food. No change in dosing for elderly. May be associated with onset or worsening of symptoms of congestive heart failure.
		Pioglitazone	Actos		30 minutes	Initially, 15 or 30 mg daily. Max dose 45 mg for monotherapy, 30 mg for combination therapy. Can be taken with or without food.
DPP-IV inhibitors	Prolongs the action of naturally occurring GLP-1 increases pancreatic insulin output, slows glucose absorption in the gut, increase satiety and can cause weight loss	Sitagliptin	Januvia	0.5–1.0%	Peak plasma concentration reached in 1–4 hours postdose	100 mg daily. Can be used in combination with metformin, sulfonylureas, and thiazolidinediones.

Note: DPP-IV = dipeptidyl peptidase IV inhibitor; GI = gastrointestinal; GLP-1 = glucagon-like peptide 1.

*On August 23, 2010 restrictions were placed on Avandia in response to data that suggest an elevated risk of cardiovascular events, such as heart attack and stroke. In summer 2013, those restrictions were lifted. See U.S. Food and Drug Administration: www.fda.gov/Safety/MedWatch/SafetyInformation/SafetyAlerts-forHumanMedicalProducts/ucm226994.htm for details. The REMS was removed in 2014.

Source: Adapted from Fick D, Semla T, Beizer J, Brandt N, Dombrowski R, DuBeau CE, Steonman M. American Geriatrics Society updated Beers criteria for potentially inappropriate medication use in older adults. *Journal of the American Geriatrics Society* 2012; 60(4):614–615

Table 5.3 Selecting Oral Antidiabetic Therapy

Agent or class of drug	Patient characteristics
α-Glucosidase inhibitors	Milder disease presentation Predominant symptom is postprandial hyperglycemia No gastrointestinal comorbidities Serum creatinine <2 mg/dl
DPP-4 inhibitor	Poor control with sulfonylureas and metformin Linagliptin can be used in renal impairment Cautious use in patients taking digitalis
Metformin	Obese, normal weight Normal kidney function (GFR >60 ml/minute/1.73 m²) Can use a half dose if eGFR is between 30 and 60 ml/minute/1.73 m² Normal liver function No class 3 or 4 CHF or acute illness
Sulfonylureas or glinides	Normal weight *Note:* ■ Sulfonylureas are contraindicated in severe liver or renal disease ■ Repaglinide or nateglinide is useful when older sulfonylureas result in hypoglycemia and in patients with postprandial hyperglycemia or erratic eating patterns ■ Glyburide should not be used in older adults
Thiazolidinediones	Obese, signs of insulin resistance No active liver disease or ALT >2.5 times normal No symptomatic heart failure (Class III/IV) *Note:* Can be used in renal insufficiency.

Note: CHF = congestive heart failure; DPP-4 = dipeptidyl peptidase-4; GFR = glomerular filtration rate.

Source:
American Diabetes Association. Standards of medical care in diabetes—2014. *Diabetes Care* 2014;37(Suppl. 1):S14–S80.
Gates BJ, Walker KM. Physiological changes in older adults and their effect on diabetes treatment. *Diabetes Spectrum* 2014;27(1):20–28.
Inzucchi SE, Bergenstal RM, Buse JB, et al. Management of hyperglycemia in type 2 diabetes: a patient-centered approach. Position statement of the American Diabetes Association (ADA) and the European Association for the Study of Diabetes (EASD). *Diabetes Care* 2012;35:1364–1379.
Kirkman MS, Briscoe VJ, Clark N, Flores H, et al. Diabetes in older adults. *Diabetes Care* 2012;35:1–15.
White JR, Campbell RK, Eds. *ADA/PDR–Medications for the Treatment of Diabetes.* Montvale, NJ, Thomson Reuters, 2008.

Sulfonylureas, also known as insulin secretagogues, have been on the market long enough that they are almost all generic and reasonably priced. With this class of drugs, however, the risk of hypoglycemia in the LTC population is a limiting factor. Clinicians should consider carefully before prescribing sulfonylureas to the older adult. There are a number of drugs in this class (see Chapter 7). Glimepiride is a long-acting agent that has both renal and hepatic clearance, which makes it a safer consideration if other comorbid conditions are present. It is convenient in that it may be given once a day before breakfast. If hypoglycemia occurs, however, it also may be prolonged and require several treatments of fast-acting glucose over several hours.[5,13,15–17] Of the sulfonylureas, glyburide has the highest risk for hypoglycemia; it should not be prescribed for older adults.[18] If the resident is taking a drug from the sulfonylurea–insulin secretagogue class, the postprandial glucose reading is the most effective report on effectiveness.

A newer category of medications that primarily targets postprandial glucose levels is the dipeptidyl peptidase 4 (DPP-4) inhibitor class. Because these oral agents have a low side-effect profile and renal dosing, they are promising for older adults with diabetes. Drugs in this class are glucose dependent and effective if intrinsic glucagon-like polypeptide 1 (GLP-1) is present. These drugs prevent the breakdown of GLP-1, which causes a glucose-dependent "nudge" to the β-cells to prevent mealtime glucose from rising. DPP-4 inhibitors also suppress pancreatic α-cell secretion of glucagon. In short, these drugs work to prevent meal-related glucose from rising too high. Because they represent the "incretin" effect and shut off when the glucose returns to normal, the risk of hypoglycemia is rare unless used in combination with sulfonylureas or insulin. This drastically reduced risk of hypoglycemia is important to reduce fall risk in the elderly. Four DPP-4 inhibitors are currently available: sitagliptin, saxagliptin, linagliptin, and alogliptin. Because these drugs target postmeal blood glucose levels, checking the postprandial glucose will give valuable information about their effectiveness.

Clinical Note

Incretin Hormones (Incretins)

- Incretins are secreted in the intestines when carbohydrate is ingested.
- Incretins travel to the pancreas and stimulate insulin secretion and decrease glucagon secretion.
- Glucagon-like polypeptide-1 (GLP-1) is an incretin.
- GLP-1 is rapidly degraded by the enzyme dipeptidyl-peptidase-4 (DPP-4)
- Medications related to the incretin system.

    ❏ GLP-1 agonists (have same action as GLP-1)

    - Exenatide
    - Exenatide long-acting
    - Liraglutide

    ❏ DPP-4 inhibitors (prevent degradation of GLP-1)

    - Sitagliptin
    - Saxagliptin
    - Linagliptin
    - Alogliptin

Some injectable medications are similar to the DPP-4 inhibitors, but they have side effects of earlier satiety and weight loss. These injectable medications—exenatide, long-acting exenatide, and liraglutide—are GLP-1 agonists. They bind to the pancreatic β-cell receptors, which allows them to provide postprandial benefit even when no native GLP-1 is present. Exenatide is dosed in micrograms (not milligrams) and is given by injection twice daily before the two largest meals of the day. A similar drug, liraglutide, is dosed in milligrams. It is a longer lasting formulation that can be given only once a day regardless of mealtimes. A newer, form of exenatide (Bydureon), an extended-release formulation, is mixed with microspheres (conceptually similar to dissolvable sutures) and injected just once a week. Nausea is a common complaint when these drugs are initiated, especially exenatide twice daily. When initiating treatment, nausea can be reduced by having the resident eat slowly and stop eating when they feel full. The slow release and titration of the extended release formulation of exenatide, however, tends to significantly reduce the occurrence of nausea. The "thermostat" or incretin effect on insulin secretion of these injectables reduces hypoglycemia to nearly nonexistent, especially when they are combined with metformin. The long-acting medication combination improves both postprandial and fasting glucose levels. If the injection can be given once daily without respect to meals, this class is a logical consideration to reduce glucose levels, reduce potential for hypoglycemia, increase satiety (feelings of fullness), and aid in weight loss. Ultimately, the resident benefits from the action of the drug, and nursing time is saved. Exenatide and liraglutide are approved for use with basal insulin. This combination of basal insulin and a GLP-1 agonist addresses the need for insulin targeting fasting glucose and GLP-1 targeting postmeal glucose with minimal risk of hypoglycemia.

No medication is perfect, and although the risk for adverse effects is low, patients using these drugs face a risk for pancreatitis. Severe unrelenting abdominal pain should be evaluated. Clinicians should be aware that liraglutide and exenatide extended release have a black-box U.S. Food and Drug Administration (FDA) warning related to medullary thyroid carcinoma and multiple endocrine neoplasia syndrome.[2] Although these potential drug effects are rare, and the time of exposure before triggering this problem may make this a moot point for the elderly population, careful resident and family histories should be reviewed before initiating GLP-1 agonist treatment.[19-23] Overall, the DPP-4 inhibitors would be a logical initial medication to consider for frail, thin elders who are fairly newly diagnosed and do not need to lose weight. On the other hand, for residents with long-standing T2D who need help with weight loss, the GLP-1 agonist should be considered. Although these drugs are relatively new and more expensive, if hypoglycemia can be prevented, fall risk reduced, and staff medication delivery time reduced, use of these medications likely will have a good return on investment.

The α-glucosidase inhibitors (AGIs)—acarbose and miglitol—reduce carbohydrate absorption in the gut and subsequently lower postmeal glucose levels. When used as monotherapy, the AGIs do not cause hypoglycemia. If a drug from this class is added to diabetes therapy that includes insulin or insulin secretagogues, hypoglycemia can occur. Because the drug is designed to slow carbohydrate absorption, treatment for hypoglycemia must take the form of glucose tablets or gel. Although the AGIs work well at reducing postmeal glucose levels, these drugs have such a high risk of gastrointestinal side effects, including bloating and flatulence, that they are not well tolerated by most people.[15–17]

The two thiazolidinediones (TZDs)—pioglitazone (Actos) and rosiglitazone (Avandia)—are oral agents that promote insulin sensitization primarily by working intracellularly to increase the signaling mechanisms that promote glucose transport. In essence, these drugs work to improve the effectiveness of endogenous insulin. They have a postprandial glucose benefit, but their side effects make them a concern for the elderly population. The side effects of fluid retention and edema increase the risk of CHF. In fact, TZDs are contraindicated when preexisting CHF (New York Class III or IV) is present. Recent FDA investigations of the potential relationship with rosiglitazone and cardiac problems have made this TZD even more worrisome for use in elders with T2D.[13,15–17,21,24] The FDA lifted the Risk Evaluation and Mitigation Strategies (REMS) on rosiglitazone in the summer of 2013. Pioglitzaone became generic in 2013, helping with cost considerations. Fracture risk in postmenopausal women and concern about bladder cancer with pioglitazone, however, have made this class difficult to justify in LTC.

The newest class of drugs to treat diabetes is the sodium-dependent glucose transporter 2 (SGLT-2) inhibitors. Canagaflozin (Invokana), the first in class in the U.S. was released to the market in early 2013, and dapaglifloxin (Farxiga) was approved in 2014. This class of drugs works by promoting excretion of glucose into the urine. It has been tested in the geriatric population, but relatively little is known about the effect of this class of drugs in the LTC resident. Increase in osmotic diuresis with potential hyperkalemia would be cautionary considerations for frail thin elders.

Insulin Management and Glycemic Control

Most oral agents and injectables for use in T2D are dependent on internal, endogenous insulin secretion to provide glycemic benefit. The exceptions are metformin, the SGLT-2 inhibitors, and the TZDs. Over time, loss of pancreatic β-cell function is common due to the progressive nature of T2D. Eventually most residents with T2D will require insulin.[5,25,26] Insulin should be initiated sooner, rather than later. Grossly elevated glucose levels will increase the risk of both short- and long-term complications. When titrated carefully, synthetic, recombinant DNA human insulin has a low–side effect profile.

Many types of insulin are available (see Chapters 9 and 10). It is now possible to achieve near-physiologic insulin action when giving insulin. The body requires insulin action 24 hours a day. Small basal (background) amounts are used throughout the day and night to keep glucose levels stable between meals (i.e., during fasting states). A bolus of insulin is needed to provide coverage for meal carbohydrates.[5,16,27,28]

In T2D, it is not uncommon for insulin to be added to an oral medication. Basal insulin often is initiated as the first step in insulin therapy. Insulin glargine (Lantus) and detemir (Levemir) are long-acting insulin analogs without substantial peak activity. The flatter action of these insulin preparations reduce potential for hypoglycemia, particularly during the night. Neutral protamine Hagedorn

(NPH) is an older insulin preparation. It is less expensive, but may increase the risk of hypoglycemia if it is not given at the right time. For example, when given before the evening meal, NPH insulin will peak ~6 hours later, putting the resident at risk for hypoglycemia around midnight. When meal-based insulin is needed, a rapid-acting analog (e.g., lispro, aspart, or glulisine) is a good choice.[29] These analogs peak at 90 minutes and, when given and taken properly, are less likely than regular insulin to cause hypoglycemia. Glulisine breaks down from a hexamer to monomers more quickly than lispro or aspart, making it more logical to be given if meal-time insulin doses are given after the meal in relation to what the resident actually ate. Because insulin dosing is weight based, older adults, particularly frail elders may start with very modest doses.

SLIDING SCALE: THE QUICKSAND OF INSULIN MANAGEMENT

A common carryover from another era, with unproven clinical validity, is the use of the sliding-scale insulin (SSI). This approach of giving insulin at sporadic points in time based solely on the glucose at that moment still is used widely in LTC, and it is particularly dangerous for the elderly.[30] SSI uses a reactive approach of giving insulin for excessively elevated glucoses. This practice may result in severe hypoglycemia. Of 52 trials evaluated from 1966 to 2003, no benefit of SSI was reported. Medical directors in LTC and diabetes clinicians all urge that this outdated practice be stopped.[5,31,32] Of particular concern is that sliding scale approaches usually have minimal, if any, basal insulin provided. When given based on elevations in glucose levels, SSI usually is given after the hyperglycemia from meals occurs. It does not account for insulin needs based on caloric or meal intake if the glucose is normal at mealtime. And, if the blood glucose level is not measured before each meal consumed, long stretches of time without adequate insulin coverage are likely to occur. According to the AMDA, SSI is not recommended because it does not provide physiologic action and it is likely to result in increased nursing time. If it is used, it should be used temporarily, should be reevaluated within 1 week, and should be converted to fixed doses of insulin that minimize the need for correction doses.[5] Additionally, the Centers for Medicare and Medicaid (CMS) identifies SSI as an issue that carries a warning with related documentation if discovered on inspection, F-Tag 329. The Medicare State Operations Manual warns "continued or long-term need for sliding-scale insulin for non-emergency coverage may indicate inadequate blood sugar control."[12]

Starting Insulin in Long-Term Care

Anticipate needs. Basal insulin is the background insulin needed overnight and between meals. Bolus or prandial insulin is the insulin required at mealtimes. If intravenous calories are infused, insulin is needed for that as well. When miscalculations in background or prandial doses occur, blood glucose levels will be out of target range at the next capillary blood glucose check. A correction dose can be done safely before a mealtime to both prevent wide fluctuations in blood glucose levels and minimize risk for hypoglycemia.[30,32-34]

Basal insulin initiation can be achieved in several ways. ADA/European Association for the Study of Diabetes (EASD) consensus algorithm recommends starting with 10 units per day or, alternatively, 0.2 units of insulin per kilogram of body weight.[14] A quick method that does not require a calculator and results in nearly the same dose as the previous formula is body weight in pounds × 10%.[35] Using this formula, the 210-pound person would need 21 units (210 × 0.10) of insulin glargine or insulin detemir to start. The 110-pound frail elder would start on 11 units of insulin. Using the 0.2 unit per kilogram formula, you would first convert body weight from pounds to kilograms (210/2.2 = 95.46) and then multiply by 0.2 (95.46 × 0.2 = 19.1). In this case, the 210-pound person would start on ~20 units Lantus and the 110-pound frail elder would start on 10 units. While important, the starting dose is not as significant as the commitment to titrate doses until the fasting glucose is in the target range. Titration can be done by increasing the background insulin by 10% every 3–7 days, or increasing 1 unit every day until the person's target blood glucose level is reached.[14] In the LTC setting, knowing the blood glucose target is the first objective. Checking fasting blood glucose levels daily until the target is reached is the second objective. Using the blood glucose patterns to adjust the insulin dose until the target is reached is the final objective. Once the target is achieved and blood glucose levels are stable, staff can check blood glucose values periodically according to facility policy.

Differences in basal insulin preparations may have implications in frail elders. Levemir attains its longer duration by being bound to serum albumin. Poorly nourished residents may have inconsistent distribution of levemir if serum albumin levels are low. In other words, the levemir will absorb into the bloodstream normally, but once there, more insulin will be freely available. This can result in inconsistent glycemic control and in unexpected episodes of hypoglycemia. Insulin glargine does not have the same sort of dynamic. Both long-acting insulin preparations are available in pens that are easy to use and allow for more accurate dosing than the vial and syringe method.

Glucose control also depends on correct injection technique. Most insulin preparations are stable at room temperature (no more than 86°F) for 28 days. An important teaching point for direct caregivers using insulin pens is to "prime every time." A 1- to 2-unit priming dose should be dialed in to the pen before each injection. Depressing the plunger to give an "air shot" allows the caregiver to visualize a drop or stream of insulin at the tip of the needle. This provides assurance that the insulin is at the tip of the needle and will be delivered when the correct dose is dialed. Insulin is administered into the subcutaneous (fatty) layer of the skin. After penetrating the skin with the needle, the dose knob (plunger) should be held down for 5–10 seconds to allow time for all the insulin to be delivered and prevent leaking at the injection site. These days, pen needles are very thin (31 to 32 gauge) and as short as 4 millimeters but up to 12.5 millimeters long. Changing the pen needle after every injection prevents the tiny needle from getting clogged with insulin. Recent data suggest that skin thickness, in both sexes and in all ethnic groups, does not exceed 2.5 millimeters in length.[36] This means that even the tiniest short needles are safe and acceptable if that is what the resident prefers. Most acute-care institutions use pen needles with auto covers that will not allow any possible needle stick injuries after an injection has been given. LTC facilities would benefit from these auto covers as well. Although the auto-cover needles are more expensive in the short run, the institution will benefit from avoiding costs associated with needle-stick injuries to employees.

Using Pattern Management to Achieve Control

Evaluating glucose levels to determine when mealtime, bolus, or prandial insulin is needed is done most logically with pattern management. Pattern management, in a nutshell, is a method of looking for patterns in blood glucose results and using those patterns as a framework for adjusting insulin doses. Blood glucose levels tested 2 hours after meals are consumed will provide valuable information on the resident's ability to secrete sufficient internal or endogenous insulin in response to the meal eaten. Similarly, testing postprandial glucose values also will inform the provider if the dose of prandial insulin is set correctly. Evaluating several days' or a week's worth of glucose readings will allow the provider to observe patterns or trends.[35]

The fasting glucose upon awakening is the overnight report. If this level is in the resident's target range, the basal (background) insulin is set at the correct dose. Premeal glucose testing is a report on the basal insulin and does not give the best reflection of the resident's response to food eaten at the previous meal. If, for example, the 2-hour postprandial glucose levels are >180 mg/dl after dinner most evenings, there is a pattern of elevated glucose after dinner. The focus for the community-dwelling elder should be on teaching the patient to use pattern management. For the LTC resident, the tools of pattern management are similar. When a pattern demonstrates that glucose levels are out of range, the clinician needs to consider potential reasons for the readings. In the previous example, problem solving to determine the cause would include evaluating *1)* the calories or carbohydrate content of the evening meal, *2)* activity levels in the early evening, and *3)* dosages of insulin or oral agents. If food intake and activity levels are consistent, the need for prandial insulin with that meal is established. There is no need and indeed no clear information on timing of the problem with an A1C. Glucose monitoring provides much more detailed data than the A1C in this case.

Clinical Note

Using insulin in pattern management

- ■ Basal, long acting: works during the night and between meals
- ■ Prandial (meal), short/rapid acting: covers the carbohydrate in meals
- ■ Correction (rapid acting): corrects for unusual high glucose level. Using correction insulin doses frequently indicates a need to change basal and/or prandial insulin depending on glucose patterns.

Clinicians, including physicians, physician assistants, nurse practitioners, and consulting pharmacists, in the LTC environment all can use pattern management to evaluate the glycemic control of residents. It will require periods of frequent monitoring and a good flow chart (see the Sample Diabetes Management/Glucose Log in Chapter 2, Figure 2.1). At least 1 week of fasting and 2-hour postprandial glucose tests are desirable. Keep the resident's blood glucose target values in mind and use the following steps when reviewing his or her glucose records:

1. Determine the glycemic abnormality

    a. Priority 1: Identify and resolve hypoglycemia
    b. Priority 2: Fix the fasting glucose
    c. Priority 3: Fix the postprandial glucose

2. Determine the frequency of the problem
3. Evaluate the cause (food, activity, medication, etc.)
4. Take preventive action (make a change the next day, *before* the problem occurs)
5. Retest glucose levels for at least 1 week after the change[35]

Taking the Fear out of Hypoglycemia

Experiencing hypoglycemia is scary. Individuals with diabetes are often afraid—and rightly so—because, at its worst, hypoglycemia can be profound and cause coma or death. In most adults, hypoglycemia is mild and easily managed. This is not necessarily true of older adults. Although symptoms of hypoglycemia in older residents may be similar to those in younger ones, deterioration of psychomotor coordination may increase fall risk and therefore increased fracture risk. Causes of hypoglycemia include use of insulin or insulin secretagogues, diabetes duration, previous hypoglycemia, erratic meals, and activity levels. Severe renal dysfunction is also a cause of hypoglycemia, and it is of particular concern in the elderly.

Clinicians also are concerned about hypoglycemia. Hypoglycemia is known to be the limiting factor of insulin therapy. Until recently, some clinicians believed that an A1C <6.5% was desirable for all adults, regardless of age. That belief changed when the glycemic control arm of the ACCORD trial was halted early. The ACCORD trial examined the role of glycemic control in preventing CVD events. Hypoglycemia and other adverse effects were more common in older participants.[37] A previous study of healthy, functional, older adults using intensive glycemic control, demonstrated glycemic control with low rates of hypoglycemia.[38] In pooled analysis, Lee et al. found a relatively low risk of hypoglycemia when basal insulin was added to the care regimen of older adults.[39] These latter two studies, however, were not done in LTC populations.

In the LTC environment, hypoglycemia remains a limiting factor of diabetes treatment. Although residents on sulfonylureas are at risk of hypoglycemia, insulin-using residents may face an even higher risk. Cognitive or functional impairment may make identification of hypoglycemia symptoms more difficult for elderly resident or caregiver, who may mistake symptoms of hypoglycemia for other symptoms of cognitive dysfunction (i.e., confusion, tiredness). When treatment is delayed, symptoms progress and hypoglycemia worsens. Blood glucose targets should be set high enough to prevent episodes of hypoglycemia, but low enough to prevent episodes of acute hyperglycemia. The challenge is in knowing what the best limits should be.

Although it is important to minimize the frequency of hypoglycemia, it is critically important for direct caregivers to know how to recognize it and then treat it when it occurs. Symptom recognition is easier when the caregiver knows the resident well. Knowing what to expect and having rapid treatment nearby helps to take the fear out of the situation.

Treatment of hypoglycemia should be 15–20 grams of carbohydrate (see Table 5.4). Blood glucose levels should rise within 15 minutes and the resident's symptoms should diminish. At this point, the glucose level should be rechecked. If it is rising, and the next meal is >1 hour away, the resident should be given a snack that includes complex carbohydrate and protein. Fifteen to twenty grams of carbohydrate will likely keep the blood glucose levels up for ~45–60 minutes. If the glucose level does not rise, repeat the treatment with an additional 15–20 grams carbohydrate. After two treatments, if the glucose level still is not responding, administer 0.5–1.0 mg glucagon. Glucagon will need to be reconstituted and given intramuscularly. Unresponsive residents should be turned on their side if glucagon is administered as this drug may cause emesis. As soon as resident is responsive, follow initial treatment with simple sugar, such as regular soda (not diet), and then a snack. Monitor blood glucose values closely for several days.

Elders with renal insufficiency may have prolonged hypoglycemia. For these individuals, a follow-up blood glucose check 1 hour after the hypoglycemic episode would be prudent. The amount of carbohydrate actually used to treat low glucose is quite variable in LTC, as it is in the general population. Using a moderate amount of carbohydrate hopefully will prevent big spikes in blood glucose. Reducing glycemic variability may contribute to better mental and functional status.

Table 5.4 Hypoglycemia Treatment Suggestions

Common choice	Better choice	Why?
½ cup orange juice	½ cup apple juice	Less acidic and easier on gastrointestinal tract
4 glucose tabs	4 sugar cubes	Dentition may not allow chewing
	1 pack glucose gel	Buccal absorption bypasses delayed gastrointestinal absorption
½ can regular cola	½ can caffeine-free soda	Less gastrointestinal irritation
Mini candy bar	3 marshmallows	No fat to delay absorption

Source: Adapted from Fick D, Semla T, Beizer J, Brandt N, Dombrowski R, DuBeau CE, Steonman M. American Geriatrics Society updated Beers criteria for potentially inappropriate medication use in older adults. *Journal of the American Geriatrics Society* 2012; 60(4):614–615.

CONCLUSION

In general, each oral agent is expected to reduce A1C levels by ~0.5–1.0%. Insulin, alone or in combination with oral agents, can be dosed in multiple ways to achieve the best benefit and reach glycemic targets. Diabetes experts now suggest that the best therapy is aimed at reducing blood glucose by targeting the various systems involved in diabetes control.[40] It would not be uncommon to see a diabetes patient on two or three different classes of antihyperglycemic medications. Translating this to the older adult in LTC is complicated. Of significant concern is the frail older adult with multiple geriatric syndromes and complicated diabetes. Multiple medications may increase the risk of hypoglycemia, but failure to achieve reasonable targets puts the resident at risk for acute episodes of a hyperosmolar hyperglycemic state, which carries with it a high mortality risk. Until more concrete recommendations exist, individualizing therapy for each resident using the updated AGS guidelines is a reasonable strategy. Finally, all direct caregivers must be comfortable in their ability to recognize and treat hypoglycemia. Safe management depends on it.

REFERENCES

1. Kitabchi AE, Umpierrez GE, Fisher JN, Murphy MB, Stentz FB. Thirty years of personal experience in hyperglycemic crises: Diabetic ketoacidosis and hyperglycemic hyperosmolar state. *Journal of Clinical Endocrinology and Metabolism* 2008;93(5):1541–1552.
2. American Diabetes Association. A1C and eAG calculator. Available at http://www.diabetes.org/living-with-diabetes/treatment-and-care/blood-glucose-control/a1c. Accessed 12 February 2014.
3. Currie CJ, Peters JR, Tynan A, Evans M, Heine R J, Bracco OL, . . . Poole CD. Survival as a function of HbA(1c) in people with type 2 diabetes: A retrospective cohort study. [Research Support, Non-U.S. Gov't]. *Lancet* 2010;375(9713):481–489.
4. Huang ES, Liu JY, Moffet HH, John PM, Karter AJ. Glycemic control, complications, and death in older diabetic patients: the diabetes and aging study. [Research Support, N.I.H., Extramural]. *Diabetes Care* 2011;34(6):1329–1336.
5. American Medical Directors Association. *Guidelines for diabetes management in the long-term care setting.* Columbia, MD, Author, 2010.
6. Sinclair AJ, Paolisso G, Castro M, Bourdel-Marchasson I, Gadsby R, Rodriguez Mañas L. European Diabetes Working Party for Older People 2011 clinical guidelines for type 2 diabetes mellitus. Executive summary. *Diabetes and Metabolism* 2011;37(Suppl3):S27–S38.
7. U.S. Department of Veterans Affairs/Department of Defense (VA/DOD). Clinical practice guidelines: Management of diabetes mellitus in primary care, 2010. Available at www.healthquality.va.gov/Diabetes_Mellitus.asp. Accessed12 February 2014.

8. American Diabetes Association. Standards of medical care in diabetes—2013. *Diabetes Care* 2013;36(Suppl1):S11–S66.

9. American Diabetes Association. Standards of medical care diabetes—2014. *Diabetes Care* 2014;37(Suppl1):S14–S80.

10. Brown AF, Mangione CM, Saliba D, Sarkisian CA, California Healthcare Foundation/American Geriatrics Society Panel on Improving Care for Older Persons with Diabetes. Guidelines for improving the care of the older person with diabetes mellitus. *Journal of the American Geriatric Society* 2003;51(5):S265–S280.

11. Kirkman MS, Briscoe VJ, Clark N, Florez H, Haas LB, Halter JB, Swift CS. Diabetes in older adults. *Diabetes Care* 2012;35(12):2650–2664.

12. Center for Medicare and Medicaid Services. State operations manual. Appendix PP: Guidance to surveyors for long term care facilities (F329 483.25(l) Unnecessary Drugs, Implementation date 10/01/2010. Available at www.cms.gov. Accessed 12 February 2014.

13. Neumiller JJ, Setter SM, Gates BJ, Sonnett TE, Dobbins EK, Campbell K. Pharmacological management of glycemic control in the geriatric patient with type 2 diabetes mellitus. *Consultant Pharmacist* 2009;24(1):45–63.

14. Nathan DM, Buse JB, Davidson MB, Ferrannini E, Holman RR, Sherwin R, Zinman B. Medical management of hyperglycemia in type 2 diabetes: A consensus algorithm for the initiation and adjustment of therapy. *Diabetes Care* 2009;32(1):193–203.

15. Chipkin SR. How to select and combine oral agents for patients with type 2 diabetes mellitus. *American Journal of Medicine* 2005;118(Suppl5A):4S–13S.

16. Jennings PE. Oral antiyperglycemics: consideration in older patients with non-insulin dependent diabetes mellitus. *Drugs and Aging* 1997;10:323–331.

17. Johnson EL, Brosseau JD, Sobule M, Kolberg J. Treatment of diabetes in long-term care facilities: a primary care approach. *Clinical Diabetes* 2008;26(4):152–156.

18. American Geriatrics Society. Updated Beers criteria for potentially inappropriate medication use in older adults. *Journal of the American Geriatrics Society* 2012;60(4):616–631.

19. Buse JB, Rosenstock J, Sesti G, Schmidt WE, Montanya E, Brett JH, . . . Group LS. Liraglutide once a day versus exenatide twice a day for type 2 diabetes: A 26-week randomised, parallel-group, multinational, open-label trial (LEAD-6). [Comparative Study Multicenter Study Randomized Controlled Trial Research Support, Non-U.S. Gov't]. *Lancet* 2009;374(9683): 39–47.

20. U.S. Food and Drug Administration. FDA briefing materials—liraglutide, 2009. Available at www.fda.gov/ohrms/dockets/ac/o9/briefing/2009-4422b2-01-FDA.pdf. Accessed 26 October 2013.

21. Fonseca VA, Kulkarni KD. Management of type 2 diabetes: Oral agents, insulin, and injectables. [Research Support, Non-U.S. Gov't Review]. *Journal of the American Dietetic Association* 2008;108(4Suppl1):S29–S33.

22. Hinnen D, Nielsen LL, Waninger A, Kushner P. Incretin mimetics and DPP-IV inhibitors: new paradigms for the treatment of type 2 diabetes. [Case Reports]. *Journal of the American Board of Family Medicine* 2006;19(6):612–620.

23. Novo Nordisk I. *Victoza* [prescribing information]. Princeton, NJ, Author, 2010.
24. Nesto RW, Bell D, Bonow RO, Fonseca V, Grundy SM, Horton ES, . . . Kahn R. Thiazolidinedione use, fluid retention, and congestive heart failure: a consensus statement from the American Heart Association and American Diabetes Association. [Consensus Development Conference Review]. *Diabetes Care* 2004;27(1):256–263.
25. Butler AE, Janson J, Bonner-Weir S, Ritzel R, Rizza RA, Butler PC. Beta-cell deficit and increased beta-cell apoptosis in humans with type 2 diabetes. [Research Support, U.S. Gov't, P.H.S.]. *Diabetes* 2003;52(1):102–110.
26. Szoke E, Shrayyef MZ, Messing S, Woerle HJ, van Haeften TW, Meyer C, . . . Gerich JE. Effect of aging on glucose homeostasis: accelerated deterioration of beta-cell function in individuals with impaired glucose tolerance. [Research Support, N.I.H., Extramural]. *Diabetes Care* 2008;31(3):539–543.
27. Bray B. Transitioning and adjusting insulin analog therapy in elderly patients. [Review]. *Consultant Pharmacist* 2008;23(SupplB):17–23.
28. Haas LB. Optimizing insulin use in type 2 diabetes: Role of basal and prandial insulin in long-term care facilities. *Journal of the American Medical Directors Association* 2007;8(8):502–510.
29. Pandya N, Nathanson E. Managing diabetes in long-term care facilities: benefits of switching from human insulin to insulin analogs. [Research Support, Non-U.S. Gov't Review]. *Journal of the American Medical Directors Association* 2010;11(3):171–178.
30. Pandya N, Thompson S, Sambamoorthi U. The prevalence and persistence of sliding scale insulin use among newly admitted elderly nursing home residents with diabetes mellitus. *Journal of the American Medical Directors Association* 2008;9(9):663–669.
31. Clement S, Braithwaite SS, Magee MF, Ahmann A, Smith EP, Schafer RG, American Diabetes Association. Diabetes in Hospitals Writing Committee. Management of diabetes and hyperglycemia in hospitals. *Diabetes Care* 2004;27(2):553–591.
32. Hirsch IB. Sliding scale insulin—time to stop sliding. *Journal of the American Medical Association* 2009;301(2), 213-214.
33. Clement M, Leung F. Diabetes and the frail elderly in long-term care. *Canadian Journal of Diabetes* 2009;33(2):114–121.
34. Garza H. Minimizing the risk of hypoglycemia in older adults: a focus on long-term care. [Research Support, Non-U.S. Gov't Review]. *Consultant Pharmacist* 2009;24(SupplB): 18–24.
35. Hinnen D, Childs BP, Guthrie DW, Guthrie R, Martin S. Combating clinical inertia with pattern management. In *The art and science of diabetes self-management education*. C. Mensing, Ed. Chicago, IL, American Association of Diabetes Educators, 2006.
36. Hirsch LJ, Gibney MA, Albanese J, Qu S, Kassler-Taub K, Klaff LJ, Bailey TS. Comparative glycemic control, safety and patient ratings for a new 4 mm x 32G insulin pen needle in adults with diabetes. [Randomized Controlled Trial Research Support, Non-U.S. Gov't]. *Current Medical Research and Opinion* 2010;26(6):1531–1541.

37. Miller ME, Bonds DE, Gerstein HC, Seaquist ER, Bergenstal RM, Calles-Escandon J, Childress RD, Cravens TE, Cuddihy RM, Caily G, Geinglos MN, Ismail-Beigi F, Largay JF, O'Conner PJ, Paul T, Savage PJ, Schubart UK, Sood A, Genuth S. The effects of baseline characteristics, glycaemia treatment approach, and glycated haemoglobin concentration on the risk of severe hypoglycaemia: Post hoc epidemiological analysis of the ACCORD study. *British Medical Journal* 2010;340:b5444.
38. Herman WH, Ilag LL, Johnson SL, Martin CL, Sinding J, Al Harthi A, . . . Raskin PA. Clinical trial of continuous subcutaneous insulin infusion versus multiple daily injections in older adults with type 2 diabetes. [Clinical Trial Comparative Study Multicenter Study Randomized Controlled Trial Research Support, N.I.H., Extramural Research Support, Non-U.S. Gov't Research Support, U.S. Gov't, P.H.S.]. *Diabetes Care* 2005;28(7):1568–1573.
39. Lee P, Chang A, Blaum C, Vlajnic A, Gao L, Halter J. Comparison of safety and efficacy of insulin glargine and neutral protamine Hagedorn insulin in older adults with type 2 diabetes mellitus: results from a pooled analysis. [Multicenter Study Randomized Controlled Trial Research Support, Non-U.S. Gov't]. *Journal of the American Geriatrics Society* 2012;60(1):51–59.
40. DeFronzo RA. From the triumvirate to the ominous octet: A new paradigm for the treatment of type 2 diabetes mellitus. *Diabetes* 2009;58(4):773–795.

6

Self-Care: Promoting Functional Abilities among Older Adults

Elizabeth Quintana, EdD, RD, LD, CDE

INTRODUCTION

An individualized approach to managing older adults with diabetes is appropriate, keeping in mind the variability and complexity of this population. The vast majority of diabetes management is self-care. Older adults are heterogeneous in their functional status and disease. It is never too late to make changes that can help people live longer and healthier lives. People are much more inclined to make behavior changes when they see themselves as part of the solution.

Self-care measures contribute to independent function and quality of life in older adults. Health promotion activities allow people to take initiative and responsibility for maintaining their own health and functional ability. It includes both provider-initiated as well as resident-initiated behaviors for disease treatment and health maintenance. Residents with diabetes may be in long-term care (LTC) permanently or for short stays. As individuals transition from community to LTC environments, they should continue to take an active part in their day-to-day diabetes management. The ability to maintain and increase skills promotes confidence in managing their health. This is the focus of self-care.

FUNCTIONAL ABILITY

For older adults, maintaining functional ability is essential for extending their independence. Self-care activities enable older adults to achieve productive and fulfilling lives. Examples of self-care activities include regular physical activity, proper nutrition, rest and relaxation, socialization, and stress reduction. Older adults are encouraged to actively participate in their own health care as much as they are able. Occupational therapy can provide opportunities for practicing daily living activities in a supportive environment.[1]

Comprehensive geriatric assessment begins with a review of the major categories of functional ability. Table 6.1 presents the activities of daily living (ADLs) and the instrumental activities of daily living (IADLs). ADLs are personal care activities that a person must perform every day. These activities include eating, dressing, bathing, using the toilet, and controlling bladder and bowel. Persons unable to perform these activities and obtain adequate nutrition may require caregiver support 12–24 hours/day. IADLs are activities that enable a person to live independently. These activities involve preparing meals, performing routine

Table 6.1 Functional Ability

Activities of Daily Living (ADLs)

Independent ◄——— **Needs help**------------**Dependent** ———► **Does not do**

Feeding
Eats independently ---Relies on being fed

Using the toilet
Cares for self --No control of bladder
No incontinence   or bowel

Bathing
Bathes self--Does not bathe
                                                            Uncooperative when assisted

Dressing
Dresses self --Completely unable to
Selects clothing   dress or undress self

Grooming
Always groomed--Resists grooming

Ambulation
Totally independent--Bedridden

Instrumental Activities of Daily Living (IADLs)

Independent ◄——— **Needs help**-------------**Dependent** ———► **Does not do**

Preparing meals
Plans, prepares, serves--Needs to have meals
Meals independently   prepared and served

Performing housework
Maintains home---Does not participate
Occasional help with heavy work   in housework

Taking medicine
Takes medicine as prescribed----------------------------------Unable to manage medicine

Managing finances
Manages financial matters--------------------------------------Incapable of handling money

Using the telephone
Uses the telephone --Does not use the telephone

Source: Adapted from WGBH Educational Foundation and Massachusetts Institute of Technology. 2008. Checklist of Activities of Daily Living (ADL). Public Broadcasting System, WGBH Educational Foundation and the Massachusetts Institute of Technology, 2008.

Available at www.pbs.org/wgbh/caringforyourparents/caregiver/pdf/cfyp_adl_checklist.pdf. Accessed 30 January 2014.

housework, taking medicine, managing finances, and using the telephone. A commonly measure of independence is the ability to perform functional tasks necessary for daily living.[2] The LTC resident is assessed as well and can be encouraged to participate in their self-care to the extent possible.

Frailty occurs with severe limitations in ADLs. Older adults must exhibit at least three of the following conditions to be considered frail: unintentional weight loss, slow walking speed, low physical activity levels, weak grip strength, and chronic exhaustion. In many instances, frailty is complicated by the presence of chronic diseases. For example, physical strength may be impaired by diabetic neuropathy.[1,2]

Clinical Note

Frailty
Must exhibit ≥3 of the following:

- Unintentional weight loss
- Slow walking speed
- Low physical activity levels
- Weak grip strength
- Chronic exhaustion

Self-Efficacy

People who feel that they have some control of their lives tend to maintain a generally positive outlook. They fare better, both physically and mentally, than people who do not hold these beliefs. Self-efficacy can be defined as one's confidence in the ability to perform a task or deal with a problem. Because of the complexity of diabetes self-management, individuals may feel very confident about one aspect of care, but less confident about others. Fear and anxiety may affect people's beliefs about their abilities and set up barriers to performing routine tasks. These beliefs can limit older adults' abilities to carry out basic daily activities, threaten their independence, and lower their quality of life.[3]

Self-efficacy is critical in developing positive health practices. Self-efficacy and behavior can be modified when older adults are informed, educated, and counseled. Older adults may model their own behavior after observing the success of other older adults in performing the same tasks. The people who can best understand and aid people with diabetes may be those who are going through or have gone through similar experiences. Counseling could help them reappraise their capabilities, overcome any perceived barriers, and participate in self-care activities. With guidance and verbal persuasion, caregivers can encourage older adults to believe that they can succeed. Breaking down an activity in smaller steps and providing opportunities to practice each step can promote success and confidence.[4]

Hearing Impairment

Hearing impairment is one of the most widespread disabilities in older adults. It is estimated that worldwide >50% of people ≥65 years of age have some degree of hearing loss. Hearing loss can cause difficulties with communication. This, in turn, can lead to frustration, low self-esteem, withdrawal, and social isolation. Hearing problems can make people feel left out. They may withdraw from people when they cannot follow the discussion. They may be misinterpreted as being confused, uncaring, or even difficult.[5]

Hearing can be protected by turning down the sound on the television or headphones, moving away from loud noise, or using earplugs or other ear protection. Earwax or fluid build-up may block sounds. Wax blockage can be treated easily with mineral oil, baby oil, glycerin, or commercial ear drops to soften earwax. A punctured eardrum can cause hearing loss. The eardrum may be damaged by infection, pressure, or objects in the ear. Viruses and bacteria, heart condition, stroke, brain injuries, or tumors may affect hearing. Hearing problems may be caused by medications.[6]

Studies found a higher prevalence of hearing impairment among people with diabetes than among those without diabetes. The degree of hearing loss ranged from mild to moderate, causing deficits that would be difficult to detect without screening. People may not be aware of what they cannot hear. Screening for hearing loss in people at risk could lead to interventions that would improve their ability to communicate, their productivity, and their safety. There are many treatments for impaired hearing, including hearing aids, medicines, or surgery. Assistive devices can help to improve hearing. For example, telephone amplifying devices make it easier to use the phone. Alert systems work with doorbells, smoke detectors, and alarm clocks send visual signals or vibrations.[6] Table 6.2 presents tips on working with those who have a hearing impairment. In the LTC environment, residents who are hearing impaired easily feel isolated. It is important to make efforts to include them in regular activities that promote self-care.

Table 6.2 Tips for Working with the Hearing Impaired

- Find a quiet place to talk
- Stand or sit in good lighting
- Use facial expressions or gestures to give clues
- Face the person and talk clearly
- Do not hide your mouth, eat, or chew gum
- Speak a little more loudly than normal, but do not shout
- Speak at a reasonable speed
- Repeat if necessary, using different words
- Let only one person talk at a time
- Be patient
- Stay positive
- Ask how you can help

Source: Adapted from the National Institute on Aging. 2013. Hearing loss. Available at www.nia.nih.gov/health/publication/hearing-loss, Accessed 31 January 2014.

Incontinence

Incontinence is the inability to control urine or fecal elimination. Incontinence is a sensitive subject. The condition often is associated with embarrassment for the sufferer. Older adults are especially prone to incontinence. In addition to diabetes, incontinence may be associated with weakened pelvic muscles, urinary tract infections, enlarged prostate gland in men, thinning of the vaginal wall in women, or an inability to get to the toilet in time. Even drinking caffeinated beverages, such as coffee and tea, or taking prescription medications can aggravate the bladder. Therapy varies and involves the treatment of the underlying condition.[7]

Urinary incontinence can impose a personal hardship in older adults. It can affect social interactions, self-esteem, and life satisfaction. It increases the risk for anxiety, depression, and self-imposed isolation. The impact of urinary incontinence on health includes increased risk for skin rashes, dermatitis, secondary yeast infection, pressure ulcers, urinary tract infection, disrupted sleep patterns, falls, and fall-related injury.[8] In LTC, older adults are particularly vulnerable to the consequences of urinary or fecal incontinence.

For older adults, the rate of incontinence can increase when the underlying chronic conditions worsen. This may include deterioration in physical mobility or cognitive function, lack of assistance for toileting, or adverse effects of medication on the lower urinary tract, leading to incontinence or urinary retention. For example, vigorous coughing may be associated with upper-respiratory infection or the use of the blood pressure medicine angiotensin-converting-enzyme inhibitor. Chronic obstructive pulmonary disease may precipitate or aggravate urinary incontinence. Optimal management of these conditions and changes in drug therapy may provide relief from urinary incontinence.[8]

Diabetes may cause fecal incontinence by decreasing rectal sensation, leading to inappropriate internal sphincter relaxation. Incontinent people with diabetes may have high rectal sensory thresholds. This means that it requires a higher volume of rectal contents to create a sense of urgency. Diabetes with autonomic neuropathy in the intestinal tract often leads to diarrhea, which can promote incontinence.[9]

Treatments include habit training, bladder training, scheduled bathroom trips, pelvic floor muscles exercises, and fluid and diet management. In LTC, regularly scheduled toileting can reduce the risk of urinary incontinence. Bladder training can involve teaching patients to delay urination by gradually lengthening the time between bathroom trips. The double-voiding procedure requires waiting a few minutes after voiding and then urinating again. This procedure helps to drain the bladder more thoroughly. Pelvic floor muscle exercises, called Kegel exercises, strengthen the muscles that help regulate urination. Biofeedback training may strengthen the sphincter muscles and give more control over bowel movements. Medications, medical devices, and surgery also may treat incontinence.[10]

Food affects the consistency of stool and how quickly it passes through the digestive system. Watery stools are hard to control. Eating foods high in dietary fiber adds bulk and makes stool easier to control. Foods and drinks that may make the problem worse are those containing caffeine—like coffee, tea, or chocolate—which relaxes the internal anal sphincter muscles.[9]

To help identify the foods that might cause problems, have the resident keep a food diary, or keep one for them. List all the foods eaten, the amounts, and when they have an incontinent episode. After a few days, a pattern involving certain foods and incontinence might appear. After identifying the foods that seem to cause problems, cut back on them and see whether incontinence improves. Foods and drinks that typically cause diarrhea probably should be avoided or eaten less often. Typical offending foods include the following:

- Drinks and foods containing caffeine
- Cured or smoked meat such as sausage, ham, or turkey
- Spicy foods
- Alcoholic beverages
- Dairy products such as milk, cheese, or ice cream
- Fruits such as apples, peaches, or pears
- Fatty and greasy foods
- Sweeteners, such as sorbitol, xylitol, mannitol, and fructose, which are found in diet drinks, sugarless gum and candy, chocolate, and fruit juices

Table 6.3 presents some tips for adjusting the diet to help manage fecal incontinence. A registered dietitian can assist with identifying the offending foods and developing individual meal plans for older adults.

Table 6.3 Adjusting the Diet to Help Manage Fecal Incontinence

Adjustments	Rationale
Change the meals to smaller, but more frequent meals	Large meals may cause bowel contractions that lead to diarrhea. Residents can eat the same amount of food in a day, but space it out by eating several small meals.
Eat food and beverages at different times during the day	Liquid helps move food through the digestive system. To slow things down, drink the liquid ~30 minutes before or after the meal, but not with the meal.
Gradually add foods high in fiber to the meals	Fiber may make stool soft, formed, and easier to control. Fiber is found in fruits, vegetables, and grains. High-fiber foods must be added to the meal plan slowly so the body can adjust. Too much fiber all at once can cause bloating, gas, or even diarrhea. If eating more fiber makes diarrhea worse, try cutting back to two servings each of fruits and vegetables and removing skins and seeds from the food.
Eat foods that make stool bulkier	Foods that contain soluble fiber slow the rate at which the bowels empty. These foods include bananas, rice, tapioca, bread, potatoes, applesauce, cheese, smooth peanut butter, yogurt, pasta, and oatmeal.
Drink enough fluids	Fluids prevent dehydration and keep stool soft and formed. Water is a good choice. Avoid drinks with caffeine, alcohol, milk, or carbonation if they trigger diarrhea.

Source: Adapted from the National Digestive Diseases Clearinghouse. Available at http://digestive. niddk.nih.gov/diseases/pubs/fecalincontinence/fecalincontinence.pdf. Accessed 31 January 2014.

Fall Prevention

Older adults experience a high incidence of falls as well as a high susceptibility to injury from these falls. According to the Center for Disease Control and Prevention (CDC), one out of three adults ≥65 years falls each year. Older adults with diabetes have an increased risk of falls. Factors of particular concern include diabetes-related complications of peripheral neuropathy, reduced vision, and renal function. Insulin therapy is associated with increased falls possibly resulting from more severe disease or hypoglycemic episodes.[11]

Even if they are not injured, many people who fall develop a fear of falling. This fear of falling comes from the feelings of unsteadiness. A fall can prompt people to limit their physical activity. Inactivity often leads to reduced mobility and loss of physical fitness, which in turn increases their actual risk of falling. Thus, falls are risk factors for future falls. This may further perpetuate the cycle of inactivity. Further decline results from reductions in muscular and cardiovascular tone, reduced food intake, and poor nutritional status.[11]

A fall signals a decline in an individual's physical ability, which is a risk for loss of independence. Risk of falls frequently increases after acute illness. These periods are associated with prolonged bed rest, inactivity, and inadequate nutritional intake. The consequence is further muscle weakness. A decline in the ability to get around often leads to a decline in ability to perform ADLs independently. These older adults have to increase their reliance on others for assistance. Their risk of social isolation, however, also is increased.[12]

As testosterone levels naturally decrease with aging, loss of muscle mass and function in frail older men often result in poor health outcomes. They experience frequent falls, resulting in dependency and institutionalization. Although short-term testosterone therapy in frail elderly men has been associated with increased muscle mass and strength, treatment must be maintained for continued benefit.[13]

Risk factors for falls also include the use of four or more prescription medicines. The use of sedatives or hypnotics, antidepressants, and benzodiazepines is associated with falls in older adults. The Beers list identifies specific drugs or drug prescriptions (excessive dose, excessive treatment duration, inappropriate drug combination, and coexisting illness) with unfavorable benefit–risk ratio or questionable efficacy. Routine medications assessments may reduce the risk of falls. Changes in medication include reduction in number and dosages.[12]

Environmental hazards that increase the risks of falling include poor lighting, slippery or irregular walking surfaces, and a lack of supportive handrails. Most often, these falls occur in the home environment and are preventable.[14]

Visual factors are associated with falls. They include poor visual acuity, reduced contrast sensitivity, decreased visual field, cataract, and glaucoma medication.[15] Multifocal glasses may impair balance and have been shown to increase the risk of falls in several studies. In a fall prevention study, subjects used multifocal glasses with an additional pair of single-lens distance glasses for outdoors and unfamiliar settings.[16]

Individual exercise programs and teaching residents how to manage ADLs may enable residents to feel more independent and less affected by their diabetes. Physical and occupational therapy may be of benefit to older adults with specific physical disabilities. Physical therapists can advise exercise programs to improve ambulation. Older adults may benefit from routine exercise and flexibility or balance training, such as Tai Chi. Strength and endurance training may reduce the risk of falls.[15]

Occupational therapists can teach proper joint protection and energy conservation, how to use assistive devices, and how to improve joint function. Assistive devices include crutches, walking aids, shoe inserts, splints, braces, and special shoes. Using special appliances promotes comfort, independent movement, and better function. In the home, medical supplies include elevated seats for toilets, canes, walkers, grab bars, and sitting stools for bathtubs and showers.[15] Such supplies commonly are found and used in LTC facilities.

Foot wear changes may reduce falls. Functional reach and mobility test results indicated that balance for women was better with low-heeled shoes. For men, foot position awareness and stability were best with high-midsole hardness and low-midsole thickness.[15] Soft or backless slippers may not provide the level of support needed for fall prevention in vulnerable elders. Medicare will cover one pair of shoes and three pairs of inserts annually for people with diabetes and sensory peripheral neuropathy under the Medicare Therapeutic Shoe Bill. Sensory peripheral neuropathy increases fall risk as residents with this condition may have decreased sensation and proprioception.

Sleep

Insufficient sleep is associated with type 2 diabetes. Sleep duration and quality have emerged as predictors of levels of A1C, an important marker of blood glucose control. Recent research suggests that optimizing sleep duration and quality may be important means of improving blood glucose control in persons with diabetes.[17]

Many older adults with diabetes complain about sleep difficulties. They tend to feel sleepy and fall asleep earlier in the evening and awaken earlier in the morning. The elderly tend to be less tolerant of shifts in the sleep–wake cycle. Daytime napping may compensate for poor sleep at night but may disrupt the sleep–wake cycle, resulting in poor nighttime sleep. The elderly take longer to fall asleep and have difficulty staying asleep, awakening frequently during the night.[17]

People with diabetes may have a sleep disorder called sleep apnea. People with sleep apnea may make periodic gasping or "snorting" noises. During this time, their sleep becomes momentarily interrupted. Those with sleep apnea also may experience excessive daytime sleepiness, as their interrupted sleep is not restorative. Treatment of sleep apnea is dependent on its cause. If other medical problems are present, such as congestive heart failure or nasal obstruction, sleep apnea may resolve with treatment of these conditions. Gentle air pressure administered during sleep (typically in the form of a nasal continuous positive airway pressure device) also may treat sleep apnea effectively. Interruption of regular breathing or obstruction of the airway during sleep can pose serious complications for the health of the individual. Symptoms of sleep apnea should be taken seriously. Untreated sleep apnea can increase the risk of developing heart disease.[18]

Measures to promote sleep include moderate physical activity in the afternoon and avoiding stimulants such as caffeine found in coffee, tea, colas, and some medications. Sometimes a light bedtime snack, such a small glass of warm milk, might promote sleep. The older adult should try to go to bed around the same time each night and avoid naps during the day. If a person cannot fall asleep after 20 minutes, the general recommendation for the person living at home is to get out of bed and do a quiet activity, such as reading or listening to music. This is less likely to occur in LTC, but LTC is where a good assessment of sleep habits can assist the care team to develop a successful sleep hygiene program. Restless leg syndrome (RLS) is characterized by an unpleasant "creeping" or "crawling" sensation. It may feel like it is originating in the lower legs, but often it is associated with aches and pains throughout the legs. This causes difficulty falling asleep. It can be relieved by leg movements, such as walking or kicking. Abnormalities in the neurotransmitter dopamine often have been associated with RLS. In treating RLS, medications may help correct the underlying cause along with medications to promote restful sleep.[17]

Clinical Note

Sleep

- Many elderly have insufficient sleep
- Sleep apnea is more common in diabetes
- Nasal continuous positive airway pressure devices may be helpful
- Help resident develop a sleep hygiene program

Cognitive Impairment

Cognition refers to a combination of mental processes that focuses on the ability to learn new things. It also includes intuition, judgment, language, and memory. Decline in cognitive abilities contributes to decline in functional independence. Older adults experiencing cognitive decline may be unable to care for themselves or conduct necessary ADLs. LTC residents already may have some level of cognitive impairment. With normal aging, the processing speed of the brain declines and recall time increases. Increasing evidence suggests that poorly controlled diabetes may contribute to the development of cognitive impairment. Studies show that people with diabetes may not be able to effectively monitor their conditions. For example, they may not recognize the signs and symptoms of hypoglycemia (low blood glucose), and community-dwelling elders may have particular difficulty following recommended treatment recommendations.[19]

Self-management support strategies must be tailored for a person who is experiencing cognitive impairment. This is just as important in LTC environment as it is in the person's home. Adapting daily tasks requires organization, such as keeping important items in their designated place for easy access. Labeling items that look similar promotes recognition. Some blood glucose meters and pill organizers come with alarms that can be set as scheduled reminders of the next finger-stick or medication. Kitchen timers, calendars, day planners, to-do lists, and other devices can enable the older adults to carry out daily tasks.[3] These easily can be adapted for the resident's use in the LTC facility.

Even in those who already have some level of cognitive impairment, benefit still can be derived from encouraging participation in cognitively stimulating activities. Keeping the mind active as long as possible is especially important for older adults. Leisure time activities can help maintain mental sharpness. Recommended activities or hobbies that seniors can do for enjoyment include socializing, playing board games, playing musical instruments, dancing, singing, reading, and working on crossword puzzles.[3,20]

Social activity is associated with quality of life outcomes among older adults Staying connected with meaningful community activities and groups can help sustain an existing source of support, maintain continuity during a time of difficult changes, and contribute to self-esteem and sense of belonging. Research has associated positive health outcomes with engagement of older adults in activities in which they experience a sense of mastery.[18]

Social Support

Older adults require regular support and encouragement to participate in health-promoting behaviors that involve self-monitoring. This is particularly true for those living in LTC facilities. Talking with someone may help older adults cope with the demands of living with diabetes. They may benefit from the understanding that comes from friends and associates, particularly age peers, with similar health conditions. These peers can serve as both a useful source of information and as a source of comfort and empathy.[3]

Efforts include how to best elicit support and minimize negative influences from family members and friends. Capitalize on the positive intentions of other family members. Teach them how to be helpful in appropriate ways. Emphasize the importance of both activity and the need for independence in older adults' self-care. This may include specific efforts to educate and train family members about particular aspects of a self-management regimen.[21]

CONCLUSION

A comprehensive approach to working with older adults must address function, independence, comfort, and quality of life. The quality of life for older adults is associated with their social interactions, level of independence, and health status. Efforts in promoting self-care efforts are enhanced by their adaptation and resilience. Caregivers play an important role in helping older adults increase their skills and confidence in managing their diabetes and maintaining their quality of life. They can enhance the older adults' interest in their own care by better informing them of the nature of their condition and understanding their unique approaches and resistances to treatment. In doing so, caregivers gain very important partners in the geriatric workforce: the residents themselves.

REFERENCES

1. Easom LR. Concepts in health promotion: Perceived self-efficacy and barriers in older adults. *Journal of Gerontological Nursing* 2003;29(5):11–19.
2. Hooyman NR, Asuman Kiyak H. *Social gerontology: A multidisciplinary perspective.* Boston, MA, Allyn & Bacon, 2011.
3. Clark DO, Frankel RM, Morgan DL, Ricketts G, Bair ML, Nyland KA, Callahan CM. The meaning and significance of self-management among socioeconomically vulnerable older adults. *Journal of Gerontology: Social Sciences* 2008;63B(5):S312–S319. Available at http://psychsocgerontology.oxfordjournals.org/content/63/5/S312.full. Accessed 30 January 2014.
4. Lee L-L, Arthur A, Avis M. Using self-efficacy theory to develop interventions that help older people overcome psychological barriers to physical activity: a discussion paper. *International Journal of Nursing Studies* 2008;45:1690–1699.
5. Bainbridge KE, Hoffman HJ, Cowie CC. Diabetes and hearing impairment in the United States: Audiometric evidence from the National Health and Nutrition Examination Survey, 1999 to 2004. *Annals of Internal Medicine* 2008;149(1):1–10.
6. Frisina ST, Mapes F, Kim SH, Frisina DR, Frisina RD. Characterization of hearing loss in aged type II diabetics. *Hearing Research* 2006;211:103–113.
7. Coll-Planas L, Denkinger MD, Nikolaus T. Relationship of urinary incontinence and late-life disability: implications for clinical work and research in geriatrics. *Zeitschrift für Gerontologie und Geriatrie* 2008;41:283–290.
8. Lekan-Rutledge D. Urinary incontinence strategies for frail elderly women, 2004. Available at www.medscape.com/viewarticle/488559. Accessed 30 January 2014.
9. Bliss DZ, Norton C. Conservative management of fecal incontinence: An evidence-based approach to controlling this life-altering condition. *American Journal of Nursing* 2010;110 (9):30–39.
10. Stevens TK, Soffer EE, Palmer RM. Fecal incontinence in elderly patients: Common, treatable, yet often undiagnosed. *Cleveland Clinic Journal of Medicine* 2003;70(5):40–49.
11. Centers for Disease Control and Prevention. Falls among older adults: An overview, 2010. Available at www.cdc.gov/HomeandRecreationalSafety/Falls/adultfalls.html. Accessed 30 January 2014.
12. Woolcott JC, Richardson KJ, Wiens MO, Patel B, Marin J, Khan KM, Marra CA. Meta-analysis of the impact of 9 medication classes on falls in elderly persons. *Archives of Internal Medicine* 2009;169(21):1952–1960.
13. Barclay L. Testosterone effects on frailty not maintained at 6 months, 2010. Available at www.medscape.com/viewarticle/731992. Accessed 31 January 2014.
14. World Health Organization. *Active aging: A policy framework.* Geneva, Switzerland, Author, 2002. Available at http://whqlibdoc.who.int/hq/2002/who_nmh_nph_02.8.pdf. Accessed 31 January 2014.
15. American Geriatric Society/British Geriatric Society. Clinical practice guidelines for the prevention of falls in older persons, 2010. Available at www.medcats.com/FALLS/frameset.htm. Accessed 31 January 2014.

16. Haran MJ, Cameron ID, Ivers RQ, Simpson JM, Lee BB, Tanzer M, Porwal M, et al. Effect on falls of providing single lens distance vision glasses to multifocal glasses wearers: VISIBLE randomised controlled trial. *British Medical Journal* 2010;340:2265–2277. Available at www.medscape.com/viewarticle/724889_print. Accessed 31 January 2014.

17. Centers for Disease Control and Prevention. Sleep and chronic disease, 2010. Available at www.cdc.gov/sleep/about_sleep/chronic_disease.htm. Accessed 31 January 2014.

18. Cochen V, Arbus C, Soto CME, Villars H, Tiberge M, Montemayor T, Hein C, et al. Sleep disorders and their impact on healthy, dependent, and frail older adults. *Journal of Nutrition, Health and Aging* 2009;13:322–329. Available at http://download.springer.com/static/pdf/610/art%253A10.1007%252Fs12603-009-0030-0.pdf?auth66=1391307595_1713637a5d30c659e9cdb160704d287c&ext=.pdf. Accessed 31 January 2014.

19. Day KL, McGuire LC, Anderson LA. The CDC Healthy Brain Initiative: Public health and cognitive impairment. *Generations* 2009;33:11–17. Available at http://findarticles.com/p/articles/mi_7543/is_200904/ai_n39232440. Accessed 31 January 2014.

20. Rockwood K. What would make a definition of frailty successful? *Age and Ageing* 2005;34:432–434.

21. Gallant MP, Spitze GD, Prohaska TR. Help or hindrance? How family and friends influence chronic illness self-management among older adults. *Research on Aging* 2007;29:375–409.

BIBLIOGRAPHY

Merck Manual of Geriatrics. Assessment domains: Sleep disorders, 2006. Available at www.merck.com/mkgr/mmg/sec1/ch4/ch4b.jsp#ind01-004-0294. Accessed 18 October 2010.

7

Key Concepts for Nutrition Therapy in Older Adults

Carrie Swift, MS, RD, BC-ADM, CDE

INTRODUCTION: THE NUTRITION CARE PLAN

R easons for admission to a long-term care (LTC) environment vary from short-term stays for physical rehabilitation to end-of-life comfort care, or long-term stays related to physical or cognitive impairments requiring assistance in activities of daily living. Multiple factors affect nutrition status in older adults in the LTC setting (see Table 7.1). A comprehensive nutrition assessment is necessary to provide optimal patient care and meet regulatory requirements.[1] An individualized nutrition care plan, integrated into each resident's overall plan of care is needed to reach successful outcomes and maximize nutrition status.[1] Admitting diagnoses and goals for the resident should be considered when developing the nutrition care plan for the older adult with diabetes in LTC. An interdisciplinary team approach is necessary to integrate the nutrition care plan into the diabetes management plan for residents with diabetes. Specific nutrition interventions should be individualized based on multiple factors, including, life expectancy, comorbidities, and patient preference.

MALNUTRITION IN OLDER ADULTS

Unintentional weight loss resulting from protein-energy malnutrition or dehydration is common among older adults in LTC. Food intake generally declines even in healthy older adults; this often is referred to as "anorexia of aging." Physiologic age-related changes typically include a decreased sense of taste and smell, and early satiety related to a more rapid transit of food from the fundus to the antrum of the stomach combined with increased levels of cholecystokinin.[2] The resulting decrease in desire to eat and drink puts older adults at high risk of malnutrition and dehydration. The actual prevalence of protein-energy malnutrition in LTC facilities varies widely and ranges from 25 to 85% depending on the population observed and the definition of malnutrition used. The high prevalence of malnutrition in LTC facilities may be attributed partly to the transfer of malnourished, older adults from acute care hospitals to LTC after an acute illness.[2]

Diagnosing malnutrition in older adults can be quite difficult. Unintentional weight loss is generally one of the most important indicators of nutritional risk in the LTC setting and is linked with poor outcomes in older adults.[2] Although the importance of monitoring weight is undeniable, obtaining accurate height and weight measures in LTC remains challenging.

DOI: 10.2337/9781580404730.07

Table 7.1 Factors Affecting Nutrition Status in Older Adults in Long-Term Care

- Poor appetite
- Cognitive impairment
- Depression
- Altered taste sensation
- Decreased sense of smell
- Swallowing difficulties
- Oral or dental issues
- Impaired thirst mechanism
- Constipation diarrhea, nausea, or vomiting
- Polypharmacy
- Ability to self-feed
- Mealtime environment
- Ethnic, cultural, or religious food practices
- Food preferences
- Isolation during meals (e.g., eating alone in room rather than in the dining room)

Source: Adapted from Suhl and Staum, 2009; American Dietetic Association. Position of the American Dietetic Association: Individualized nutrition approaches for older adults. *Journal of the American Dietetic Association* 2010;110:1549–1553.

Suhl E, Staum E. Medical nutrition therapy for older adults: What do we need to do differently? On the Cutting Edge 2009;30(2):20–25.

NUTRITION STATUS DOCUMENTATION

The Centers for Medicare and Medicaid Services requires documentation in a periodic resident assessment instrument known as the Minimum Data Set (MDS).[3] Conditions that specifically affect a resident's ability to maintain nutrition and hydration status are documented in Section K: "Swallowing/Nutritional Status," although other sections of the MDS provide information relevant to nutrition status as well (MDS 3.0) (see Table 7.2). When a resident is identified with inadequate nutrition intake, documentation is required that the resident is at risk and then the appropriate Care Area Assessment(s) needs to be triggered based on the findings. Nutrition supplements, closer monitoring of food eaten, changes in foods offered based on resident preference, or texture modifications are potential interventions to improve food intake. Documentation of nutrition approaches used to improve oral intake should be included in the resident's medical record.

Older adults may prefer foods with stronger flavor because of alterations in taste and smell. Aging decreases the sense of smell, which affects the ability to

Table 7.2 MDS 3.0 Section K: Swallowing/Nutritional Status

- Signs and symptoms of possible swallowing disorder: Loss of liquids/solids from mouth when eating or drinking; holding food in mouth/cheeks or residual food in mouth after meals; coughing or choking during meals or when swallowing medications; complaints of difficulty or pain with swallowing

- Height

- Weight

- BMI

- Decreased sense of smell

- Weight loss: No; yes, on physician-prescribed weight-loss regimen; yes, not on a physician-prescribed weight-loss regimen

- Nutritional approaches: Parenteral/intravenous feeding; feeding-tube; mechanically altered diet; therapeutic diet

- Percent intake by artificial route: Proportion of total calories the resident received through parenteral or tube feedings ≤25%; 26–50%; ≥51%; average fluid intake per day by parenteral or tube feedings ≤500 ml/day; ≥501 ml/day

Source: Adapted from Centers for Medicare and Medicaid Services. Resident assessment user's manual version 3.0, 2010. Available at www.ahcancal.org/facility_operations/Documents/RAI_3.0/MDS%203%200%20Chapter%203%20Section%20K%20V1.02%20May%2028,%202010.pdf. Accessed 15 March 2013.

distinguish the taste of food. Presentation and food selection may play a more significant role in the eating experience than the actual taste of the food.[2] Swallowing disorders are common among LTC residents and often contribute to protein-energy malnutrition in older adults. Modifying texture of foods and consistency of fluids offered is a fundamental aspect of managing swallowing disorders.[4] An interprofessional team approach to the management of these disorders is desirable; recommended team members include a physician, nurse, speech pathologist, occupational therapist, and registered dietitian (RD). Texture modified diets and thickened liquids can be unappetizing, which may contribute to further decline in oral intake. Using appropriate seasoning to improve taste and making modified texture foods visually appealing may lead to improved intake in some residents with swallowing disorders.

Use of Liberalized Diets in LTC

Culture changes in LTC have placed an emphasis on moving away from institutionalized care to a more home-like environment with personalized care. The goal for this paradigm shift is to improve the resident's quality of care and quality of life. As a component of these culture change initiatives, there has been an increased awareness in the need to offer a wider variety of food choices, allowing for personal food preferences and providing dining options in the LTC setting. The practice of ordering therapeutic diets has not kept pace with these initiatives. Even though increasing evidence discourages the use of therapeutic diets for older adults, these diets continue to be prescribed.[5] Although intended to improve health, therapeutic diets may negatively affect the variety and flavor of food offered to residents with diabetes because of restrictions needed to meet therapeutic requirements.

Diets that are restrictive inadvertently may lead to decreased food intake, unintentional weight loss, and undernutrition, which is the opposite of the desired outcome. The Academy of Nutrition and Dietetics (formerly, the American Dietetic Association) holds the position that "the quality of life and nutritional status of older adults residing in health care communities (LTC) can be enhanced by individualization to less-restrictive diets." More liberal diets have been associated with improvement in food and beverage intake in the LTC population.[6] For many older adults, the benefits gained from liberalizing the meal plan outweigh any potential health risks. Possible benefits to the resident include increased quality of life, higher satisfaction with meals, improved nutrition status, and enhanced enjoyment of eating. Additionally, providing choices in food selection, dining options, and mealtimes may help residents maintain a sense of dignity, control, and autonomy.[6]

Importantly, no evidence supports the use of "no-concentrated-sweets" or "no-sugar-added" diets in the LTC setting. These diets do not reflect current diabetes nutrition guidelines and they needlessly restrict sucrose.[7] Calories should not be restricted to less than daily needs to control blood glucose. This puts the resident at undue risk of malnutrition. Older nursing home residents with diabetes should be offered a regular, unrestricted menu that is consistent in amount of carbohydrate for meals and snacks.[6,8] Balancing food intake with physical activity and diabetes medication, when needed, are the cornerstones of achieving and maintaining blood glucose control.

Clinical Note

Use of liberalized meal plans:

- Allow for food preferences
- Are culturally appropriate
- Improve food and beverage intake
- Improve quality of care
- Improve quality of life
- Help maintain residents' dignity, control, and autonomy

Consistent Carbohydrate

The consistent carbohydrate meal plan has been implemented in many hospitals and LTC settings. To be effective, the amount of carbohydrate content should be consistent from day to day at breakfast, lunch, dinner, and snacks with no set calorie level. Table 7.3 provides an example of a single day's meal plan. The

Table 7.3 Sample Menu: Regular Diet, Consistent Carbohydrate

Menu item	Serving size	Carbohydrate content (grams)
Breakfast		
Oatmeal	3/4 cup	20
Sliced Bananas	1/2 cup	15
Whole Wheat Toast	1 slice	15
Margarine	1 teaspoon	0
Jelly	1 teaspoon	4
Scrambled Eggs	2	3
1% Milk	6 ounces	8
Coffee	6 ounces	0
Sucralose (Splenda)*	1 packet	0
Total carbohydrate		**65 grams**
Lunch		
Tuna Salad Sandwich on Whole Wheat Bread	1 sandwich	30
Vegetable Noodle Soup	1 cup	15
Tossed Salad	3/4 cup	0
Ranch Dressing	2 Tablespoons	0
Chocolate Ice Cream	1/2 cup	15
Iced Tea	8 ounces	0
Sugar*	1 packet	3
Total Carbohydrate		**63 grams**
Dinner		
Roast Turkey	3 ounces	0
Mashed Potatoes & Gravy	1/2 cup	15
Whole Wheat Bread	1 slice	15
Margarine	2 teaspoons	0
Green Beans	1/2 cup	3
Applesauce with Cinnamon	1/2 cup	15
Vanilla Wafers	4 each	11
Coffee	6 ounces	0
Total Carbohydrate		**59 grams**

(Continued)

Table 7.3 Sample Menu: Regular Diet, Consistent Carbohydrate (Continued)

Menu item	Serving size	Carbohydrate content (grams)
HS Snack		
Light Strawberry Yogurt	6 ounces	19
Graham Cracker Squares	2 each	10
Total Carbohydrate		**29 grams**

Note:

*No-calorie sugar substitutes such as Splenda, Equal, and Truvia may be used to help maintain a consistent carbohydrate intake. Small amounts of added sugar may have minimal impact on blood glucose levels. Because an average sugar packet contains ~3–4 grams carbohydrate, it would have little to no effect on blood glucose.

purpose of the consistent carbohydrate plan is to meet individual nutrition needs while facilitating metabolic control.[9] Although it is recommended that the majority of carbohydrate in this meal plan comes from whole grains, fruit, vegetables, legumes, and dairy; sucrose-containing foods may be included. Sugars do not have an additional impact on blood glucose when substituted for isocaloric amounts of other carbohydrate sources.[7] A good starting carbohydrate amount for women is 45–60 grams of carbohydrate per meal and for men is 60–75 grams of carbohydrate per meal. If snacks are needed, 15–30 grams of carbohydrate is reasonable.[10] Assessing individual nutrition needs and preferences, however, will help determine the recommended carbohydrate provided and what adjustments to the meal plan are desirable. Consistency in carbohydrate intake allows for blood glucose patterns to be identified more easily identified to aid in the assessment of medication effectiveness. Adjusting medications to manage blood glucose, lipids, and blood pressure rather than restricting food intake is preferable to decrease the risk of malnutrition and enhance the enjoyment of eating for older adults.[8]

Starting a consistent carbohydrate (CHO) meal plan

- Females: 45–60 g CHO/meal
- Males: 60–75 g CHO/meal
- Snacks: 15–30 g CHO/snack

More flexibility in the meal plan and potentially improved diabetes control may be achieved for residents on insulin who receive mealtime, rapid-acting insulin. Insulin dose requirements should be based on "basal" and "nutritional" needs. The basal, or background insulin dose, is the amount of insulin required by the body when the individual is not eating. The nutritional insulin or mealtime (prandial) insulin is the amount of insulin needed to cover the carbohydrate in the meal, and it should not be withheld for a normal premeal blood glucose result.[11] Correction dosing may be used, as appropriate, for elevated premeal blood glucose. For residents with poor appetites, injecting the dose of rapid-acting insulin immediately after a meal may be a better option than taking mealtime insulin before eating. This allows for dosing based on actual carbohydrate eaten, which may result in more accurate dosing with reduced risk of hypoglycemia. Sliding-scale insulin as a sole source of insulin is not recommended.[9] Because of circumstances, such as understaffing, limited resources, and policies prohibiting mealtime insulin regimens, mealtime insulin dosing is not possible at some LTC facilities. Combination insulin therapy, for example, premixed insulin, may be used to cover basal and nutritional needs in those settings (see Chapter 10).

There seems to be a misconception that LTC residents no longer need diabetes education. In fact, education for the resident and family members regarding recommended food choices for diabetes management should be included in the nutrition care plan to improve understanding of the meal plan and goals for diabetes nutrition therapy. An important teaching point is that all sources of carbohydrate will elevate blood glucose, not just foods containing sugar. Older adults with diabetes may have difficulty shifting the focus away from sugars to the amount of total carbohydrate eaten, especially those with long-standing diabetes who previously learned a more sucrose-restrictive approach.[12] Understanding that residents with diabetes can eat desserts and other sugar-containing foods in the portions offered on the menu helps alleviate misunderstanding about residents receiving the "wrong diet" or that they are "cheating." Healthful, nutrient-dense carbohydrate such as whole grains, fruit, starchy vegetables, and low-fat milk and yogurt should continue to be encouraged and offered at each meal.

The message that total amount of carbohydrate eaten—rather than sugar content, or percentage of the meal eaten—is the largest determinant of postmeal blood glucose is an important concept for LTC staff as well. With additional training regarding carbohydrate content of menu items, nursing assistants can learn to document carbohydrate intake as well as percentage of the meal eaten. For example, if the majority of the food at a meal is primarily protein and fat—steamed broccoli, tossed salad, and oven-fried chicken—hypoglycemia may occur even with meal documentation indicating adequate intake of ≥75%. If the 75% of the meal eaten consists of carbohydrate-containing foods—milk, mashed potatoes, and a dinner roll—the effect on the blood glucose could be quite different. Accurate estimation of carbohydrate consumed may lead to improved accuracy of the mealtime insulin dosing. Potential benefits include hypoglycemia prevention and better overall blood glucose control for residents. Additional training helps improve understanding of appropriate meal substitutions and the potential glycemic effect of foods brought in from outside the facility by family members. Ongoing training to facility food service employees and nursing staff regarding menu offerings and the carbohydrate content of foods served is essential to fully implement this concept.

Hyperglycemia

Prolonged hyperglycemia may lead to serious consequences in LTC residents. Hyperosmolar hyperglycemic state (HHS) is a life-threatening condition that occurs when hyperglycemia and dehydration slowly worsen until both conditions are extreme. HHS is seen most commonly in older adults with type 2 diabetes (T2D), especially when the diabetes is undiagnosed.[13]

Because older adults do not have typical symptoms of hyperglycemia, HHS can go undetected in LTC. Polydipsia usually is absent because of the reduction in thirst associated with advanced age, leading to inadequate supplemental fluid intake.[14] Hyperglycemia may present as confusion, incontinence, or diabetes related complications in older adults.[14] Careful monitoring and emphasizing the importance of fluid intake to prevent dehydration may decrease the development of HHS in residents with diabetes. Maintaining adequate fluid intake can be especially challenging in individuals with swallowing disorders who find thickened liquids unpalatable. Offering appropriate fluids throughout the day and involving staff, family members, and the residents themselves is critical to the success of this effort. (For more information about HHS, see Chapter 5.)

Hypoglycemia

Hypoglycemia is defined as a blood glucose <70 mg/dl, with or without symptoms.[15] Older adults with diabetes are more prone to hypoglycemia than younger adults with diabetes due to multiple factors, including poor or erratic nutritional intake, mental status changes, polypharmacy, impaired renal function, and other comorbid conditions.[16] In the LTC setting, the risk of hypoglycemia should be weighed against the potential benefits of tighter glycemic control in older adults. Even in high-risk, frail older adults, it is important to avoid acute hyperglycemic complications of diabetes, such as dehydration, poor wound healing, and HHS.[17]

The risk of severe hypoglycemia for individuals treated with insulin and oral insulin secretagogues increases dramatically with age. Furthermore, use of medications with anticholinergic properties or age-related changes in the counterregulatory effect may cause the familiar adrenergic hypoglycemic symptoms of shakiness, anxiety, hunger, sweating, and pallor to be lost.[18] Instead of the typical symptoms, hypoglycemia may first present with neuroglycopenic symptoms, such as abnormal mentation, confusion, difficulty speaking, and irritability. In the older adult with multimorbidities, these symptoms may be misinterpreted as altered mental status or dementia.[18] Thus, ongoing assessment of cognitive function is an important consideration when individualizing a nutrition care plan, and setting diabetes treatment goals for older adults in LTC facilities.

Hypoglycemia is understandably one of the most feared complications of diabetes, by health care professionals and individuals living with diabetes alike. That fear may result in the overtreatment of hypoglycemia leading to hyperglycemia. For example encouraging multiple snacks or drinking large amounts of juice in response to hypoglycemia may significantly elevate blood glucose rather than just treating the hypoglycemia. Consuming 15–20 grams of glucose is the preferred

Table 7.4 15–15 Rule for Treatment of Hypoglycemia

1. Check blood glucose.

    If blood glucose is 50–69 mg/d, give 15 grams carbohydrate.*

    If blood glucose is <50 mg/dl, give 30 grams carbohydrate.**

2. Recheck blood glucose after 15 minutes.

    If not >70 mg/dl, give another 15 grams of carbohydrate.

3. If it is >1 hour until the next mealtime, provide a snack.

Note: Do not treat hypoglycemia with foods containing fat (e.g., whole milk, candy bar, chocolate, peanut butter). Fat may delay the rise in the blood glucose, slowing down the effect of the carbohydrate.

*Sources of 15 grams of carbohydrate include the following:
  4 glucose tablets
  1 tube of glucose gel
  4 ounces fruit juice
  8 ounces fat-free or 1% milk

**If a resident is unable to take oral carbohydrate due to confusion or unresponsiveness, or is unconscious, glucagon is indicated for treatment. Facilities should implement a protocol for prevention and treatment of hypoglycemia.

method of treatment for hypoglycemia in conscious individuals, although any form of glucose-containing carbohydrate may be used.[17]

Glucose tablets or gels provide a standardized dose of glucose and generally are less likely to result in overtreatment of hypoglycemia. Any kind of fruit juice (4 ounces) or fat-free milk (8 ounces) may be used to treat hypoglycemia (see Table 7.4). These items commonly are available to LTC staff and may be more palatable to older adults. If the resident has difficulty swallowing thin liquids, glucose gel may be the preferred treatment. Thickened fruit juice, or fat-free or low-fat regularly sweetened, smooth-textured yogurt or puddings also may be used. Foods such as candy bars, cookies, cakes, and whole milk should be discouraged as a treatment of hypoglycemia because of the higher fat content of these foods. Fat may slow and then prolong the acute glycemic response delaying the effect of the carbohydrate on raising the blood glucose.[17]

Although not used often, a particular class of drugs for diabetes, the α-glucosidase inhibitors, inhibit carbohydrate digestion to control blood glucose. Residents taking these medications will need to use glucose tablets or gel for treatment of hypoglycemia.[19] Drugs in this class include acabose and miglitol. These drugs do not cause hypoglycemia unless they are used in combination with insulin secretagogues (e.g., glipizide or glyburide, or insulin).

Regardless of type of treatment, rechecking the blood glucose 15 minutes after treatment is particularly important in the older adult who does not have clear symptoms of hypoglycemia. If the blood glucose remains <70 mg/dl, the original treatment should be repeated. When the blood glucose is normal, a meal or snack should be provided to prevent a recurrence of hypoglycemia.[17] Nutrition supplements designed for individuals with diabetes, such as Glucerna™ or Boost Glucose Control™, are not appropriate for first-line treatment of hypoglycemia, but they may be used to prevent hypoglycemia or following treatment.

Weight Management

Many individuals with T2D are overweight and are insulin resistant. Weight loss is a commonly recognized strategy to decrease insulin resistance and improve the health of people with diabetes. Weight loss in overweight and obese older adults with diabetes, however, remains controversial. The American Geriatrics Society emphasizes medical nutrition therapy as an important component of treatment for older adults with diabetes.[20,21] A modest weight loss of 5–10% of body weight may be indicated for some obese older adults. Although benefits in risk reduction may still be seen with weight loss, with respect to mortality, findings suggest that weight maintenance should be the goal even among healthy, obese older adults in the community setting.[22] Several explanations are offered for this seemingly contradictory recommendation. When obesity occurs after the age of 65 years, excess adipose tissue may serve as a calorie reserve during illness or stress, and some protection against osteoporotic fractures also may be gained.[22] Weight loss recommendations, especially due to the higher risk of undernutrition in the LTC setting, should be considered cautiously and individualized when it comes to obese older adults. Unintentional weight loss of >10% of body weight in <6 months should be addressed as part of the nutrition assessment.

NUTRITION STRATEGIES FOR SUCCESS: EVERYONE HAS A PART

Food Service

Food safety is of critical importance in the LTC setting. Serving food at the proper temperatures—hot food served hot and cold food served cold—helps prevent foodborne illness and increases residents' satisfaction with the meals. Dietary managers are generally responsible for seeing that appropriate safety and sanitation practices are used in food preparation and service areas. Serving meals in a pleasant dining-room setting with table service can help ensure a positive mealtime experience for residents. Offering choices for entrées and snacks, honoring food preferences, and meeting ethnic and religious food practices whenever possible aids in increasing resident and family satisfaction with meal service. Appropriate fluids should be offered with meals and frequently throughout the day. Small portions of desserts may be offered to all residents so they can be incorporated more easily into consistent carbohydrate menus. Offering nonnutritive sweeteners such as sucralose (Splenda) and aspartame (Equal) with meals may help some residents achieve consistent carbohydrate intake. Carbohydrate content of menu and snack items should be posted in the dining room and printed material should be made available to staff, residents, and family members. A better understanding of the menu items helps allow for alternate meal choices and substitutions of items based on individual food preferences and potential effect on the blood glucose. Offering special occasion menu selections for the resident to choose is a nice way to acknowledge a resident's birthday and celebrate them in a personal way.

Role of food service departments

- Serve food at appropriate temperature
- Use appropriate safety and sanitation measures
- Facilitate pleasant meal-time settings
- Post carbohydrate (or nutritional) content of menu and snack items
- Offer special occasion menus

Nursing Staff

Nursing staff play a vital role in the mealtime eating experience for residents to help meet treatment goals. The following strategies can be used to help residents optimize food intake:

- Encourage residents to eat in the dining room for socialization rather than eating alone in their rooms.
- Help set a positive atmosphere during mealtimes and allow residents the time to eat at their own pace; this can make a significant difference in overall meal intake for some residents.
- If residents are not eating well—<75% of meal consumed, or when carbohydrate intake is inadequate—encourage food substitutions with a similar amount of carbohydrate, based on individual food preference. Reduce the mealtime insulin dose when needed rather than force meals or snacks.
- Give rapid-acting insulin immediately after a meal, based on actual carbohydrate consumed, to residents with inconsistent carbohydrate intake or poor appetite.
- Observe interaction with other residents and change seating location in the dining room for compatible table companions.
- Identify when feeding assistance is needed and offer appropriate assistance.
- Ensure that snacks and fluids are offered during activities.
- Encourage consumption of low-carbohydrate or carbohydrate-free beverages between meals to maintain hydration status.
- Offer any supplemental nutrition beverages between meals, not immediately before, or in place of meals to increase caloric intake.
- Obtain accurate weights of residents on a scheduled basis.
- Make referrals to the RD as soon as it is observed that a resident is not meeting nutrition goals to help initiate early nutrition intervention when needed.

Registered Dietitians

RDs develop individual nutrition care plans for residents based on nutrition status, personal preferences, and medical treatment goals. RDs collaborate with interdisciplinary clinical staff, the resident, family members, dietary managers, diet technicians, and food service staff to carry out the nutrition care plan. RDs are involved in developing and implementing nutrition-related policies and procedures for the facility. RDs should provide ongoing education to clinical staff, family members, and residents to improve understanding of individual nutrition care plans and use of less-restrictive diets to achieve nutrition goals.[6] Observing and interacting with residents during meals provides valuable information and lets the residents know their feedback is important. Mealtimes may present "teachable moments" to share information with staff, family members, and residents. When everyone involved has a better understanding of the nutrition care plan and diabetes management goals, they will be more likely to actively participate in reaching the goals.

Family Members

LTC staff should encourage family members to visit during mealtimes and assist with feeding as appropriate. All staff members can encourage input from family members regarding food preferences, including ethnic, religious, or cultural foods, to individualize meals for the resident. Family members can help gather input from the resident and help with recall about foods the resident enjoys. Discuss alternate food sources, and let family members know how to notify staff if they are bringing in food for the resident. Food safety requirements should be emphasized and a consistent message delivered about foods brought in from outside the facility.

Residents

The residents play a vital role to the success of diabetes management plans and nutrition care plans. Every effort should be made to include each resident in the decision-making process related to their individual plan of care.

CONCLUSION

Many factors affect nutrition status of older adults with diabetes in the LTC setting, undernutrition and malnutrition are common. No evidence supports the use of the "no-concentrated-sweets" or "no-sugar-added" diets. Use of liberalized diets in the LTC setting should be encouraged. Offering a regular, consistent carbohydrate meal plan to residents with diabetes is recommended. Adequate hydration is a key strategy in preventing extreme hyperglycemia in older adults with diagnosed (or undiagnosed) T2D. Weight management in older adults should be approached with caution due to associated risks. Hypoglycemia should be prevented whenever possible, without causing excessive hyperglycemia. When hypoglycemia does occur, overtreatment should be avoided. The residents, family members, and LTC staff members all play key roles in meeting the nutrition therapy and diabetes management goals of older adults in LTC.

REFERENCES

1. Thomas DR. Nutrition assessment in long-term care. *Nutrition in Clinical Practice* 2008;23(4):383–387.
2 Thomas DR., Morley JE, Kamel H. Nutritional deficiencies in long-term care: Parts I, II, III. *Annals of Long-Term Care* 2004;(Suppl6)(10):325–332. Available at www.annalsoflongtermcare.com/attachments/1079364363-NutritionLTC.pdf. Accessed 25 March 2013.
3. Centers for Medicare and Medicaid Services. Resident assessment user's manual version 3.0, 2010. Available at www.ahcancal.org/facility_operations/Documents/RAI_3.0/MDS%203%200%20Chapter%203%20Section%20K%20V1.02%20May%2028,%202010.pdf. Accessed 15 March 2013.
4. Garcia JM, Chambers E. Managing dysphagia through diet modifications. *American Journal of Nursing* 2010;110(11):26–33.
5 Feldman SM, Rosen R, DeStasio J. Status of diabetes management in the nursing home setting in 2008: a retrospective chart review and epidemiology study of diabetic nursing home residents and nursing home initiatives in diabetes management. *Journal of the American Medical Directors Association* 2009;10(5):354–360.
6. American Dietetic Association. Position of the American Dietetic Association: Individualized nutrition approaches for older adults. *Journal of the American Dietetic Association* 2010;110:1549–1553.
7. American Diabetes Association. Nutrition therapy recommendations for the management of adults with diabetes. *Diabetes Care* Evert AB, Boucher JL, Cypress M, Dunbar SA, Franz MJ, Mayer-Davis EJ, Neumiller JJ, Urbanski P, Yancy W: Nutrition therapy recommendations for management of adults with diabetes. *Diab Care* 2014;37 (suppl 1) S120–S123.
8. American Diabetes Association. Nutrition Recommendations and Interventions for Diabetes. *Diabetes Care* 2008;31(S1);S61–S78.
9. Clement S, Braithwaite SS, Magee MF, Ahmann A, Schafer RG, Hirsch IB. Management of diabetes and hyperglycemia in hospitals. *Diabetes Care* 2004;27:553–591.
10. Diabetes Care and Education Practice Group of the Academy of Nutrition and Dietetics. Carbohydrate counting: A tool to help manage your blood glucose. Patient handout, 2011. Available at http://dbcms.s3.amazonaws.com/media/files/84fbc534-f57f-4c01-9ebf-a65b207ae2e0/ADA_Carbohydrate%20counting_FINAL.pdf. Accessed 24 March 2013.
11. Swift CS, Boucher JL. Nutrition care for hospitalized individuals with diabetes. *Diabetes Spectrum* 2005;18(1):34–38.
12. Swift CS. Promoting healthy eating among older adults with diabetes. *Topics in Geriatric Rehabilitation* 2010;26(3):214–220.
13. Trence DL. Hyperglycemia. In *The art and science of diabetes self-management education: A desk reference*. C. Mensing, Ed. Chicago, IL, American Association of Diabetes Educators, 2011, p. 591–595.
14. Chau D, Edelman SV. Clinical management of diabetes in the elderly. *Clinical Diabetes* 2001;19(4):172–175.
15. U.S. Department of Health and Human Services. Hypoglycemia. National Institutes of Health, National Diabetes Information Clearinghouse, 2008.

NIH Publication No. 09–3926. Available at http://diabetes.niddk.nih.gov/dm/pubs/hypoglycemia/hypoglycemia_508.pdf. Accessed 10 March 2013.

16. Wallace JI. Management of diabetes in the elderly. *Clinical Diabetes* 1999;17(1):19–25.

17. American Diabetes Association. Standards of medical care in diabetes—2014. *Diabetes Care* 2014;37(S1):S14–S80.

18. Briscoe VJ, Davis SN. Hypoglycemia in type 1 and type 2 diabetes: Physiology, pathophysiology, and management. *Clinical Diabetes* 2006;24(3):115–121.

19. Sisson EM, Cornell S. In *The Art and Science of Diabetes Self-Management Education: A desk reference*. C. Mensing, Ed. Chicago, IL, American Association of Diabetes Educators, 2011, p. 417-457.

20. Brown AF, Mangione CM, Saliba D, Sarkisian CA, California Healthcare Foundation/American Geriatrics Society Panel on Improving Care for Older Persons with Diabetes. Guidelines for improving the care of the older person with diabetes mellitus. *Journal of the American Geriatric Society* 2003;51(5):S265–S280.

21. Moreno G, Mangione CM, Kimbro L, Vaisberg E, American Geriatrics Society Expert Panel on the Care of Older Adults with Diabetes Mellitus. *Guidelines for improving the care of older adults with diabetes mellitus*. 2nd ed. New York, NY, American Geriatrics Society, 2013.

22. Miller SL, Wolfe RR. The danger of weight loss in the elderly. *Journal of Nutrition Health and Aging* 2008;12(7):487–491.

8

Physical Activity and Diabetes: Considerations for Older Adults in Long-Term Care Facilities

Meghan Warren, PT, MPH, PhD

INTRODUCTION

This chapter reviews the importance of physical activity in the older population with type 2 diabetes (T2D) with a focus on those in long-term care (LTC) facilities. An additional purpose is to provide evidence-based guidelines on exercise testing and prescription in this population. There is a paucity of research on effective interventions in older people living in LTC facilities, so much of the included evidence was completed in community-dwelling elderly. When available, research for those living in LTC is included.

Before reviewing the evidence, it is necessary to define several terms that are used throughout the chapter. Although the terms "physical activity" and "exercise" often are used interchangeably, there are distinct definitions for each:

- Physical activity is defined as "any bodily movement produced by the contraction of skeletal muscles that results in a substantial increase over resting energy expenditure."[1] Physical activity therefore can include household, transportation, occupational, and leisure activities.
- Exercise is "a type of physical activity consisting of planned, structured, and repetitive bodily movements done to improve or maintain one or more components of physical fitness."[1]

Most exercise activities fall into one of four categories:

1. Aerobic or endurance exercise, which refers to continuous or intermittent rhythmic movement of the large muscles of the body to improve cardio-respiratory endurance.
2. Resistance or strength training, which includes exercises that cause muscles to move or hold against a force or weight to improve muscular strength, power, and endurance.
3. Flexibility exercises, which are exercises that preserve or increase range of motion of a joint.
4. Balance training, which refers to exercises designed to reduce the risk of falls.[2]

This chapter primarily focuses on aerobic and resistance exercises. The definition of old age is not consistent in the literature. The current physical activity guidelines[3] use ≥65 years to define "old age," although these guidelines may be

DOI: 10.2337/9781580404730.08

relevant for adults 50–64 years old with functional limitations or chronic conditions. Consistent with this definition, most of the evidence presented in this chapter is limited to studies in samples ≥65 years, which also reflects the age demographic of the population in LTC.[4]

BENEFITS OF PHYSICAL ACTIVITY IN OLDER ADULTS WITH DIABETES

Age is a primary risk factor for diabetes.[2] Among the several factors that are thought to contribute to the increase in insulin resistance (decreased insulin sensitivity) and higher incidence of diabetes seen in older adults is the increasing sedentary lifestyle that occurs with aging.[5,6] This association has been shown to occur independent of body weight changes,[7] as well as occurring with increased body weight and increased fat mass.[8] These changes in body composition are a common consequence of aging.[2,8–10] Finally, age-related declines in maximal aerobic capacity and muscle function (strength power, endurance, and control) can increase the risk of metabolic diseases like diabetes.[11,12]

Although age is a primary risk factor for diabetes, regular physical activity can modify the risks[2] with favorable changes in circulating levels of glucose. These beneficial effects have been shown with both aerobic and resistance exercise[13,14] and have been shown both acutely and chronically (with training). With exercise, there is increased glucose uptake by the skeletal muscle, which has been shown to be both insulin facilitated and insulin independent.[15,16] This increase in glucose uptake by skeletal muscle decreases the amount of circulating glucose, and the hyperglycemia that is seen with diabetes, favoring overall glycemic control.[14,17–20]

A meta-analysis completed by Boulé et al.[21] examined the effects of structured exercise interventions for at least 8 weeks compared with nonexercise control on glycosylated hemoglobin (A1C), a long-term marker of glycemic control. This meta-analysis included 14 randomized and nonrandomized studies with 504 participants with a mean age of the participants of 55 ± 7.2 years. The exercise interventions included both aerobic (*n* = 12 studies) and resistance (*n* = 2) exercise interventions, which were conducted an average of 3.4 times per week for 15 weeks. At baseline, there were no significant differences in A1C between the two pooled groups; post intervention, A1C was significantly lower in the exercise group compared with the control group (7.65 vs. 8.31%, *p* < 0.001), indicating better long-term glycemic control; this was independent of any changes in body weight.

Although the average age in the previous meta-analysis is not considered "old age," similar results have been reported in other studies including older people. In a 6-month randomized trial on the effect physical activity prescription (PAP) on body composition and cardiometabolic risk factors, positive effects were reported.[22] The PAP intervention included one session of individualized counseling resulting in a written PAP; an agreement, including the patient's own goals to gradually increase physical activity to recommended levels of physical activity. The study included 91 adults aged 68 years who were randomized to the PAP (*n* = 41) or a standard care (one-page sheet on the importance of physical activity) control (*n* = 50). After 6 months, A1C decreased significantly more in the

PAP group compared with the control group ($p = 0.001$). In another study of 58 older adults (mean age 65 ± 7 years) with impaired glucose tolerance (IGT), a single-session exercise program along with a pedometer with goals for steps per day was compared with usual care (sheet on the importance of physical activity in people with IGT).[23] The pedometer goals included 3,000 steps/day for sedentary people (~30 minutes of walking) and 9,000 steps/day for those completing at least 6,000 steps/day at baseline (adding ~30 minutes of walking/day); those with > 9,000 steps/day at baseline were encouraged to increase activity as able. Fasting glucose decreased significantly in the intervention group compared with the usual care group at 3 months (–0.37 mmol/l, 95% confidence interval [CI] –0.63 to –0.11 mmol/l), 6 months (–0.30 mmol/l, –0.57 to –0.03 mmol/l), and 12 months (–0.32 mmol/l, –0.59 to –0.003 mmol/l). Two-hour glucose also showed significant decrease in the intervention versus the control group at 3 and 12 months. Taken together, these studies show there is substantial support that exercise and physical activity can have positive effects of glycemic control in older adults with diabetes.

Physical activity confers benefits in older adults with diabetes beyond glycemic control. Regular activity has shown favorable changes in cardiovascular fitness,[24-26] lipids,[22,27,28] body weight,[22,25,27-29] body composition,[26,27,30] and blood pressure.[13,27,28,31] Because of all of these improvements, including better glycemic control, cohort studies have shown reduced risk of cardiovascular disease (CVD) in those with IGT (T2D and metabolic syndrome) between 35% and 55% who maintained an active lifestyle.[32,33] This reduction in cardiovascular risk is especially important because of a two-times increased risk of a serious cardiovascular event (i.e., myocardial infarction or cerebrovascular accident) and a higher immediate and long-term mortality rate after cardiovascular events in people with IGT compared with the general population.[34]

Physical activity may increase feelings of well-being,[13] and result in favorable reductions in depression.[35] Physical activity also has been shown to reduce the functional decline that occurs with aging,[36] and decrease fall risk.[37] In addition, physical activity may help prevent or delay some of the systemic complications from diabetes, such as neuropathy, retinopathy, and nephropathy.[20]

In relatively high-functioning men and women ages 70–79 years, Seeman et al.[38] examined the association between modifiable risk factors, including exercise, and physical functioning over 2.5 years of follow-up. This study found that moderate or strenuous exercise (intensity adapted from previous studies)[39,40] predicted better physical performance, independent of sociodemographic (e.g., gender, age, and education) and health status characteristics (e.g., BMI, cognitive performance, presence of high blood pressure, diabetes, or cancer). In LTC facilities, this may be especially of interest to increase the number of residents with high physical performance and functional independence.

The benefits of physical activity for older adults with diabetes to improve glycemic control and ameliorate risk factors for other conditions are consistent and convincing. It is important, therefore, to examine the evidence to determine whether older adults can improve fitness with an exercise program. The effect on most physiologic variables (e.g., maximal heart rate) with aging is one of decline.[2] Numerous studies, however, have shown that older adults can derive physiologic and neuromuscular benefits from exercise and physical activity. A meta-analysis of 41 trials ($n = 2,012$ participants) found a 16% improvement in maximal aerobic capacity (VO_{2max}) with aerobic exercise training compared with nonexercising controls.[41] Trials with resistance exercise have shown even greater relative increases (28%).[42] Although the absolute amount of improvement tends to be less in older adults compared with younger adults, the relative increases in VO_{2max},[41] muscle strength, endurance, and size appears to be similar,[42,43] supporting the beneficial effects of physical activity and exercise in older adults.

PREVALENCE OF PHYSICAL ACTIVITY IN OLDER ADULTS

Despite the benefits of physical activity and exercise already discussed, older adults report low levels of physical activity. In the 2009 Behavioral Risk Factor Surveillance Survey, a nationwide telephone survey of community-dwelling adults, 40.3% of adults >65 years reported meeting the physical activity guidelines (at least 30 minutes of moderate physical activity ≥5 days/week, or at least 20 minutes of vigorous physical activity for ≥3 days/week).[6] This is lower than younger age-groups, reflecting other studies that have shown a decline in energy expenditure due to physical activity with increasing age.[5] Even lower levels of physical activity are reported when older adults with diabetes were examined. Based on data from the National Health and Nutrition Examination Survey (NHANES III), only 32% (95% CI 27–38%) of the people ≥65 years with diabetes reported meeting the physical activity guidelines, and 38% (95% CI 35–43%) reported participating in no leisure-time physical activity.[44]

People with diabetes also report significant limitations in physical function, which can further lead to a sedentary lifestyle and physical inactivity. In 2008, the percent of adults with diabetes who reported a limitation with walking a quarter mile was 50.4 ± 1.9% (percent ± standard error [SE]) for adults 65–74 years old and 63.3 ± 2.4% for adults ≥75 years.[45] Limitations also were reported with climbing up 10 steps (41.6 ± 1.9% and 53.8 ± 2.3% for 65–74 years and ≥75 years, respectively), standing for 2 hours (53.0 ± 1.9% and 67.2 ± 2.3% for 65–74 years and ≥75 years, respectively), and stooping, bending, or kneeling (60.7 ± 1.8% and 66.4 ± 2.2% for 65–74 years and ≥75 years, respectively).

Estimates for physical activity among those adults living in LTC are scarce, but most of the evidence concluded that a sedentary lifestyle is the norm. MacRae et al.[46] reported large amounts of inactivity in 95 ambulatory nursing home residents, with >85% of the observations representing either lying or sitting. When physical activity (versus inactivity) was measured, it was very low. In a German study of 47 ambulatory female nursing home residents, only 34% of the females were active for >2 hours/ week,[47] which is less than the current physical activity guidelines of 150 minutes (2.5 hours) per week.[3] The intensity of activity was not specified, but evidence shows that residents of nursing homes have lower intensity of physical activity compared with community-dwelling seniors as measured by walking speed.[48] After adjusting for age, the community sample (*n* = 28) walked significantly faster (*p* < 0.0001) than the nursing home sample (*n* = 26) at self-selected slow (0.95 ± 0.20 meters per second [m/s] vs. 0.42 ± 0.17 m/s), normal (1.27 ± 0.20 m/s vs. 0.64 ± 0.28 m/s), and fast (1.61 ± 0.21 m/s vs. 0.80 ± 0.35 m/s) paces, indicating that physical activity in LTC may be of lower intensity. In a study of 93 nursing home residents, ~70% of women and ~30% of men reported rare or no participation in physical activity strenuous enough to "work up a sweat," and ~20% of men and <5% of women reported participating in physical activity sufficient to "work up a sweat" often.[49] Details on the responses "often" and "rarely" were not described, nor were the intensity of physical activity necessary to "work up a sweat," so care should be used with interpretation, but this study does confirm other studies showing low levels of physical activity or exercise in residents of LTC facilities.

Estimates for physical activity in assisted-living facilities are even more scarce, but they show low levels of physical activity as well. A study was recently completed including 171 residents in four assisted-living facilities.[50] Physical activity was measured using the Physical Activity Survey for Long-Term Care (PAS-LTC), as well as an accelerometer, a way to objectively measuring the amount and intensity of activity. On the basis of data collected from the PAS-LTC, the participants engaged in 162.9 ± 81.4 (mean ± standard deviation) minutes of activity over a 24-hour period; most of the time in activity was spent in personal care (e.g., bathing and dressing). The participants reported a daily average of 8.5 ± 17.6 minutes of exercise, and 16.5 ± 38.9 minutes of recreational activity. Objectively measured (i.e., accelerometry), data showed that much of the activity was low intensity with only 13.0 ± 3.5 minutes/day of moderate intensity physical activity (accelerometry counts >1,041 counts/minute).[51] None of the participants achieved the amount of physical activity recommended in the current guidelines.[3] Most of the participants were independent with transferring (92%) and ambulation (81%).

The amount of physical activity among older adults with diabetes living in LTC is lacking. It is not difficult to infer, from the information in older adults with diabetes and older adults living in LTC already presented, that the average physical activity in people with diabetes living in LTC would be very low.

Barriers to Physical Activity in Long-Term Care

Because of the benefits of physical activity and exercise, it is important for older adults to remain physically active. But from the data presented on the prevalence of physical activity, it is clear that older adults are primarily sedentary, and this is especially true in LTC facilities. Therefore, understanding some of the barriers to physical activity may help to mitigate these barriers to allow activity to enhance glycemic control and confer other benefits. Many of these barriers are interrelated and are not specific to adults with diabetes living in LTCs; rather, they affect all people living in LTC facilities. So addressing the barriers needs to be a multifactorial process.

One consideration to physical activity among people in LTC is related to the possible reason for admission to the facility—functional decline and lack of independence with activities of daily living (ADL), which include bathing, dressing, toileting, transferring, or eating. This functional decline would be especially true in skilled nursing facilities, and they may be less of a consideration in assisted-living facilities. As expected, healthy individuals were more likely to be physically active than those with medical conditions and those with lower levels of function.[52] Therefore, those with lower functional levels and those with many medical conditions—two things commonly seen in older adults—are more likely living a sedentary lifestyle. In 2004, only 1.6% of all nursing home residents were independent with all ADL, whereas 51.1% required assistance with all five ADL, and a significant percent were totally dependent (e.g., 22.9% for transferring and 38.4% for bathing).[4] The amount of assistance required for locomotion (i.e., ambulation or wheelchair propulsion) for residents of nursing homes is reported in the National Nursing Home Survey[53] and the percentages of residents by level of assistance is displayed in Table 8.1.

The lack of independence with functional mobility may prevent or limit a resident's physical activity options. A small study (*n* = 12) examining factors affecting adherence to an exercise program found that despite the fact that individuals required assistive locomotion devices (i.e., wheelchair, walker), using one had no effect on activity levels.[54] Most of the participants, however, were independent with locomotion using the device.

Table 8.1 Percent of Nursing Home Residents by Level of Assistance with Locomotion, U.S., 2004

Activity[a]		Age			
		65–74 years	75–84 years	>85 years	Total
Walking in room	Independent or supervision	32.7	29.0	24.9	27.3
	Assistance required[b]	20.8	27.0	30.5	28.1
	Unknown	43.9	42.9	43.7	43.5
Walking in corridor	Independent or supervision	30.3	26.8	22.4	25.0
	Assistance required	20.1	26.3	29.7	27.4
	Unknown	46.8	45.7	47.1	46.6
Locomotion[c] on unit	Independent or supervision	46.7	39.9	34.1	37.8
	Assistance required	47.6	55.7	62.6	58.1
	Unknown	3.9	3.0	2.5	2.8
Locomotion off the unit	Independent or supervision	41.0	32.7	27.3	31.0
	Assistance required	50.2	58.9	65.2	60.9
	Unknown	6.8	7.1	6.7	6.9

Note:
[a] Percentages do not add to totals when residents are excluded who did not do activity in the past 7 days.
[b] Assistance required = limited or extensive assistance or total dependence.
[c] Locomotion includes ambulation and wheelchair use.

Source: Centers for Disease Control and Prevention. National Nursing Home Survey, 2004. Available at www.cdc.gov/nchs/nnhs.htm. Accessed 7 January 2011.

Additionally, several studies have found a strong association between social support and physical activity in older adults.[54–56] This association also has been shown with ADL limitations, which may further limit an individual's ability to participate in physical activity. Moritz et al.[57] analyzed data from 1,856 older adults in the Yale Health and Aging Project and examined the association between social isolation and ADL limitations. Social isolation was defined as "no monthly visual contact with friends or relatives" and was positively associated with ADL limitations, odds ratio (95% CI) for males 1.9 (1.1–3.0) and for females 1.9 (1.3–2.9). This social support could come from other members in an exercise program or from family or friends. Unfortunately, in LTC, there is often a lack of social support. Drageset et al.[58] interviewed 227 long-term nursing home residents and found that 56% of the residents reported loneliness and that social support and loneliness were related. Likewise, a Canadian survey of older adults living in at a LTC facility found that only 50% of the individuals reported having visitors "often" or "very often" and 39% of the individuals would like more visitors.[59] These studies provide evidence that older adults in LTC facilities are lacking social support, are lonely, and would accept further social support, which may result in more physical activity.

A further barrier to physical activity in LTC facilities is medical conditions that may limit the adult's ability to be physically active without modifications. An example of this is arthritis, the most common cause of disability among adults with self-reported disabilities.[60] Data from the U.S. National Health Interview Survey (NHIS) from 2007–2009 reported 45.4% (95% CI 43.9–46.9%) of adults ≥65 year with doctor-diagnosed arthritis reported arthritis-attributable activity limitation,[61] which was defined as any limitation in any daily activity because of arthritis or joint symptoms. The results of this study show that there are significant limitations among adults with arthritis, and these limitations may limit a person's ability to participate in physical activity. Although results from the National Nursing Home Survey reported only 3% of nursing home residents had a primary arthritis diagnosis and 19% had any arthritis diagnosis at admission,[62] this is probably an underrepresentation of the diagnosis among nursing home residents. The NHIS reported a prevalence of doctor-diagnosed arthritis of 50% among community-dwelling adults ≥65 years;[61] it is not unreasonable to assume that a similar prevalence would be found in residents of nursing homes.

A final barrier to physical activity in LTC may be environmental restrictions/designs. The presence of facilities available for physical activity has been shown to increase the amount of physical activity completed. A survey of 800 independent living, assisted living, and nursing home facilities was conducted to examine this association.[63] This study found a consistent, albeit modest, association between outdoor (e.g., walking paths) and indoor (e.g., indoor exercise room) physical activity facilities and participation in physical activity, although the overall number and percentages were small. For example, the presence of walking paths was related to more residents in assisted living facilities walking as part of a walking club (5% vs. 1% in facilities without walking paths). For indoor physical activity facilities, the availability of an indoor exercise room was related to more residents of nursing homes participating in aerobic exercises (6% vs. 2% in facilities without indoor exercise rooms). The same association between facilities for activity and participation in physical activity has also been shown in several studies of community-dwelling older people.[64-67]

Two recent studies examined the resident's perception of barriers and influences to physical activity in LTC facilities.[68,69] Both of these studies interviewed residents and reported the barriers that were similar to those discussed previously, although the following different barriers were reported:

1. Health status and physical frailty
2. Environmental restriction
3. Future health concerns and fear of injury or falling
4. Past sedentary lifestyle and intergenerational influences
5. Insufficient understanding about physical activity

Both the barriers published in quantitative literature as well as the resident's perception of barriers can be addressed through education, as well as modifications to physical activity programs, and administrative changes and design aspects. For example, a recent publication stated benches that are located 75–100 feet apart encourage residents to use a sidewalk around the building for exercise.[70]

Barriers to physical activity in LTC residents

- Dependence with ADLs, physical frailty
- Lack of social support, loneliness
- Medical conditions, e.g., arthritis
- Environmental restrictions/designs
- Residents' fear of falling
- Residents' lack of knowledge
- Residents' past sedentary lifestyle

RECOMMENDATIONS FOR PHYSICAL ACTIVITY AND EXERCISE FOR OLDER ADULTS WITH DIABETES LIVING IN LONG-TERM CARE FACILITIES

Before beginning any exercise program, older adults with diabetes should undergo a thorough medical evaluation to identify diabetes-related complications and risk for cardiac complications, as well as to help identify precautions or contraindications for exercise, including modification or the need for supervision. This evaluation should include screening of the cardiovascular, nervous, renal, and visual systems because of the high prevalence of these conditions in individuals with diabetes.[1]

1. Cardiovascular system: a screening may include 10-year risk of coronary heart disease events[71] or established risk stratification measures.[1] Additional cardiac testing may be required, including resting electrocardiogram (ECG) and ankle-brachial index for peripheral arterial disease, although further testing may be required in the presence of calcified arteries.[72]

2. Neurologic system: screening tests may include deep tendon reflexes, proprioception, and assessment of protective sensation using a Semmes-Weinstein monofilament.[31,73]
3. Renal system: screening may identify individuals with reduced exercise capacity, but specific recommendations for physical activity do not exist for individuals with nephropathy.[31]
4. Visual system: eye examinations should follow the recommended schedule from the American Diabetes Association (ADA) to screen for retinopathy.[74]

Exercise Testing

There is consensus among ADA, American College of Sports Medicine (ACSM), and U.S. Preventative Services Task Force on the use of a graded exercise test (GXT) with ECG for adults with diabetes before starting a physical activity program. For adults who are asymptomatic for CVD, are at low risk (<10% over a 10-year period) for cardiac events, and want to begin a low-moderate physical activity program, exercise testing is not required,[1,14,75] because of the risks involved with the test and the high number of false positives in predicting coronary death in asymptomatic people.[76,77] The current ADA position paper on physical activity and exercise[14] recommends a GXT without ECG monitoring for low-risk individuals with diabetes to assist with exercise prescription and assess functional capacity, rather than to determine cardiac ischemia threshold. A variety of treadmill, cycle ergometry, and field protocols for exercise testing have been published,[1] and the most appropriate protocol should be based on individual factors.

Conversely, for individuals with diabetes who have ≥10% risk of a cardiac event over a 10-year period or those who would like to begin a vigorous-intensity exercise program, the ADA and ACSM recommend a medically supervised GXT with ECG monitoring before beginning a physical activity program.[1,14,78] Individuals who are unable to perform a GXT, those with an abnormal ECG with an exercise test, or those with an autonomic neuropathy may require additional medical testing for cardiac ischemia before initiating a physical activity or exercise program.[1]

Exercise Prescription

A physical activity or exercise program is recommended by several professional organizations (i.e., ACSM, ADA), as well as the U.S. government, for all individuals with diabetes, except those for whom exercise is contraindicated.[1,3,13,14,36,79] The recommendations are summarized in Table 8.2. Although there are no specific recommendations for older adults living in LTC, the recommendations for older adults (≥65 years) would be appropriate. It is interesting to note the similarities of the recommendations in Table 8.2 between those <65 years old, older adults >65 years, and adults with diabetes. These minimal activity recommendations were developed to reduce chronic disease risk, optimize overall health, and enhance glycemic control, and result in ~1,000 kilocalories/week of energy expenditure. For the many people with diabetes for whom weight loss is a goal, additional energy expenditure of at least 2,000 kilocalories/week, coupled with dietary control, would be recommended.[80] Weight loss, however, may not be a goal, even for overweight residents in LTC (see Chapter 7).

A standard exercise prescription for people with and without diabetes should include both aerobic and resistance activities.[1,13,31] In addition to a conditioning phase (i.e., the primary aerobic or resistance activity), the components of an exercise session should include the following:

1. A 5–10 minute aerobic warm-up at low (<40% oxygen consumption reserve [VO_2R] or heart rate reserve [HRR]) progressing up to moderate (40–60% VO_2R/HRR) intensity The purpose of the warm-up is to gradually increase the body temperature and transition the body from rest to the additional physiologic, biochemical, and biomechanical demands placed on it during the conditioning phase. The formula to calculate target VO_2 or HR for all exercise or activity is as follows:

$$\text{Target } VO_2 \text{ or } HR = [(VO_{2max} \text{ or } HR_{max} - VO_{2rest} \text{ or } HR_{rest}) * \% \text{ intensity}] + VO_{2rest} \text{ or } HR_{rest}$$

Where HR_{max} can be estimated by 220 – age, VO_{2max} can be estimated or measured using aGXT, % intensity is the percent of VO_2R or HRR, HR_{rest} is resting HR, and VO_{2rest} is 3.5 ml/kg/minute.

2. Stretching for 5–10 minutes, which can occur after the warm-up or cool down. Stretching should focus on the muscles used during the conditioning phase.

3. A 5- to 10-minute cool down should be structured similarly to the warm-up. The purpose is to gradually return heart rate and blood pressure to pre-exercise levels, and assist in the removal of metabolic by-products from the exercising muscles.

The conditioning phase of an exercise prescription for any individual with diabetes should consider four parameters: mode (type), intensity (volume), frequency, and duration.[1]

Mode (Type). Mode or type refers to the specific exercise or activity completed. An exercise prescription should include both aerobic and resistance activities as both are included in the current guidelines, and both have been shown to be effective in increasing glucose uptake and ameliorating insulin resistance.[13,14]

An exercise prescription includes:

- Aerobic exercise (walking, swimming, arm ergometry)
- Resistance exercise—stress all muscle groups (weights, machines, resistance bands)
- Intensity—energy expenditure required
- Frequency—number of sessions/time period

Aerobic Activities or Exercise. Because of the ease and convenience, and lack of specialized equipment needed, walking is a common mode of exercise prescribed for adults with diabetes.[81] Several comorbid conditions commonly present in individuals with diabetes, such as peripheral neuropathy or degenerative arthritis, may limit the appropriateness of walking as the mode of exercise;[13,14] non-weight-bearing exercise, such as swimming, bicycling, or arm ergometry, could be acceptable alternatives.

A mode of exercise that has been shown to increase overall well-being[82] and have a high level of adherence[83] among older adults is tai chi, which can be modified for different fitness levels or levels of functional independence and can be completed in groups or individually.[84] In adults with at least one cardiovascular risk factor, 12 weeks of tai chi was found to decease resting and submaximal systolic blood pressure,[85] as well as increase balance, muscular strength, and endurance.[86] Therefore, it is useful to assess the effectiveness of this unique activity on glycemic control in individuals with diabetes.

Table 8.3 summarizes three randomized controlled trials (RCT) and Table 8.4 summarizes five pre–post experimental studies on the effect of tai chi on measures of glucose control (A1C and fasting blood glucose [FBG]). None of the RCT showed any statistically significant differences when compared with a nonexercising or sham exercise control, despite tai chi interventions of 16 weeks for two studies, and 24 weeks for one study. Although these results show no support for the use of tai chi, a final conclusion should be made cautiously because of methodologic limitations in the studies. For example, the Lam et al.[84] study determined that 40 participants per group was required to detect a statistically significant difference in A1C if one was present. This study finished with 44 participants (n = 24 in tai chi group and n = 20 in control group), potentially exposing this study to Type II error (i.e., failing to detect a statistical significance when one is actually present). Additionally, in the Tsang et al.[87] study, the rate of perceived exertion (RPE) using a 6–20 scale for the group randomized to tai chi was 11 ± 2, which is lower than the commonly accepted RPE values for moderate intensity activity.[1] The frequency and duration for tai chi in all of the RCTs was twice weekly for 60 minutes (120 minutes/week), which does not meet the current guidelines of 150 minutes/week of aerobic exercise.[3] This may contribute to the lack of significant findings, especially when coupled with the lower intensity. Some of the pre–post trials did find statistically significant improvements in AIC but not in FBG (Table 8.4). The studies with significant results were those with a frequency and duration >150 minutes per week. So a higher frequency of exercise may be necessary to achieve benefits in glycemic control. Although the preliminary evidence does not look promising, more research is needed to elucidate the effect of tai chi as a mode of exercise for individuals with diabetes.

Resistance Exercise. Historically, resistance training either was not included in recommendations for individuals with diabetes or was a secondary recommendation.[13,88] Recent studies have prompted a change in the relative importance of resistance training, as studies have shown a greater improvement in glycemic control and insulin sensitivity with resistance compared with aerobic exercise.[89,90] Resistance exercises are now part of all current exercise recommendations,[1,3,13,14]

Table 8.2 Recommendations for Physical Activity from Professional Organizations and U.S. Government to Promote Health, Reduce Chronic Disease Risk, and Enhance Glycemic Control (Diabetics)

Reference	Aerobic			Resistance		
	Intensity	Frequency	Duration	Volume (sets/repetitions)	Type	Frequency
Healthy adults						
2007 ACSM/AHA[79]	3–6 METs (moderate) >6 METS (vigorous)	5 days/week (moderate) 3 days/week (vigorous)	30 minutes/day (moderate); can be performed in 10-minute bouts 20 minutes/day (vigorous)	1 set 8–12 RM	8–10 exercises involving major muscle groups	2 days/week
2008 Physical Activity for Americans[3]	3–6 METs (moderate) >6 METS (vigorous)	150 minutes/week (moderate); can be performed in 10-minute bouts 75 minutes/week (vigorous) Completed throughout the week		1–3 sets 8–12 RM	Work the major muscle groups of the body	2 days/week
2010 ACSM[1]	40–60% VO$_2$R (moderate) ≥60% VO$_2$R (vigorous)	3–5 days/week	20–30 minutes (can be performed in 10-minute bouts)	2–4 sets 8–12 RM	Target agonist and antagonist muscle groups	2–3 days/week; 48 hours in between
Older adults (≥ 65 years)						
2007 ACSM/AHA[44]	5–6/10 effort (moderate) 7–8/10 effort (vigorous)	5 days/week (moderate) 3 days/week (vigorous)	30 minutes/day (moderate); can be performed in 10-minute bouts 20 minutes/day (vigorous)	1 set 10–15 RM	8–10 exercises involving major muscle groups	2 days/week

	Intensity	Frequency/Duration	Duration	Sets/Reps	Resistance	Frequency
2008 Physical Activity for Americans[3]	5–6/10 effort (moderate) 7–8/10 effort (vigorous)	150 minutes/week (moderate); can be performed in 10-minute bouts 75 minutes/week (vigorous) Completed throughout the week		1–3 sets 8–12 RM	Work the major muscle groups of the body	2 days/week
Adults with type 2 diabetes						
2000 ACSM Position Stand[13]	40–70% VO_{2max}	3–5 days/week	10–15 min progressing to 30 minutes; can be performed in 10-minute bouts	1 set 10–15 RM	8–10 exercises involving major muscle groups	2 days/week
2004 ADA Statement[14]	40–60% VO_{2max} or 50–70% HR_{max} (moderate) >60% VO_{2max} or >70% HR_{max} (vigorous)	3 days/week with no more than 2 consecutive days without activity 150 minutes/week (moderate) 90 minutes/week (vigorous)		3 sets 8–10 RM	Work the major muscle groups of the body	3 days/week
2010 ACSM[1]	50–80% VO_2R/HRR RPE 12–16/20	3–7 days/week 15-minutes/week; can be performed in 10-minutes bouts		2–3 sets 8–12 reps 60–80% of 1 RM	8–10 exercises involving major muscle groups	2–3 days/week

Note: ACSM = American College of Sports Medicine; AHA = American Heart Association; ADA = American Diabetes Association; MET = metabolic equivalent (oxygen consumption relative to a resting state[91]); VO_2R = VO_2 reserve; HRR = heart rate reserve; RPE = rate of perceived exertion on a 6–20 scale; RM = repetition maximum

Source: Reprinted with permission from Warren M. Physical activity: Exercise prescription for the older adult with type 2 diabetes. *Topics in Geriatric Rehabilitation* 2010;26(3):221–232.

Table 8.3 Randomized Controlled Trials Comparing the Effect of Tai Chi Versus a Control Group on Measures of Glucose Control

Study	Sample size Age[a]		Intervention		Outcome			
	Tai Chi	Control	Tai Chi	Control		Tai Chi	Control	*p*[b]
Lam, Dennis, et al. 2008	$n = 24$ 63.2±6.8y	$n = 20$ 60.7±12.2y	60-minutes session, 2 days/week for 3 months then 1 day/week for 3 months	Tai chi after intervention period	A1C (%)	Pre: 8.4 ± 1.2[a] Post: 8.1 ± 1.4	Pre: 8.7 ± 1.3 Post: 8.5 ± 1.5	0.86
Tsang, Orr, et al. 2008	$n = 17$ 66±7.43y	$n = 20$ 65±8.05y	60-minute session, 2 days/week for 16 weeks	60-minute session, 2 days/week for 16 weeks; sham exercise (calisthenics, gentle stretching)	AIC (%) mean change	−0.07 ± 0.4[a]	0.12 ± 0.3	0.13
Orr, Tsang, et al. 2006	$n = 17$ 65.9±7.4y	$n = 18$ 64.9±7.8y	65-minute session, 2 days/week for 16 weeks	65-minute session, 2days/week for 16 weeks; sham exercise (e.g., seated calisthenics, stretching)	FBG[c] (mmol/l)	Pre: 7.6 (3.9–15.6)[d] Post: 7.5 (5.7–12.5)	Pre: 7.9 (5.6–13.9) Post: 7.4 (5.4–15.4)	0.2

Note:
[a] Mean ± standard deviation.
[b] *p*-value comparing between-group differences.
[c] Fasting blood glucose.
[d] Median (range).

Sources: Lam P, Dennis SM, et al. Improving glycaemic and BP control in type 2 diabetes. The effectiveness of tai chi. *Australian Family Physician* 2008;37(10):884–887; Tsang T, Orr R, et al. Effects of tai chi on glucose homeostasis and insulin sensitivity in older adults with type 2 diabetes: A randomised double-blind sham-exercise-controlled trial. *Age & Ageing* 2008;37(1):64–71; Orr R, Tsang T, et al. Mobility impairment in type 2 diabetes: Association with muscle power and effect of tai chi intervention. *Diabetes Care* 2006;29(9):2120–2122.

Table 8.4 Nonrandomized Trials (Pre–Post Studies) Examining the Effect of Tai Chi on Measures of Glucose Control

Study	Sample size Age[a]	Tai Chi	Outcomes[a]	Pre	Post	p
Shen, Feng, et al. 2007	n = 25 53.9 ± 9.5 years	60-minute session 2 times/week for 12 weeks	A1C (%)	9.1 ± 1.4	8.1 ± 2.0	0.104[b]
Song, Ahn, et al. 2009	n = 62 (31 adherent with tai chi and 31 nonadherent 64 ± 8.0 years	60-minute session 2 times/week with 20-minute session 3 times/week at home for 6 months	A1C (%)	Adherent: 7.31 ± 1.12 Nonadherent: 7.19 ± 1.18	6.83 ± 0.59 7.31 ± 1.23	0.02[d]
			FBG[c] (mg/dl)	Adherent: 151.70 ± 61.81 Nonadherent: 144.22 ± 46.74	127.86 ± 31.70 166.26 ± 72.23	0.006[d]
Yeh, Chuang, et al. 2009	n = 30 56.7 ± 10.8 years	60-minute session 3 times/week for 12 weeks	A1C (%) FBG (mg/dl)	7.59 ± 0.32 165.3 ± 53.2	7.16 ± 0.22 152.6 ± 48.8	0.047[b] 0.12[b]
Yeh, Chuang, et al. 2007	n = 32 57.9 ± 14.1 years	60-minute session 3 times/week for 12 weeks	A1C (%) FBG (mg/dl)	7.74 ± 1.93 164.56 ± 53.3	7.28 ± 1.35 150.53 ± 46.02	0.026[b] 0.08[b]
Hung, Liou, et al. 2009	n = 28 58.1 ± 13.4 years	60-minute session 3 times/week for 12 weeks	FBG (mg/dl)	160.6 ± 53.8	142.6 ± 44.0	Not reported

Note:
[a] Mean ± standard deviation
[b] *p*-value for within-group differences
[c] Fasting blood glucose
[d] *p*-value for comparing those who adhered to the tai chi program (≥ 80% of sessions attended) versus those who did not (<80% of sessions attended)

Sources: Hung JW, Liou CW, et al. Effect of 12-week tai chi chuan exercise on peripheral nerve modulation in patients with type 2 diabetes mellitus. *Journal of Rehabilitation Medicine* 2009;41(11):924–929; Shen CL, Feng D, et al. Effect of tai chi exercise on type 2 diabetes: A feasibility study. *Integrative Medicine Insights* 2007;2:15–23; Song R, Ahn S, et al. Adhering to a t'ai chi program to improve glucose control and quality of life for individuals with type 2 diabetes. *Journal of Alternative and Complementary Medicine* 2009;15(6):627–632; Yeh SH, Chuang H, et al. tai chi chuan exercise decreases A1C levels along with increase of regulatory T-cells and decrease of cytotoxic T-cell population in type 2 diabetic patients. *Diabetes Care* 2007;30(3):716–718; Yeh SH, Chuang H, et al. Regular tai chi chuan exercise improves T cell helper function of patients with type 2 diabetes mellitus with an increase in T-bet transcription factor and IL-12 production. *British Journal of Sports Medicine* 2009;43(11):845–850.

although they may be contraindicated for those with proliferative diabetic retinopathy to minimize the risk of vitreous hemorrhage or retinal detachment.[31] Recommendations from all organizations include the statement that resistance training should stress all major muscle groups. The form of resistance can include free, cuff, or ankle weights; weight machines; resistance bands; or even body weight for some exercises.

Intensity (Volume). Intensity or volume is related to the effort or amount of work (energy expenditure) required to complete the activity.

Aerobic Activities or Exercises. Current recommendations include moderate (e.g., 40–60% VO_2R/HRR) to vigorous (60–80% VO_2R/HRR) intensity.[1,3,13,14] Oxygen consumption often is expressed in metabolic equivalents (METs) with moderate intensity including activities between 3.0 and 6.0 METs and vigorous intensity >6.0 METs.[91] A meta-analysis including seven studies ($n = 256$ participants with diabetes) of aerobic exercise reported a stronger relationship between changes in A1C and exercise intensity ($r = -0.91$, $p = 0.002$) than with exercise volume ($r = -0.46$, $p = 0.26$), which includes intensity, frequency, and duration.[92] This study provides some evidence suggesting that high intensity may be more beneficial than low to moderate intensity for glycemic control. Unfortunately, many individuals with diabetes, especially older adults, may not have adequate fitness levels for vigorous intensity activity, so moderate intensity would be most appropriate.[31,93] With lower intensity (moderate), a longer duration is necessary to allow for equivalent energy expenditure.

For individuals who may not have a normal heart rate and blood pressure response with activity (i.e., autonomic neuropathy), it may be appropriate to determine the intensity using alternative methods like RPE with 12–16 (on a 6–20 scale) corresponding to moderate- to vigorous-intensity exercise.[1](American College of Sports Medicine 2010) Additionally, the current U.S. government recommendations use of a relative intensity scale for aerobic exercise for older adults.[3] For this scale, 0 is defined at rest and 10 is defined as all-out effort; moderate-intensity activity is therefore between 5 and 6 and vigorous intensity is between 7 and 8.

Resistance Exercises. The recommended intensity or volume of resistance exercise varies by professional organization, but it ranges from an 8- to 12-repetition or 10- to 15-repetition maximum,[1,31,36] meaning that after 8–12 (or 10–15) repetitions, the individual is unable to complete another repetition. Recommendations on the number of sets for each exercise also varies, with ACSM recommending a single set of each exercise in a position statement from 2000,[13] but in 2010 recommending two to three sets.[1] The ADA recommends three sets.[14] The number of sets therefore should reflect a prescription that an individual will be compliant with and is able to complete with available equipment. Proper technique should be emphasized and the amount of weight lifted should be lowered if the individual is unable to maintain proper form. Instruction in resistance should stress an avoidance of the Valsalva maneuver and prolonged isometric contractions, especially in those with substantial retinopathy or cardiovascular risk.[13,31]

Frequency. Frequency indicates the number of training sessions in a given period of time.

Aerobic Activities or Exercise. The recommended frequency is a minimum of 3 days/week or 150 minutes/week.[1,31] Because the enhanced insulin sensitivity from an exercise bout lasts between 24 and 72 hours,[15,16] it is recommended that some type of activity be performed every day with no more than 2 consecutive days without activity.[13,14,93] A meta-analysis that found positive effects of aerobic exercise on glycemic control had a mean of 3.4 sessions/week,[21] supporting the current recommendations.

Resistance Exercise. Most recommendations include 2 times/week of resistance exercises, although some organizations recommend up to 3 times/week. All recommend resistance exercises on nonconsecutive days[36,79] to reduce the risk of injury and minimize muscle soreness.

Duration. Duration refers the length of the activity within an activity or exercise session. The duration of the exercise session is related directly to the energy expenditure. In many individuals with diabetes, the duration is related inversely to the intensity of the exercise.[13]

Aerobic Activities or Exercise. Minimal duration is 10 minutes, when multiple (at least three) sessions are performed throughout the day for a total of 30 minutes/day.[1,3,36] The mean duration of aerobic sessions in a meta-analysis that showed a positive effect on glycemic control was 49 minutes/session,[21] so a longer duration of exercise may be more beneficial, and the current recommendations should be considered to be a minimum.

MONITORING AND PROGRESSING EXERCISE PROGRAMS

Several complications can arise during an activity or exercise program because of autonomic neuropathy.[31] During aerobic exercise, autonomic neuropathy may lead to a blunted heart rate and blood pressure response,[1] especially with vigorous-intensity exercise. Blood pressure and heart rate should be monitored, especially when starting or progressing the exercise; RPE also should be used to monitor exercise response. Because individuals with an autonomic neuropathy may have difficulty with thermoregulation, exercise should be avoided in extreme hot and cold environments, and adequate hydration should be maintained. Finally, the signs and symptoms of silent ischemia should be monitored because the individuals with diabetes and autonomic neuropathy may be unable to perceive angina.

For individuals for whom it is appropriate to use walking as a mode of exercise, proper footwear is essential to prevent blisters, and polyester or polyester blend socks, and silica-gel or air insoles should be utilized to keep feet dry and protected. The individual's feet also should be checked after exercise for blisters and other potential areas of skin breakdown.[1,31] For older adults, this may require assistance to complete. The ability of older people with diabetes (ages 65–91 years) to locate and touch artificial lesions on the individual's toes, and first and fifth metatarsal heads was examined in 28 individuals.[94] For the artificial lesions placed on the toes, 79% of the participants could locate the lesions; however, 39% were unable to reach and touch the lesions. Furthermore, although 54% of the participants could touch the lesions on the metatarsal heads, only 14% of the participants had sufficient joint flexibility or visual acuity to allow for inspection of the lesions. This study shows the inability of older people with diabetes to complete this essential screening.

Any exercise program should start gradually to minimize risk of injury and increase the likelihood that the individual will be compliant with the program.[1] Initially, progression should focus on frequency and duration rather than intensity.[13] After the desired frequency and duration are achieved, small increases in intensity can occur with frequent supervision and monitoring to ensure safety. Because of the musculoskeletal[95-97] and cardiorespiratory[98] deconditioning occurring in individuals with diabetes, a progression from a sedentary lifestyle to meeting the activity recommendation may take 6–12 weeks.[93] The rate of progression will be different for each individual and depends on several factors, including age, functional capacity, medical and clinical status, and personal preference and goals.[1]

Possible Resources

www.sitandbefit.org—An award-winning exercise program for nonambulatory persons shown on the Public Broadcasting System.
http://www.projectenhance.org/enhancefitness.aspx—An evidence-based exercise program currently available in 30 states. Will help train trainers.
    Level 1, nonambulatory
    Level 2, ambulatory

Additional Considerations with Physical Activity or Exercise Programs

Although the timing of an exercise program is not part of the current recommendations, it may be important if individuals are taking insulin or oral hypoglycemic agents.[1] For these individuals, hypoglycemia (blood glucose levels <3.9 mmol/l [70 mg/dl][99]) is the most common adverse event associated with physical activity, although still rare.[1,13,78] Exercise typically is not recommended during peak insulin action because of the risk of hypoglycemia, characterized by weakness, abnormal sweating, anxiety, tingling in the mouth and fingers, and hunger, among others.[1] Recent evidence, however, showed that aerobic exercise was safe in 43 men (n = 31 taking hypoglycemic agents) with diabetes in the fasted state,[100] and did not result in substantial hypoglycemia. The most beneficial time for exercise may be during the postprandial state to facilitate glucose uptake and suppress endogenous glucose production.[93] Blood glucose levels should be monitored to determine an individual's response to exercise,[1] especially when initiating or progressing an exercise program. Changes in medication dose may be warranted to minimize hypoglycemia, and this may be preferable to increasing energy intake, especially in those for whom weight loss is part of the management of diabetes.

Individuals with diabetes frequently require medications for CVD management, including β-blockers and angiotensin-converting-enzyme (ACE) inhibitors.[14] For most individuals, there will be no limitations with physical activity when taking any of the medications, but other considerations are important to understand. β-Blockers can block symptoms and recovery from hypoglycemia through an inhibition of gluconeogenesis.[101] β-Blockers also can reduce maximal exercise capacity, but this probably is not an issue as most individuals with diabetes would not be exercising at a high enough intensity to have a significant effect. ACE inhibitors frequently are used for hypertension management and to prevent or delay diabetic nephropathy; these drugs often are used in individual with diabetes in the absence of hypertension.[101] ACE inhibitors, however, may modestly increase insulin sensitivity, and their use was associated with an increased risk of serious hypoglycemia in some individuals.[102]

Individuals with diabetes have a higher prevalence of several musculoskeletal conditions compared with individuals without diabetes. Differences in prevalence previously have been reported with Dupuytren's disease (20% in individuals with diabetes vs. 3% in those without diabetes), adhesive capsulitis (16% vs. 0%), carpal tunnel syndrome (11% vs. 8%), and flexor tenosynovitis (20% vs. 2%).[103] Differences between those with an without diabetes also have been reported with limited joint mobility[104] and diffuse idiopathic skeletal hyperostosis.[105] The etiology for the higher prevalence seen in individuals with diabetes is not clear, although evidence indicates that abnormal collagen deposition may occur, altering the structural matrix and mechanical properties of tissues. Individuals with diabetes also have musculoskeletal conditions that typically do not occur in individuals without diabetes, such as Charcot foot.[106] All of the musculoskeletal conditions are associated with poor glycemic control,[107] further supporting the need for a physically active lifestyle. An individual's joint structure and function should be evaluated by a physically therapist before initiating an exercise program, with appropriate modifications as indicated.

CONCLUSION

Physical activity has both acute and chronic effects for individuals with diabetes in terms of glycemic control, overall health, and minimizing complications that arise. The long-term benefits are significant, underscoring the need for regular participation in a physical activity or exercise program.

Unfortunately, individuals with diabetes are primarily sedentary, and this is especially apparent in LTC facilities. In addition to the barriers to physical activity and exercise in LTC facilities discussed in this chapter, the lack of activity in part may be due to a lack of understanding by individuals and health care professionals on safe and appropriate exercise recommendations. This chapter reviewed the current, evidence-based recommendations for exercise testing and prescription for aerobic and resistance exercise. It is hoped that professionals who work in LTC settings can utilize this information to prescribe safe and effective exercise to assist in the management of diabetes.

REFERENCES

1. American College of Sports Medicine. *ACSM's guidelines for exercise testing and prescription.* Philadelphia, PA, Lippincott Williams & Wilkins, 2010.
2. Chodzko-Zajko WJ, Proctor DN, et al. Exercise and physical activity for older adults. *Medicine & Science in Sports & Exercise* 2009;41(7):1510–1530.
3. U.S. Department of Health and Human Services. 2008 Physical Activity Guidelines for Americans, 2008. Available at www.health.gov/paguidelines/default.aspx. Accessed 1 September 2009.
4. Jones AL, Dwyer LL, et al. The National Nursing Home Survey: 2004 overview. National Center for Health Statistics. *Vital Health Statistics* 2009;13(167): 3;17-18.
5. Westerterp KR. Daily physical activity and ageing. *Current Opinion in Clinical Nutrition & Metabolic Care* 2000;3(6):485–488.
6. Centers for Disease Control and Prevention (CDC). *Behavioral risk factor surveillance system survey data.* Atlanta, GA, U.S. Department of Health and Human Services, Centers for Disease Control and Prevention, 2009.
7. Blair SN, Brodney S. Effects of physical inactivity and obesity on morbidity and mortality: current evidence and research issues. *Medicine & Science in Sports & Exercise* 1999;31(11Suppl):S646–S662.
8. Ryan AS. Insulin resistance with aging: effects of diet and exercise. *Sports Medicine* 2000;30(5):327–346.
9. Nair KS. Aging muscle. *American Journal of Clinical Nutrition* 2005; 81(5):953–963.
10. Scheen AJ. Diabetes mellitus in the elderly: Insulin resistance and/or impaired insulin secretion? *Diabetes & Metabolism* 2005;31(Spec No 2):5S27–5S34.
11. Janssen I, Ross R. Linking age–related changes in skeletal muscle mass and composition with metabolism and disease. *Journal of Nutrition, Health & Aging* 2005;9(6):408–419.
12. Racette SB, Evans EM, et al. Abdominal adiposity is a stronger predictor of insulin resistance than fitness among 50–95 year olds. *Diabetes Care* 2006;29(3):673–678.
13. Albright A, Franz M, et al. American College of Sports Medicine position stand. Exercise and type 2 diabetes. *Medicine & Science in Sports & Exercise* 2000;32(7):1345–1360.
14. Sigal RJ, Kenny GP, et al. Physical activity/exercise and type 2 diabetes. *Diabetes Care* 2004;27(10):2518–2539.
15. Gulve EA. Exercise and glycemic control in diabetes: benefits, challenges, and adjustments to pharmacotherapy. *Physical Therapy* 2008;88(11):1297–1321.
16. Rockl KS, Witczak CA, et al. Signaling mechanisms in skeletal muscle: acute responses and chronic adaptations to exercise. *IUBMB Life* 2008;60(3):145–153.
17. Goodyear LJ, Kahn BB. Exercise, glucose transport, and insulin sensitivity. *Annual Review of Medicine* 1998;49:235–261.
18. Wasserman DH, Davis S, et al. Fuel metabolism during exercise in health and diabetes. In *The Handbook of Exercise in Diabetes.* Ruderman N, Devlin JT, Kriska A, Eds. Alexandria, VA, American Diabetes Association, 2002, p. 63–99.

19. Toledo FG, Menshikova EV, et al. Effects of physical activity and weight loss on skeletal muscle mitochondria and relationship with glucose control in type 2 diabetes. *Diabetes* 2007;56(8):2142–2147.
20. Hayes C, Kriska A. Role of physical activity in diabetes management and prevention. *Journal of the American Dietetic Association* 2008; 108(4Suppl1):S19–S23.
21. Boule NG, Haddad E, et al. Effects of exercise on glycemic control and body mass in type 2 diabetes mellitus: a meta-analysis of controlled clinical trials. [See comment]. *Journal of the American Medical Association* 2001;286(10):1218–1227.
22. Kallings LV, Sierra Johnson J, et al. Beneficial effects of individualized physical activity on prescription on body composition and cardiometabolic risk factors: Results from a randomized controlled trial. *European Journal of Cardiovascular Prevention & Rehabilitation* 2009;16(1):80–84.
23. Yates T, Davies M, et al. Effectiveness of a pragmatic education program designed to promote walking activity in individuals with impaired glucose tolerance: a randomized controlled trial. *Diabetes Care* 2009;32(8): 1404–1410.
24. Ligtenberg PC, Hoekstra JB, et al. Effects of physical training on metabolic control in elderly type 2 diabetes mellitus patients. *Clinical Science* 1997;93(2):127–135.
25. Bjorgaas M, Vik JT, et al. Relationship between pedometer-registered activity, aerobic capacity and self-reported activity and fitness in patients with type 2 diabetes. *Diabetes, Obesity & Metabolism* 2005;7(6):737–744.
26. Giannopoulou I, Ploutz-Snyder LL, et al. Exercise is required for visceral fat loss in postmenopausal women with type 2 diabetes. *Journal of Clinical Endocrinology & Metabolism* 2005;90(3):1511–1518.
27. Balducci S, Leonetti F, et al. Is a long-term aerobic plus resistance training program feasible for and effective on metabolic profiles in type 2 diabetic patients? *Diabetes Care* 2004;27(3):841–842.
28. Fritz T, Wandell P, et al. Walking for exercise—does three times per week influence risk factors in type 2 diabetes? *Diabetes Research & Clinical Practice* 2006;71(1):21–27.
29. Di Loreto C, Fanelli C, et al. Validation of a counseling strategy to promote the adoption and the maintenance of physical activity by type 2 diabetic subjects. [See comment]. *Diabetes Care* 2003;26(2):404–408.
30. Ibanez J, Izquierdo M, et al. Twice-weekly progressive resistance training decreases abdominal fat and improves insulin sensitivity in older men with type 2 diabetes. *Diabetes Care* 2005;28(3):662–667.
31. American Diabetes Association. Physical activity/exercise and diabetes. *Diabetes Care* 2004;27(Suppl1):S58–S62.
32. Bassuk SS, Manson JE. Epidemiological evidence for the role of physical activity in reducing risk of type 2 diabetes and cardiovascular disease. *Journal of Applied Physiology* 2005;99(3):1193–1204.
33. Orchard TJ, Temprosa M, et al. The effect of metformin and intensive lifestyle intervention on the metabolic syndrome: The Diabetes Prevention Program randomized trial.[See comment]. *Annals of Internal Medicine* 2005;142(8):611–619.

34. Buse JB, Ginsberg HN, et al. Primary prevention of cardiovascular diseases in people with diabetes mellitus: A scientific statement from the American Heart Association and the American Diabetes Association. *Circulation* 2007;115(1):114–126.
35. Vasterling JJ, Sementilli ME, et al. The role of aerobic exercise in reducing stress in diabetic patients. *The Diabetes Educator* 1988;14(3):197–201.
36. Nelson ME, Rejeski WJ, et al. Physical activity and public health in older adults: recommendation from the American College of Sports Medicine and the American Heart Association. *Medicine & Science in Sports & Exercise* 2007;39(8):1435–1445.
37. American Geriatrics Society Expert Panel on the Care of Older Adults with Diabetes Mellitus. Guidelines abstracted from the American Geriatrics Society guidelines for improving the care of older adults with diabetes mellitus: 2013 update. *Journal of the American Geriatrics Society* 2013;61(11):2020–2026.
38. Seeman TE, Berkman LF, et al. Behavioral and psychosocial predictors of physical performance: MacArthur studies of successful aging. *Journal of Gerontology A: Biological Sciences & Medical Sciences* 1995;50(4):M177–M183.
39. Paffenbarger RS Jr, Wing AL, et al. Physical activity as an index of heart attack risk in college alumni. *American Journal of Epidemiology* 1978;108(3):161–175.
40. Taylor HL, Jacobs DR Jr, et al. A questionnaire for the assessment of leisure time physical activities. *Journal of Chronic Diseases* 1978;31(12):741–755.
41. Huang G, Gibson CA, et al. Controlled endurance exercise training and VO2max changes in older adults: a meta-analysis. *Preventive Cardiology* 2005;8(4):217–225.
42. Lemmer JT, Hurlbut DE, et al. Age and gender responses to strength training and detraining. *Medicine & Science in Sports & Exercise* 2000;32(8):1505–1512.
43. Clarke MS. The effects of exercise on skeletal muscle in the aged. *Journal of Musculoskeletal Neuronal Interactions* 2004;4(2):175–178.
44. Nelson KM, Reiber G, et al. Diet and exercise among adults with type 2 diabetes: Findings from the third national health and nutrition examination survey (NHANES III). *Diabetes Care* 2002;25(10):1722–1728.
45. Centers for Disease Control and Prevention and National Diabetes Surveillance System. n.d. Available at www.cdc.gov/diabetes/statistics/index.htm. Accessed 15 December 2010.
46. MacRae P G, Schnelle JF, et al. Physical activity levels of ambulatory nursing home residents. *Journal of Aging & Physical Activity* 1996;4(3):264–278.
47. Schmid A, Weiss M, et al. Recording the nutrient intake of nursing home residents by food weighing method and measuring the physical activity. *Journal of Nutrition Health & Aging* 2003;7(5):294–295.
48. Cyarto EV, Myers AM, et al. Pedometer accuracy in nursing home and community-dwelling older adults. *Medicine & Science in Sports & Exercise* 2004;36(2):205–209.
49. Dermott M, McDaniel JL, et al. Is physical activity associated with appetite? A survey of long-term care residents. *Journal of Nutrition for the Elderly* 2009;28(1):72–80.
50. Resnick B, Galik E, et al. Perceptions and performance of function and physical activity in assisted living communities. *Journal of the American Medical Directors Association* 2010;11(6):406–414.

51. Copeland JL, Esliger DW. Accelerometer assessment of physical activity in active, healthy older adults. *Journal of Aging & Physical Activity* 2009;17(1):17–30.
52. Jette AM, Rooks D, et al. Home-based resistance training: predictors of participation and adherence. *Gerontologist* 1998;38(4):412–421.
53. Centers for Disease Control and Prevention. National nursing home survey, 2004. Available at www.cdc.gov/nchs/nnhs.htm. Accessed 7 January 2011.
54. Ingrid B, Marsella A. Factors influencing exercise participation by clients in long-term care. *Perspectives* 2008;32(4):5–11.
55. McAuley E, Jerome GJ, et al. Predicting long-term maintenance of physical activity in older adults. *Preventive Medicine* 2003;37(2):110–118.
56. Kang HS, Ferrans CE, et al. Aquatic exercise in older Korean women with arthritis: identifying barriers to and facilitators of long-term adherence. *Journal of Gerontological Nursing* 2007;33(7):48–56.
57. Moritz DJ, Kasl SV, et al. Cognitive functioning and the incidence of limitations in activities of daily living in an elderly community sample. *American Journal of Epidemiology* 1995;141(1):41–49.
58. Drageset J, Kirkevold M, et al. Loneliness and social support among nursing home residents without cognitive impairment: A questionnaire survey. *International Journal of Nursing Studies.* 2001;48(5):611-619.
59. Kennett D, Cezer D. *Extendicare Lakefield resident satisfaction survey–Fall 2003.* Peterborough, Ontario, Trent University, 2004.
60. Brault MW, Hootman JM, et al. Prevalence and most common causes of disability among adults—United States, 2005. *Morbidity and Mortality Weekly Report* 2009;58(16):421–426.
61. Cheng YJ, Hootman JM, et al. Prevalence of doctor-diagnosed arthritis and arthritis-attributable activity limitation—United States, 2007–2009. *Morbidity and Mortality Weekly Report* 201059(39):1261–1265.
62. Abell JE, Hootman JM, et al. Prevalence and impact of arthritis among nursing home residents. *Annals of the Rheumatic Diseases* 2004;63(5):591–594.
63. Joseph A, Zimring C, et al. Presence and visibility of outdoor and indoor physical activity features and participation in physical activity among older adults in retirement communities. *Journal of Housing for the Elderly* 2006;19(3/4):141–165.
64. Brownson RC, Housemann RA, et al. Promoting physical activity in rural communities: walking trail access, use, and effects. *American Journal of Preventive Medicine* 2000;18(3):235–241.
65. Carnegie MA, Bauman A, et al. Perceptions of the physical environment, stage of change for physical activity, and walking among Australian adults. *Research Quarterly in Exercise & Sport* 2002;73(2):146–155.
66. Brownson RC, Baker EA, et al. A community-based approach to promoting walking in rural areas. *American Journal of Preventive Medicine* 2004;27(1):28–34.
67. Sharpe PA, Granner ML, et al. Association of environmental factors to meeting physical activity recommendations in two South Carolina counties. *American Journal of Health Promotion* 2004;18(3):251–257.
68. Weeks LE, Profit S, et al. Participation in physical activity: influences reported by seniors in the community and in long-term care facilities. *Journal of Gerontological Nursing* 2008;34(7):36–43.

69. Chen YM. Perceived barriers to physical activity among older adults residing in long-term care institutions. *Journal of Clinical Nursing* 2010;19(3–4):432–439.

70. Regnier V, Denton A. Ten new and emerging trends in residential group living environments. *Neurorehabilitation* 2009;25:169–188.

71. National Heart Lung and Blood Institute and National Cholesterol Education Program. Risk assessment tool for estimating 10-year risk of developing hard CHD (myocardial infarction and coronary death). n.d. Available at http://cvdrisk.nhlbi.nih.gov/calculator.asp. Accessed 10 January 2011.

72. American Diabetes Association. Peripheral arterial disease in people with diabetes. *Diabetes Care* 2003;26(12):3333–3341.

73. Yuzhe F, Felix JS, et al. The Semmes Weinstein monofilament examination as a screening tool for diabetic peripheral neuropathy. *Journal of Vascular Surgery* 2009;50(3):675–682.e1.

74. Gimeno-Orna JA, Faure-Nogueras E, et al. Ability of retinopathy to predict cardiovascular disease in patients with type 2 diabetes mellitus. *American Journal of Cardiology* 2009;103(10):1364–1367.

75. U.S. Preventive Services Task Force. Screening for coronary heart disease: recommendation statement. *Annals of Internal Medicine* 2004;140:569–572.

76. Gibbons LW, Mitchell TL, et al. Maximal exercise test as a predictor of risk for mortality from coronary heart disease in asymptomatic men. *American Journal of Cardiology* 2000;86(1):53–58.

77. Fowler-Brown A, Pignone M, et al. Exercise tolerance testing to screen for coronary heart disease: A systematic review for the technical support for the U.S. Preventive Services Task Force. *Annals of Internal Medicine* 2004;140:W9–W24.

78. American Diabetes Association. Standards of medical care in diabetes—2009. *Diabetes Care* 2009;32(Suppl1):S13–S61.

79. Haskell WL, Lee IM, et al. Physical activity and public health: Updated recommendation for adults from the American College of Sports Medicine and the American Heart Association. *Medicine & Science in Sports & Exercise* 2007;39(8):1423–1434.

80. American College of Sports Medicine. Position stand. Appropriate intervention strategies for weight loss and the prevention of weight gain in adults. *Medicine & Science in Sports & Exercise* 2001;33:2145–2156.

81. Johnson ST, Boule NG, et al. Walking: A matter of quantity and quality physical activity for type 2 diabetes management. *Applied Physiology, Nutrition, & Metabolism* 2008;33(4):797–801.

82. Kutner NG, Barnhart H, et al. Self-report benefits of tai chi practice by older adults. *Journal of Gerontology B: Psychological Sciences and Social Sciences* 1997;52(5):P242–P246.

83. La Forge R. Mind-body fitness: encouraging prospects for primary and secondary prevention. *Journal of Cardiovascular Nursing* 1997;11(3):53–65.

84. Lam P, Dennis SM, et al. Improving glycaemic and BP control in type 2 diabetes. The effectiveness of tai chi. *Australian Family Physician* 2008;37(10):884–887.

85. Taylor-Piliae RE, Haskell WL, et al. Hemodynamic responses to a community-based tai chi exercise intervention in ethnic Chinese adults with

cardiovascular disease risk factors. *European Journal of Cardiovascular Nursing* 2006;5(2):165–174.

86. Taylor-Piliae RE, Haskell WL, et al. Improvement in balance, strength, and flexibility after 12 weeks of tai chi exercise in ethnic Chinese adults with cardiovascular disease risk factors. *Alternative Therapies in Health & Medicine* 200612(2):50–58.

87. Tsang T, Orr R, et al. Effects of tai chi on glucose homeostasis and insulin sensitivity in older adults with type 2 diabetes: a randomised double-blind sham-exercise-controlled trial. *Age & Ageing* 2008;37(1):64–71.

88. American Diabetes Association. Diabetes mellitus and exercise. *Diabetes Care* 2002;25(Suppl1):S64-S68.

89. Cuff DJ, Meneilly GS, et al. Effective exercise modality to reduce insulin resistance in women with type 2 diabetes. *Diabetes Care* 2003;26(11):2977–2982.

90. Cauza E, Hanusch-Enserer U, et al. The relative benefits of endurance and strength training on the metabolic factors and muscle function of people with type 2 diabetes mellitus. [See comment]. *Archives of Physical Medicine & Rehabilitation* 2005;86(8):1527–1533.

91. Ainsworth BE, Haskell WL, et al. Compendium of physical activities: an update of activity codes and MET intensities. *Medicine & Science in Sports & Exercise* 2000;32(9Suppl):S498–S504.

92. Boule NG, Kenny GP, et al. Meta-analysis of the effect of structured exercise training on cardiorespiratory fitness in type 2 diabetes mellitus. *Diabetologia* 2003;46(8):1071–1081.

93. Praet SF, van Loon LJ. Optimizing the therapeutic benefits of exercise in type 2 diabetes. *Journal of Applied Physiology* 2007;103(4):1113–1120.

94. Thompson FJ, Masson EA. Can elderly patients cop-operate with routine foot care? *Age & Ageing* 1992;21:333–337.

95. Volpato S, Blaum C, et al. Comorbidities and impairments explaining the association between diabetes and lower extremity disability: The Women's Health and Aging Study. *Diabetes Care* 2002;25(4):678–683.

96. Andersen H, Nielsen S, et al. Muscle strength in type 2 diabetes. *Diabetes* 2004;53(6):1543–1548.

97. Sayer AA, Dennison EM, et al. Type 2 diabetes, muscle strength, and impaired physical function: the tip of the iceberg? *Diabetes Care* 2005;28(10):2541–2542.

98. Fang ZY, Sharman J, et al. Determinants of exercise capacity in patients with type 2 diabetes. *Diabetes Care* 2005;28(7):1643–1648.

99. American Diabetes Association. Defining and reporting hypoglycemia in diabetes. *Diabetes Care* 2005;28(5):1245–1249.

100. Gaudet-Savard T, Ferland A, et al. Safety and magnitude of changes in blood glucose levels following exercise performed in the fasted and the postprandial state in men with type 2 diabetes. *European Journal of Cardiovascular Prevention & Rehabilitation* 2007;14(6):831–836.

101. Katzung BG, Masters SB, et al. *Basic and clinical pharmacology.* 11th ed. New York, NY, McGraw Hill Medical, 2009.

102. Shorr RI., Ray WA, et al. Antihypertensives and the risk of serious hypoglycemia in older persons using insulin or sulfonylureas. *Journal of the American Medical Association* 1997;278(1):40–43.

103. Cagliero E, Apruzzese W, et al. Musculoskeletal disorders of the hand and shoulder in patients with diabetes mellitus. *American Journal of Medicine* 2002;112(6):487–490.
104. Chapple M, Jung RT, et al. Joint contractures and diabetic retinopathy. *Postgraduate Medical Journal* 1983;59(691):291–294.
105. Kiss C, Szilagyi M, et al. Risk factors for diffuse idiopathic skeletal hyperostosis: a case-control study. *Rheumatology* 2002;41(1):27–30.
106. Arkkila PE, Gautier JF. Musculoskeletal disorders in diabetes mellitus: An update. *Best Practice & Research in Clinical Rheumatology* 2003;17(6):945–970.
107. Smith LL, Burnet SP, et al. Musculoskeletal manifestations of diabetes mellitus. *British Journal of Sports Medicine* 2003;37(1):30–35.

9

Fundamentals of Medication Management for the Older Adult with Diabetes in Long-Term Care

Donald K. Zettervall, RPH, CDE

INTRODUCTION

Management of diabetes in the elderly offers challenges far more complicated than simply keeping blood glucose levels within acceptable limits. Most seniors whether living at home, in assisted-living facilities (ALFs) or in skilled nursing facilities (SNFs), usually will present with multiple health conditions requiring multifaceted drug therapies that not only are complicated in and of themselves but also are affected directly by the health of the residents, their other conditions, and therapies used to treat those conditions. Data published by the Centers for Disease Control and Prevention (CDC) showed that 65% of seniors >64 years have taken three or more prescription medications in the past month.[1]

Within the long-term care (LTC) setting, as many as 30% of residents will have diabetes, with most having type 2 diabetes (T2D).[2,3] Of those residents with diabetes, 80% have cardiovascular disease, 56% have hypertension, and 69% have two more other chronic conditions.[4] In addition, residents with a long history of diabetes also may have the common long-term complications of diabetes: the neuropathies, retinopathy, nephropathy, peripheral vascular disease, and depression. Residents may have conditions associated with aging itself, such as decline in kidney function, which often limits drug therapy options; arthritis, which increases pain and discomfort; constipation; incontinence; weight loss; and cognitive decline. With this complex backdrop, it is not uncommon to care for residents taking as many as 12 or more different prescription medications, each with different dosing instructions and effectiveness that is difficult to measure. Additionally, therapies can require large copays and be collectively expensive, thus putting added strain on health care dollars.

Drug therapy in the senior population is especially prone to medication misuse. In the home environment, seniors often become confused about instructions, are unable to afford copays, or may even perceive they no longer need a given therapy because of a lack of obvious improvement in a condition or conversely because of improvement in a condition. Medication misuse alone can lead to unnecessary and costly hospitalizations and the loss of independence with entry into LTC. According to the CDC, 76% of emergency room visits are related to medications in some way.[5] Given the number of medications seniors with diabetes need to take, these statistics are especially troublesome.

DOI: 10.2337/9781580404730.09

Continuity of care is an issue that must be considered in a population that may have many specialty health care providers. Seniors frequently are hospitalized and spend time in an SNF or rehabilitation facility before returning home, or to an LTC facility. In each setting, the senior with diabetes may be under the care of different prescribers for short or prolonged periods of time. It is not uncommon for an older adult to be under the care of a hospitalist while in an acute care setting, under the care of a medical director, attending physician, or a nurse practitioner, while in subacute care or LTC, and a generalist when back at home. Subspecialist clinicians add to the complexity at various points throughout the continuum, depending on the individual's various comorbid conditions. These prescribers often have differing opinions about therapies and how aggressive treatments should be for diabetes in a population that is inherently frail with a potentially short life expectancy.

Regardless of the setting, the prescriber, or the caregiver, four basic principles should be considered with respect to medication therapy. These principles are as follows:

1. Whenever possible, therapies should be optimized to improve quality of life.
2. All therapy approaches should be assessed for potential risk and, whenever possible, changed to minimize that risk.
3. Therapy should be aimed at treating to a goal that provides positive outcomes and provides a realizable benefit to the resident.
4. Therapy should be simplified to use as few medications or doses as possible.

Drug therapy in the older adult population is complex, so utilization and ongoing involvement of a pharmacist should be encouraged. The services of consultant pharmacists are readily available in LTC environments. The elderly resident in an ALF, or discharged from an SNF to home, can obtain these services through their local pharmacy provider as part of the Medicare-covered Medication Therapy Management (MTM) program.[6] Each Part D sponsor is required to incorporate a Medication Therapy Management Program (MTMP) into their plan's benefit structure. Annually, sponsors must submit an MTMP description to the Centers for Medicare and Medicaid Services (CMS) for review and approval. A CMS-approved MTMP is one of several required elements in the development of sponsors' bids for the upcoming contract year.[6]

Key Issues Requirements for Medication Therapy Management Programs

Under 423.153(d), a Part D sponsor must have established a MTM program that achieves the following:

■ Ensures optimum therapeutic outcomes for targeted beneficiaries through improved medication use.

- Reduces the risk of adverse events.
- Is developed in cooperation with licensed and practicing pharmacists and physicians.
- Describes the resources and time required to implement the program if using outside personnel and establishes the fees for pharmacists or others.
- Can be furnished by pharmacists or other qualified providers.
- Distinguishes between services in ambulatory and institutional settings.
- Is coordinated with any care management plan established for a targeted individual under a chronic care improvement program.

Utilizing a pharmacist's expertise in the everyday management of diabetes and related conditions has been shown to significantly improve resident care, outcomes, and quality of life.[7-11] One study that specifically focused on diabetes demonstrated significant positive outcomes and reduced costs within a time frame of <1 year.[8] This short time frame shows that benefits that can be realized quickly will benefit a population considered to have a short life expectancy and decrease costs for payers.

Pharmacists working in the LTC setting routinely perform medication regimen reviews, and the principles used can serve as a model for other health professionals. The medication regimen review process ensures that therapies and dosage forms are appropriate for the individual and the diagnoses, that there are no duplications, and that positive benefits are being realized from the therapy. The review process starts with an assessment of preexisting conditions and current therapies and then compares them to new diagnoses. With a population often being seen by multiple providers for multiple conditions, it is not uncommon for one prescriber to continue medications that were started by other prescribers, even if the prescriber does not know why the medications were prescribed, or the prescriber may think the current medication is effective for a condition that they may not be comfortable treating. When this medication continuation occurs, therapy duplication can result because of dose increases for current medications or for additional medications being prescribed for the same condition by multiple prescribers. Establishing communication with all of the resident's caregivers is essential, especially when a resident enters or is discharged from a facility. The medication assessment process includes obtaining a comprehensive medication list from the resident, caregiver, discharging facility, or pharmacy provider. An updated list of medications always should be provided to the resident upon discharge, with instructions to discontinue and dispose of any medications not on the list that may be at home. Residents also should be encouraged to bring the updated list to all future medical appointments with all prescribers.

If residents are just entering or returning to an ALF, they will be expected to manage their own medications. Health care providers who interact with residents in these settings should be assessing the residents' medication use on a routine basis. This assessment can be done using some of the following techniques:

1. Have the resident provide all currently prescribed medication bottles.

    a. Review date and quantity of all medications. Compare this to the instructions on the label and the doses remaining.

    b. Compare the medications in the resident's possession to the current medication list on record.

    c. Ask the resident if they know what each medication is for, and how and when they take it.

    d. Look for therapy duplications, especially from different prescribers and medications not on current orders.

2. If any discrepancies are discovered, try to determine the cause and notify the primary prescriber(s).

    a. Causes of discrepancies may include family members bringing old medications from home, other prescribers being unaware of currently prescribed medications, or residents forgetting or omitting doses to save money.

3. The resident should be instructed which medications to take, their appropriate use, and why they are taking them.
4. All medications not listed on the current orders should be destroyed.

Clinical Note

Medication Regimen Review

    1. Assessment of preexisting conditions and current therapies

    2. Comparison of results of #1 to new diagnoses

    3. Monitor for effectiveness.

MONITORING EFFECTIVENESS: MORE THAN BLOOD GLUCOSE

Monitoring for effectiveness and adverse effects of medications should be done on a timely and routine basis. In fact, monitoring is part of the Minimum Data Set (MDS) review conducted by pharmacists who are assessing therapy. Monitoring for effectiveness will help minimize the possibility of misdiagnosing adverse medication effects as symptoms of "old age" or other conditions. Residents also may be unable to recognize or notify caregivers of symptoms. When current symptoms are not identified correctly as being caused by a medication, a "prescribing cascade" can result. The prescribing cascade occurs when the effects from one medication lead to the addition of another medication, which in turn, can cause more adverse effects leading to a third medication and so on. Given the multimorbidities of the elderly in the LTC setting, and the number of medications being prescribed for those conditions, this prescribing cascade can be especially problematic. One example of this prescribing cascade, often seen with diabetes residents, results from side effects associated with the medication metoclopramide (Reglan), a medication frequently used to treat gastroparesis. In the elderly, because side effects of metoclopramide often mimic symptoms of Parkinson's disease, levodopa or carbidopa therapies are prescribed. The drugs for Parkinson's disease, in actuality, are unnecessary and could be avoided if the metoclopramide is discontinued.[9,10]

Of greater concern, and a far more common example, is the adverse effect of glucose-lowering medications with respect to hypoglycemia. Hypoglycemia has become so commonplace that it often is accepted as a consequence of diabetes treatment. Unfortunately, there is also a significant fear of hypoglycemia, and an ever-present desire to avoid hypoglycemia at all costs. This avoidance attitude within the LTC setting can compromise residents' care and, more important, can decrease their quality of life on the premise that it is "safer" to maintain higher blood glucose levels than to tighten glycemic control and risk hypoglycemia.

Hypoglycemia is a significant risk and attempts should be made to minimize occurrences. When a resident experiences frequent episodes of hypoglycemia, the prescribing cascade often begins. Treatments are prescribed to treat or prevent hypoglycemia. These treatments include routine use of snacks, especially at bedtime, or increased calorie intake to prevent hypoglycemia. Increased caloric intake then leads to episodes of hyperglycemia. Similarly, when episodes of hypoglycemia are detected, glucose gels, glucose tablets, and even glucagon injections are given routinely and frequently as therapy. These approaches, although considered standard protocols, often lead to prolonged episodes of hyperglycemia. A classic example of the prescribing cascade occurs when hypoglycemia is overtreated. The resulting hyperglycemia is documented and treated with increased doses of oral agents to lower glucose levels or, worse yet, sliding-scale insulin.

When a resident with diabetes has frequent or reoccurring episodes of hypoglycemia, staff should recall that hypoglycemia results from the glucose-lowering effects of medication. For example, a resident who receives glyburide twice a day is experiencing multiple episodes of hypoglycemia between 2:00 and 4:00 P.M. Staff observes that on these occasions the resident refused to eat or consumed significantly less lunch than normal. Although it was the decreased consumption at lunch that triggered the hypoglycemia, it is the morning dose of glyburide that actually is responsible for the hypoglycemic event. In this case, glyburide may not be appropriate for this resident given inconsistencies in meal consumption. Changing to a rapid-acting insulin secretagogue such as nateglinide or repaglinide at each meal might be a more appropriate choice for this resident. These medications are similar to glyburide in that they increase insulin release from the pancreas, but they have a shorter duration of action; one that is approximately the same as the time for digestion, and therefore the glucose-lowering effects are more targeted. These rapid-acting secretagogues can be administered after the meal if a resident has unpredictable eating patterns and also can be withheld when the resident does not eat.

There is a general misconception that all glucose-lowering medications can cause hypoglycemia. In fact, only two classes of medication therapies for diabetes will directly cause hypoglycemia on a regular basis. These are the insulin secretagogues (sulfonylureas and glinides) and insulin. If hypoglycemia is occurring on a regular basis, the causal medication or dose should be determined and adjusted accordingly. Treatment of hypoglycemia when it occurs is important, but clinicians should not prescribe extra or routine snacks to prevent routinely occurring hypoglycemia.

These adverse effects, including hypoglycemia, also present when inappropriate dosage forms are prescribed for the elderly resident who has difficulty swallowing. Commonly, medications are crushed and mixed with applesauce or pudding and then given to the resident. A number of currently available medications, however, are not indicated or approved for dosing in this manner.

Most long-acting medications fall into this category, including long-acting diabetes medications. Common prefixes or suffixes for sustained-release, controlled-release, or controlled-delivery products include 12-hour, 24-hour, CC, CD, CR, ER, LA, SA, Slo-, SR, XL, XR, or XT. Medications containing these labels should not be crushed. If a long-acting glucose- lowering medication, such as glipizide XL, is crushed and ingested, higher levels of the drug will be available in the bloodstream, and this will cause hypoglycemia at first and then, hours later, when the drug wears off, hyperglycemia will occur. Additionally, tablets that have enteric coatings should never be crushed. Certain drugs can be irritating to mucosal linings, are degraded by stomach acid, or simply taste terrible. Encasing the tablet in an enteric coat delays release of the medication until it reaches the stomach or small intestine, where the risk or irritation is less, taste is not a factor, or the medication can be absorbed without degradation. Prefixes for these types of medications include EN- and EC-.

The elderly are especially prone to adverse effects of medications. The Beers criteria is a resource of medications that are not recommended for use by the elderly because of their high potential for adverse effects. Using these medications is not prohibited, but residents who receive Beers-listed medications should be carefully monitored for benefit versus risk and adverse effects.[15] Use of Beers listed medications in the elderly may also place the facility at risk for F-Tag citations from state surveyors for inappropriate therapy.

MEDICATION ERRORS

Because of the number of medications prescribed for diabetes residents, another area of concern is the likelihood of medication errors. Any time a medication is given incorrectly, regardless of the cause, it is an error. An example is a resident who is prescribed rapid-acting insulin before meals.

If this resident receives the injection during a morning medication pass at 7:00 A.M. and the food tray does not arrive until 8:30 A.M., the resident is likely to experience a severe episode of hypoglycemia. Even though the medication nurse does not have control over the food arrival time, the resultant hypoglycemia can be considered a medication error because rapid-acting insulin should not be given >15 minutes before the meal.[16–18]

A common and costly medication error occurs when residents who experience repeated episodes of hypoglycemia do not receive correct treatment. In many cases, these residents are given glucagon injections when they do not warrant glucagon use. Glucagon should be used *only* if a resident is unresponsive or is to receive nothing by mouth. Using glucagon when a resident is capable of consuming treatment by mouth can be considered a medication error, even though a glucagon injection may be perceived as easier to administer than trying to have a resident take glucose gel, tablets, or juices by mouth. The effectiveness of glucagon is reduced if the resident is experiencing chronic hypoglycemia, is in a state of starvation, or has had prolonged period of fasting because of diminished glycogen stores in the liver.[19] Glucagon is an extremely expensive treatment. When given, the facility must absorb >$100 per injection. The cost of glucose gels, tablets, or juice, which is minimal, is very effective in raising the glucose level of the resident who is conscious and cooperative.[20] The need for a unit in a facility to have its glucagon replaced on a regular basis is an indication to evaluate appropriate hypoglycemia protocols. Frequent use of glucagon may suggest the need for in-service staff training and also may indicate the need for diabetes medication therapies to be adjusted.

Clinical Note

Glucagon

- An IM or IV injectable that raises blood glucose levels by stimulating glucose production by the liver

- Only use if resident is unresponsive or NPO

- Turn resident on side after injection as glucagon can cause emesis

- If glucagon is being used frequently, resident's insulin regimen should be reviewed and changed.

Virtually all of the diabetes-related hypoglycemia within the LTC setting results from using insulin and insulin secretagogues, drugs that actively lower glucose levels. Glucose levels normally vary from meal to meal, so having a protocol in place to address therapy with respect to a resident's caloric consumption is beneficial. When insulin and insulin secretagogues are used and hypoglycemia is a significant and reoccurring problem, the protocols should allow for either more flexible dosing to accommodate the resident's eating on a meal-to-meal basis, or changes in therapy need to be made that will minimize the risk for hypoglycemic episodes rather than continually treating a recurring problem.

CHOOSING THE RIGHT DIABETES MEDICATION

Knowing when to change or add a glucose-lowering medication is one of the most important skills in managing therapy in the elderly resident with diabetes. The process should first and foremost account for the resident's quality of life.[21]

For example, frequent episodes of hypoglycemia or severe hyperglycemia, as well as persistent hyperglycemia, all decrease the resident's quality of life and indicate the need for a change in therapy. The choice of which antihyperglycemic medication to use will depend on several factors, including the following:

Resident-Specific Factors

■ Frailty of the resident, comorbid conditions, diabetes complications, or contraindications: For example, long-acting insulin secretagogues would be inappropriate for the frail resident with a history of hypoglycemia or hypoglycemic unawareness. Metformin would be inappropriate for the resident with congestive heart failure or poor kidney function (i.e., an estimated glomerular filtration rate [eGFR] <30 and should be used with caution with an eGFR >30, but <60).

■ Life expectancy: Prescribers often consider use of aggressive glucose control to be inappropriate in a hospice resident. In this case, a more appropriate approach goal for therapy might be to simply start with a goal of keeping glucose levels <180 mg/dl to limit symptoms of hyperglycemia.

■ Resident and family preferences: If a resident eventually will be discharged, consideration should be made as to the resident's ability to continue the current therapy at home. For example, if insulin is required, using insulin pens versus syringes, and allowing the resident to self-administer the insulin, with nurse supervision, for a few days before discharge will help ensure safety and continuity of care. A resident's family may expect the same level of glucose control as other "younger" family members. When glucose targets are determined that are higher than those generally recommended, the family should be informed as to why.

Facility or Prescriber Factors

■ Current standards of care and clinical practice guidelines as defined by agencies and organizations concerned with the specific resident population.

  ■ American Diabetes Association (ADA)
  ■ American Geriatric Society (AGS)
  ■ American Medical Directors Association (AMDA)
  ■ Minimum Data Set (MDS-3.0)
  ■ The Joint Commission (TJC) accreditation

Within the LTC setting, adherence to any number of different clinical recommendations may be expected. As a general rule, if the prescriber utilizes therapies that will stabilize blood glucose levels to between 100 and 180 mg/dl, all standards of care will be met regardless of their source. As indicated in several other chapters, the ideal glucose level for the frail elder has yet to be established. The ADA Standards of Medical Care 2014,[22] however, has recommended using a table presented in a consensus report from a conference on the care on diabetes in older adults (see Chapter 5, Table 5.1).

■ Attitudes of the prescribers and staff: Often the greatest obstacle for appropriate therapy is resistance to change. If a new approach to therapy can improve a resident's quality of life, prescribers should be encouraged to utilize that therapy. Updating and involving staff in the decision-making process helps to increase dialog and decrease resistance. Routine in-service trainings should be available, especially when flexible therapies are utilized that require staff-initiated dosage adjustments based on day-to-day changes in resident status.

■ The burden the new medication will have on staff: Insulin often is seen as being too great a burden on staff because of the increased need for glucose testing, frequent injections, and timing of meals. In reality, the burden on staff ultimately may be reduced if insulin pens are used rather than syringes, if less hypoglycemia is occurring, and if greater flexibility in dosing around meals is ordered. Once blood glucose levels are stabilized, even the number of glucose tests can be reduced.

Protocols and decision pathways are valuable tools that ensure appropriate therapy utilization and provide consistent diabetes management approaches regardless of the prescriber. Protocols maintain continuity of care and can reduce prescriber phone calls by eliminating multiple or conflicting orders that change frequently or are difficult for staff to interpret.

Clinical Note

Should fasting (premeal) or postprandial glucose levels be targeted?

■ If A1C >8%, target fasting
■ If A1C <8%, target postprandial

TRANSLATING GLUCOSE GUIDELINES INTO PROTOCOLS

The American Diabetes Association has several recommendations for glucose control that are meant for the general population. Older adults who are functional, are cognitively intact, and have significant life expectancy should receive diabetes care using goals developed for younger adults. The ADA has suggested A1C values of <7%, which translates to an estimated average glucose level of ~154 mg/dl. A less-stringent A1C goal may be appropriate for residents with a history of severe hypoglycemia, limited life expectancy, advanced microvascular or macrovascular complications, and extensive comorbid conditions, as well as for those with longstanding diabetes in whom the general goal is difficult to attain. Hyperglycemia leading to symptoms or risk of acute hyperglycemia complications, however, should be avoided in all residents.[22] The fact that hyperglycemia, increased urination, and dehydration all begin at glucose levels >180 mg/dl suggests it is reasonable to initially target the upper limits of glucose to this level to improve quality of life and minimize risks.

Translating A1C targets into blood glucose targets in the senior population is slightly more difficult. For the general diabetes population, the ADA recommends target fasting blood glucose of 70–130 mg/dl, with peak postprandial glucose levels remaining <180 mg/dl.[11] Maintaining these glucose targets would provide the target A1C levels of <7% as recommended by the ADA for the general population. Doing so, however, could significantly increase the risk of hypoglycemia, especially if the fasting targets are used. To ensure continuity of care with respect to target glucose levels, it may be advisable to use the targets recommended for hospitalized residents. In this case, the recommendation is for fasting glucose levels is <140 mg/dl, while postprandial peak glucose levels remain at a target of <180–200 mg/dl.[22] If these targets are reached and maintained, corresponding A1C values should be within an acceptable range as recommended in the ADA framework of considering glycemic targets in older adults[23] and adopted by the ADA Standards of Medical Care, 2014.[22]

Choosing therapies to reach target glucose levels should not be based only on overall efficacy in lowering A1C but also on a systematic targeting of blood glucose. This targeting will minimize the risk for hypoglycemia while improving overall glucose control. A1C results can be used to determine both the number of glucose medications required and the necessity of utilizing insulin therapy.

Pens Versus Vials

Storage and expiration of medication is a frequently overlooked aspect of therapy that leads to increased costs for facilities in the form of expired medications. The best example of this unnecessary cost is with insulin therapy. Most vials of insulin should be discarded 28 days after opening, with the exception being insulin detemir, which has a discard date of 42 days after opening. Storing the vial in the refrigerator while in use does not extend the discard date. In fact, injection of cold insulin is uncomfortable, which means refrigeration of opened insulin vials is not only unnecessary but also causes patient discomfort. As a general rule, a resident who is using <30 units of any one type of insulin per day from a vial will have significantly higher costs for insulin because of the wasteful discarding of expired, unused insulin.

One method to significantly reduce costs associated with insulin use, especially when the stay may be relatively short or the resident is covered under Medicare Part A, is through the use of insulin pen devices. When used correctly, insulin pens have many advantages over vials, including the following:

- More accurate and faster dosing mechanism using a dial system.
- Less medical waste in sharps containers because of a smaller self-contained needle requiring sharps disposal.
- Less unused insulin to be discarded because of a smaller amount of insulin to use before expiration.

Each pen contains only 3 ml (300 units) of insulin and, with newer insulin formulations, has the same expiration as a 10 ml (1,000 unit) vial. Therefore, even a resident using just 10 units of insulin per day of U-100 insulin will have little to no unused insulin to discard because of expiration. In the retail setting, insulin pens are dispensed as five pens per box or 15 ml of insulin versus 10 ml in vial form. Unopened pens should be stored under refrigeration and each pen should be discarded according to its expiration after its first use (see Table 9.1).

An LTC facility need not order full boxes of pens. Prescribers can and should be encouraged to only order the number of pens required for the resident's stay.

Table 9.1 Storage and Expiration of Insulin Preparations

	Recommended Insulin Storage			
Insulin Type	**Refrigerated (36°F-46°F)**		**Room Temperature (59°F-86°F)**	
VIAL	**Opened**	**Unopened**	**Opened**	**Unopened**
Humalog, Humulin, Novolog, Novolin, Apidra	28 days	until expiration date	28 days	
Lantus 10ml	28 days	until expiration date	28 days	
Levemir 10ml	42 days	until expiration date	42 days	
PENS/Cartridges	**Not is use**		**In use**	
Humalog	until expiration date		28 days	
Humulin R (available in cartridge only)	until expiration date		28 days	
Humulin N	until expiration date		14 days	
Humulin 70/30	until expiration date		10 days	
Humalog Mix 75/25	until expiration date		10 days	
Novolog 3ml cartridge & Flexpen	until expiration date		28 days	
Novolog Mix 70/30 3ml cartridge & Flexpen	until expiration date		14 days	
Novolin R 3ml cartridges	until expiration date		28 days	
Novolin N 3ml cartridge & Innolet	until expiration date		14 days	
Novolin 70/30 3ml cartridge & Innolet	until expiration date		10 days	
Levemir 3ml cartridge, Innolet & Flexpen	until expiration date		42 days	
Apidra	until expiration date		28 days	
Lantus	until expiration date		28 days	

This is especially true if the resident is in a rehabilitation facility for a short duration, the patient is a hospice resident, or the facility is paying for the medication. Ordering smaller quantities will reduce the need to discard unused or expired insulin. For example, assume an insulin vial costs $180. This would translate to $0.18 per unit of insulin. A box of pens might appear to cost considerably more at $300 per box ($60 per pen), translating to $0.20 per unit of insulin. If a resident requires only 10 units/day of insulin, however, each month

Table 9.2 Cost Differences Between Insulin Vials and Pens

Units/day	Insulin cost Purchased Used		Units/mo Discarded	$ lost per mo
10 units	Vial $180	$50	720	$130
280 u prior to exp	Pen $60	$56	20	$4
20 units	Vial $180	$101	440	$79
560 u prior to exp	Pens $120	all	0	0
30 units	Vial $180	$151	160	$29
840 u prior to exp	Pens $180	all	0	0

Note: Assuming an average wholesale price (AWP) for a vial of insulin is $180. The cost per unit would be $0.18 compared with its insulin pen option at $60 per pen or $0.20 per unit.

$130 worth of unused insulin will be discarded from an expired vial. Using a pen, no insulin would be unused. The breakeven point for pens versus vials tends to be at around 30 units/day, but even with higher dosing, use of insulin pens saves nursing time for dosing, decreased sharps volume, and can increase dosing accuracy (see Table 9.2).

Hypertension

The ADA has recommended blood pressure levels of <140/80 mmHg for individuals with diabetes.[22] If these recommendations are used as the basis for hypertension therapy decisions, the goal of treatment should be to maintain blood pressure as close to recommended values as possible. Aggressively treating blood pressure, however, can lead to more orthostatic hypotension, which can significantly increase the risk of falls in elderly residents.

In the U.K. Prospective Diabetes Study, improved blood pressure control (mean blood pressure of 144/82 mmHg), in addition to improved glucose control, reduced the risk of stroke, heart failure, and diabetes-related death as well as diabetes-related microvascular complications.[24] More recent studies have shown that attaining blood pressures of <150/80 mmHg in residents >80 years of age demonstrated a reduction in fatal or nonfatal stroke of 30%, and a 39% reduction in the rate of death from stroke. It also resulted in a 23% reduction in the rate of death from cardiovascular causes, a 64% reduction in the rate of death from heart failure, and a 21% reduction in the rate of death from any cause.[25] There is no question that blood pressure control is important and can decrease the progression of diabetic nephropathy. It remains controversial, however, as to how aggressive to be in the frail elderly. The recent studies indicate that although we may strive for the ideal goal of <140/80 mmHg to obtain optimal outcomes, it may not be necessary to reach this goal if it places the resident at significant risk.

Angiotensin-converting enzyme (ACE) inhibitors are considered to be the treatment of choice whenever possible for hypertensive residents with diabetes. In addition to reducing blood pressure, ACE inhibitors have been shown to

Table 9.3 Antihypertensive Agents

Category	Generic name	Brand name™	Minimum daily dose	Maximum daily dose	Special considerations for class of drugs
Angiotensin-converting enzyme (ACE) inhibitors	benazepril	Lotensin™	10 mg QD	40 mg QD or divided	May cause cough. May increase potassium concentrations. Caution if creatinine >1.5.
	captopril	Capoten™	25 mg QD QD divided dose	100 mg divided dose	
	enalapril	Vasotec™	5 mg QD	40 mg QD or divided	
	fosinopril	Monopril™	10 mg QD	40 mg QD or divided	
	lisinopril	Prinivil™, Zestril™	10 mg QD	40 mg QD	
	moexipril	Univasc™	7.5 mg QD	30 mg QD or divided	
	perindopril	Aceon™	4 mg QD	8 mg QD	
	quinapril	Accupril™	10 mg QD	80 mg QD or divided	
	ramipril	Altace™	2.5 mg QD	20 mg QD or divided	
	trandolapril	Mavik™	1 mg QD	4 mg QD	
Angiotensin II receptor blockers	candesartan	Atacand™	8 mg QD	32 mg QD or divided	May cause dizziness and upset stomach.
	eprosartan	Teveten™	400 mg QD	800 mg QD or divided	Caution if creatinine >1.5.
	irbesartan	Avapro™	150 mg QD	300 mg QD	
	losartan	Cozaar™	25 mg QD	100 mg QD or divided	
	olmesartan	Benicar™	20 mg QD	40 mg QD	
	telmisartan	Micardis™	20 mg QD	80 mg QD	
	valsartan	Diovan™	80 mg QD	320 mg QD	

(Continued)

Table 9.3 Antihypertensive Agents (Continued)

Category	Generic name	Brand name™	Minimum daily dose	Maximum daily dose	Special considerations for class of drugs
Thiazides and related diuretics	bedroflumethia-zide	Naturetin™	2.5 mg QD	20 mg QD	May increase blood glucose concentrations. Give in morning to minimize diuretic effect at night. Monitor potassium level.
	chlorothiazide	Diuril™	125 mg QD	500 mg QD or divided	
	chlorthalidone	Hygroton™	12.5 mg QD	25 mg QD	
	hydrochlorothiazide	HydroDIURIL™	12.5 mg QD	50 mg QD or divided	
	hydrochlorothiazide	Microzide™	12.5 mg QD	50 mg QD or divided	
	indapamide	Lozol™	1.25 mg QD	2.5 mg QD	
	methyclothiazide	Enduron™	2.5 mg QD	5 mg QD	
	metolazone	Mykrox™	0.5 mg QD	1 mg QD	
	metolazone	Zaroxolyn™	2.5 mg QD	5 mg QD	
Loop diuretics	bumetanide	Bumex™	0.5 mg QD	2 mg QD or divided	Monitor potassium level.
	ethacrynic acid	Edecrin™	25 mg QD	200 mg divided dose	
	furosemide	Lasix™	20 mg QD	80 mg QD or divided	
	torsemide	Demadex™	2.5 mg QD	10 mg QD	
Potassium-sparing diuretics	amiloride	Midamor™	5 mg QD	10 mg QD	
	triamterene	Dyrenium™	50 mg QD or divided	100 mg divided dose	
Aldosterone receptor blockers	eplerenone	Inspra™	50 mg QD	100 mg divided dose	
	spironolactone	Aldactone™	25 mg QD	50 mg divided dose	

Calcium-channel blockers	amlodipine	Norvasc™	2.5 mg QD	10 mg QD	May cause constipation, dizziness, upset stomach, and flushing.
					Call physician for shortness of breath, unusual heart-beat, or swelling of hands or feet.
	diltiazem	Cardizem LA™	120 mg QD	540 mg QD	
	diltiazem	Cardizem CD™	180 mg QD	420 mg QD	
	diltiazem	Dilacor XR™	180 mg QD	420 mg QD	
	diltiazem	Tiazac™	180 mg QD	420 mg QD	
	felodipine	Plendil™	2.5 mg QD	20 mg QD	
	isradipine	DynaCircCR™	2.5 mg QD	10 mg QD	
	nicardipine	Cardene SR™	60mg QD divided dose	120 mg QD divided dose	
	nifedipine	Adalat CC™	30 mg QD	60 mg QD	
	nifedipine	Procardia XL™	30 mg QD	60 mg QD	
	nisoldipine	Sular™	10 mg QD	40 mg QD	
	verapamil	Calan™	80 mg QD divided dose	320 mg divided dose	
	verapamil	Calan SR™	120 mg QD	480 mg divided dose	
	verapamil	Covera HS™	120 mg QD	360 mg QD	
	verapamil	Isoptin™	80 mg QD divided dose	320 mg divided dose	
	verapamil	Isoptin SR™	120 mg QD	480 mg QD or divided	
	verapamil	Verelan™	80 mg QD divided dose	320 mg divided dose	

(Continued)

Table 9.3 Antihypertensive Agents (Continued)

Category	Generic name	Brand name™	Minimum daily dose	Maximum daily dose	Special considerations for class of drugs
	verapamil	Verelan PM™	120 mg QD	360 mg QD	Intrinsic sympathomimetic activity. May alter blood glucose, may mask signs of low blood glucose. Call physician for slow heart rate (<60 beats per minute), confusion, or swelling of feet or legs. Can cause claudication. Do not discontinue abruptly.
β-Blockers	acebutolol	Sectral™	200 mg QD	800 mg divided dose	
	atenolol	Tenormin™	25 mg QD	100 mg QD	
	betaxolol	Kerlone™	5 mg QD	20 mg QD	
	bisoprolol	Zebeta™	2.5 mg QD	10 mg QD	
	carteolol	Cartol™	2.5 mg QD	10 mg QD	
	metoprolol	Lopressor™	50 mg QD	100 mg QD or divided	
	metoprolol	Toprol XL™	50 mg QD	100 mg QD	
	nadolol	Corgard™	40 mg QD	120 mg QD	
	penbutolol	Levatol™	10 mg QD	40 mg QD	
	pindolol	Visken™	10 mg in divided dose	40 mg divided dose	
	propranolol	Inderal™	40 mg divided dose	160 mg divided dose	
	propranolol	Inderal LA™	60 mg QD	180 mg QD	
	timolol	Blocadren™	20 mg divided dose	40 mg divided dose	
α-Blockers	doxazosin	Cardura™	1 mg QD	16 mg QD	To prevent dizziness, avoid standing up suddenly, especially with the first few doses.
	prazosin	Minipress™	2 mg in divided dose	20 mg divided dose	
	terazosin	Hytrin™	1 mg QD	20 mg QD	

Combined α- and β-blockers	carvedilol	Coreg™	12.5 mg divided dose	50 mg divided dose	May mask signs of low blood glucose levels.
	labetalol	Normodyne™	200 mg divided dose	800 mg divided dose	
	labetalol	Trandate™	200 mg divided dose	800 mg divided dose	
Direct vasodila-tors	hydralazine	Apresoline™	25 mg QD	100 mg divided dose	May cause headaches, fluid retention, or fast heart rate.
	midoxidil	Loniten™	2.5 mg QD	80 mg divided dose	
Central α-agonists	clonidine	Catapres™	0.1 mg QD	0.8 mg divided dose	Do not discontinue drug suddenly without consulting physician.
	clonidine	Catapres TTS™ (patch)	0.1 mg Q week	0.3 mg Q week	
	methyldopa	Aldomet™	250 mg divided dose	1,000 mg divided dose	
	guanfacine	Tenex™	0.5 mg QD	2 mg QD	
Peripheral anti-adrenergics	guanadrel	Hylorel™	10 mg in divided dose	75mg divided dose	May cause dizziness, nasal congestion, and depression.
	guanethidine	Ismelin™	10 mg QD	50 mg QD	
	resperine		0.1 mg divided dose	0.25 mg divided dose	

Source: National Diabetes Education Program. Visit http://ndep.nih.gov for updated tables.

Table 9.4 Comparison of Lipid-Lowering Agents

Category	Generic name	Brand name	Minimum daily dose	Maximum daily dose	Special considerations for class of drugs
HMG-CoA reductase inhibitors (statins)	atorvastatin	Lipitor™	10 mg QD	80 mg in divided doses	Main action: Lowers LDL. Also lowers TG and modestly raises HDL.
	fluvastatin	Lescol™	20 mg QD	80 mg in divided doses	Periodic testing liver enzyme concentrations.
	fluvastatin	Lescol XL™	80 mg QD	80 mg in divided doses	Notify physician if muscle aches or weakness develops.
	lovastatin	Mevacor™	10 mg QD	80 mg in divided doses	Use caution if combined with fibric acid derivatives due to the increased risk of rhabdomyolysis.
	lovastatin (extended release)	Altocor™	20 mg QD	60 mg QD	
	pravastatin	Pravachol™	10 mg QD	80 mg QD	
	rosuvastatin	Crestor™	5 mg QD	40 mg QD	
	simvastatin	Zocor™	5 mg QD	80 mg in divided doses	
Cholesterol absorption inhibitors	ezetimibe	Zetia™	10 mg QD	10 mg QD	Main action: Lowers LDL, inhibits absorption of cholesterol. If used with a statin, take together. If used with bile acid sequestrant, ezetimibe should be taken 2 hours before or 4 hours after bile acid sequestrant.
Nicotinic acid (niacin)	nicotinic acid (extended release)	Niaspan™	50–100 mg QD	2,000 mg QD	Main action: Lowers LDL increases HDL lowers TGs. Take with food. May cause flushing. May increase blood glucose levels. Periodic testing liver enzyme concentrations. Long-acting forms may be more likely to cause liver malfunction.
	nicotinic acid		250 mg/day QD	Titrated up to 1,500 mg therapeutic dose in three divided doses; maximum dose = 3,000 mg	

Category	Generic name	Brand name	Dose	Dose	Notes
Lipid combinations	lovastatin-niacin	Advicor™	20 mg/500 mg QD	40 mg/2,000 mg QD	Main action: Reduces LDL, TC, and TG increases HDL.
	simvastatin-ezetimibe	Vytorin™	10 mg/10 mg QD	80 mg/10 mg QD	Main action: Reduces LDL.
Fibric acid derivatives	fenofibrate	Tricor™	48 mg QD	145 mg QD	Main action: Lowers TG, increases HDL. Periodic liver enzyme concentrations. Adjust dose based on age and renal impairment. Notify physician if muscle aches or weakness develops.
	fenofibrate	Lofibra™	67 mg QD	200 mg QD	
	fenofibrate	Triglide™	50 mg QD	160 mg QD	
	fenofibrate	Antara™	43 mg QD	130 mg QD	
	gemfibrozil	Lopid™	1,200 mg BID	1,200 mg BID	
Bile acid sequestrants	cholestyramine	LoCHOLEST™	4 g QD	24 g in divided doses	Main action: Lowers LDL. May cause constipation and stomach upset. May need to be taken at a different time than other medications to avoid drug interactions. May increase triglycerides blood concentrations. Can be combined with other agents such as statins.
Fish Oil	Omega 3-acidethyl ester	Lovaza™	4 g QD	4 g QD	Main action: Lowers very high TGs (>500 mg/dl). May increase LDL. Periodic liver enzyme concentrations.

Source: National Diabetes Education Program. Visit http://ndep.nih.gov for updated tables.

slow the progression of microalbuminuria to macroalbuminuria and to improve endothelial dysfunction, which is common in residents with T2D. Thus, ACE inhibitors may be considered for normotensive residents with diabetes as well.[26] ACE inhibitors can cause an increase in serum creatinine of up to 35% above baseline; therefore, doses may need to be adjusted if hyperkalemia develops or the resident's eGFR is <30 ml/minute/1.73 m^2.

If a resident cannot tolerate ACE inhibitors, angiotensin-receptor blockers (ARB) have been shown to have similar benefits. ARBs are recommended over ACE inhibitors when macroalbuminuria or renal insufficiency is present. To achieve blood pressure targets, however, two or more blood pressure–lowering agents generally are required. The addition of a thiazide diuretic should be considered when eGFR is >30 ml/minute/1.73 m^2, and a loop diuretic should be considered when the eGFR is <30 ml/minute/1.73 m^2. Doses or the total number of prescriptions can be reduced if combination products are considered (see Table 9.3).

Dyslipidemia

The ADA recommends that all residents with diabetes receive treatment to attain low-density lipoprotein (LDL) cholesterol of ≤100 mg/dl, high-density lipoprotein (HDL) cholesterol levels >40 mg/dl in men and >50 mg/dl in women, and triglycerides of ≤150mg/dl in all residents. Statins, specifically simvastatin and atorvastatin, have been shown to reduce cardiovascular events in people with diabetes regardless of baseline LDL.[27-29] Therefore, statin therapy is recommended for all residents with diabetes regardless of age. The ADA recommends statin therapy for all persons with diabetes and cardiovascular disease (CVD) and people with diabetes who are >40 years of age and have at least one CVD risk factor.[22] For residents with preexisting CVD, an LDL goal of <70 is recommended; however, this sometimes is seen as too aggressive for high-risk elderly residents. One study of nursing home residents with histories of previous heart attacks and LDL cholesterol levels >125 mg/d found a 20% incidence of coronary events when subjects were treated with statins to lower LDL to <90 mg/dl versus a 48% incidence of new coronary events if treated to an LDL target of 90–99 mg/dl. In addition to coronary disease, reduction in stroke was observed in residents <90 years of age with a 47% reduction in the LDL ≤90 versus 90–99 mg/dl groups.[26] In residents who are treated with statins and unable to reach target LDL, however, a 30–40% reduction in current LDL levels can be used as an alternative goal (see Table 9.4).[22]

CONCLUSION

Appropriate management of medications in the elderly in LTC requires balance and vigilance relevant to the resident, the multiple conditions being treated, and the expectations of the family, care providers, payers, and even regulators. This is especially true with respect to glucose control. However complex the process or the pressures, there are two primary goals that should first and foremost guide the clinician when considering therapy decisions for the elderly. These goals are to *1)* do no harm and *2)* improve or maintain quality of life. Achieving the appropriate outcomes can be accomplished with less risk when there is consistency across the continuum of care. Chapter 10 discusses methods of standardizing the process of glycemic management with respect to glucose-lowering therapy decisions.

REFERENCES

1. Centers for Disease Control and Prevention. Table 95: Prescription drug use in the past month, by sex, age, race and Hispanic origin: United States, 1998–1994 and 2005–2008 (data are based on a sample of the civilian non-institutionalized population). Available at www.cdc.gov/nchs/data/hus/hus2009tables/Table095.pdf. Accessed 2 June 2012.
2. Worcester S. Adverse events in elderly mostly from common drugs. *Caring for the Ages* 2012;13:4.
3. Travis SS, Buchanan RJ, Wang S, Kim M. Analysis of nursing home residents on admission. *Journal of the American Medical Directors Association* 2004;4:320–327.
4. Haines ST. The diabetes epidemic: Can we stop the spread? *Pharmacotherpy* 203;23:1227–1231.
5. Centers for Disease Control and Prevention. National hospital ambulatory medical care survey: 2007 emergency department summary (Tables 17, 18, 19). Available at www.cdc.gov/nchs/data/nhsr/nhsr026.pdf. Accessed 13 June 2012.
6. Centers for Medicare and Medicaid Services. Medicare-covered Medication Therapy Management (MTM) program. Available at http://www.cms.gov/Medicare/Prescription-Drug-Coverage/PrescriptionDrugCovContra/MTM.html. Accessed 10 January 2014.
7. Beney J, Bero LA, Bond C. Expanding the roles of outpatient pharmacists: Effects on health services, utilization, costs, and outcomes. *Cochrane Database Syst Rev* 2000;3, CD000336.
8. Indritz ME, Artz MB. Value added to health by pharmacists. *Social Science and Medicine* 1999;48:647–660.
9. Bootman JL, Harrison DL, Cox E. The health care cost of drug-related morbidity and mortality in nursing facilities. *Archives of Internal Medicine* 1997;157:2089–2096.
10. Fouts M, Hanlon J, Pieper C, Perfetto E, Feinberg J. Identification of elderly nursing facility residents at high risk for medication-related problems. *The Consultant Pharmacist* 1997;12:1103–1111.
11. Harms SL, Garrard J. The Fleetwood Model: an enhanced method of pharmacist consultation. *The Consultant Pharmacist* 1998;13:1350–1355.
12. Garrett D, Eckel F, et al. The Asheville Project. *The Pharmacy Times* (Suppl) Oct 1998.
13. Rochon PA, Gurwitz JH. Drug therapy. *Lancet* 1995 Jul 1;346(8966):32–36.
14. Rochon PA, Gurwitz JH. Optimizing drug treatment for elderly people: the prescribing cascade. *British Medical Journal* 1997;315:1096–1099.
15. American Geriatrics Society 2012 Beers Criteria Update Expert Panel. Beers criteria. Available at http://www.americangeriatrics.org/health_care_professionals/clinical_practice/clinical_guidelines_recommendations/2012. Accessed 12 June 2012.

16. Apidra package insert. Available at http://products.sanofi.us/apidra/apidra. html. Accessed 16 February 2014.
17. Humalog package insert. Available at http://www.insidehumalog.com/ Pages/type2-humalog.aspx?WT.srch=1&WT.mc_id=33918-649952-2698. Accessed 18 February 2014.
18. Novolog package insert. Available at http://www.novolog.com/default. aspx?RequestId=781c9ac9. Accessed 16 February 2014.
19. Glucagon package insert. Available at http://www.glucagonapp.com/Pages/ index.aspx. Accessed 16 February 2014.
20. Lexi-Comp, Inc. (Lexi-Drugs™). Available at http://webstore.lexi.com/ Lexi-Drugs. Accessed 24 February 2011.
21. American Medical Directors Association (AMDA). Diabetes management in the long term care setting. Columbia, MD, AMDA, 2008, revised 2010, p. 45.
22. American Diabetes Association. Standards of medical care in diabetes—2014 *Diabetes Care* 2014;37(Suppl1):S14–S180.
23. Kirkman MS, et al. Diabetes in older adults. *Diabetes Care* 2012;35:2650–2664.
24. King P, Peacock I, Donnelly R. The UK Prospective Diabetes Study (UKPDS): clinical and therapeutic implications for type 2 diabetes. *Br J Clin Pharmacol* 1999 November; 48(5):643–648.
25. Beckett NS, Peters R, Fletcher AE, Staessen JA, Liu L, Dumitrascu D, Stoyanovsky V, Antikainen RL, Nikitin Y, Anderson C, Belhani A, Forette F, Rajkumar C, Thijs L, Banya W, Bulpitt CJ. Treatment of hypertension in patients 80 years of age or older. *New England Journal of Medicine* 2008;358:1887–1898.
26. Aronow WS, Ahn C. Incidence of new coronary events and new atherothrombotic brain infarction in older persons with diabetes mellitus, prior myocardial infarction and serum low density lipoprotein cholesterol >125 treated with statin. *Journals of Gerontology Series A: Biological* Sciences and *Medical Sciences* 2002;57:M747–M750.
27. Baigent C, Keech A, Kearney PM, Blackwell L, Buck G, Pollicino C, Kirby A, Sourjina T, Peto R, Collins R, Simes R, Cholesterol Treatment Trialists' (CTT) Collaborators. Efficacy and safety of cholesterol-lowering treatment: prospective meta-analysis of data from 90,056 participants in 14 randomised trials of statins. *Lancet* 2005;366:1267–1278.
28. Pyorala K, Pedersen TR, Kjekshus J, Faergeman O, Olsson AG, Thorgeirsson G. Cholesterol lowering with simvastatin improves prognosis of diabetic patients with coronary heart disease: a subgroup analysis of the Scandinavian Simvastatin Survival Study (4S). *Diabetes Care* 1997;20:614–620.
29. Collins R, Armitage J, Parish S, Sleigh P, Peto R, Heart Protection Study Collaborative Group. MRC/BHF Heart Protection Study of cholesterol-lowering with simvastatin in 5963 people with diabetes: a randomised placebo-controlled trial. *Lancet* 2003;361:2005–2016.

10

Diabetes Medications and Long-Term Care Insulin Therapy

Donald K. Zettervall, RPH, CDE

INTRODUCTION

The management of diabetes therapy and medications in general for an elderly population tends to be a much more subjective endeavor than in the general population. This is because therapies seldom are studied in the very old, and this is especially true of those residing within assisted-living and skilled nursing facility (SNF) environments where the median age is currently >83 years old.[1] Taking into account factors such as caregiver fears of hypoglycemia associated with tighter control, the existence of multiple comorbid conditions, multiple medications, diminished functionality, and the prospect of a relatively short life expectancy, the clinical recommendations for this population tend to be less stringent with respect to glucose targets than in the general population. As such, there is a tendency and justification for discontinuing medications that are perceived to have minimal impact on outcomes to reduce costs and the burden of care.

Changes associated with the implementation of outcome-focused health care reform, particularly those involving the transition of care for Medicare beneficiaries, are affecting the decision process for managing therapy in the elderly. For example, hospitals risk being financially penalized if a Medicare beneficiary is readmitted to the hospital within 30 days of discharge. As a result, hospitals now have a vested interest in establishing closer relationships with the post–acute care facilities to which they send residents, and they are looking for facilities that are willing to implement protocols and approaches to therapy that are similar to the hospitals' or that ensure a best practice approach to managing diabetes to minimize risk for readmission.

The purpose of this chapter is not to discuss the philosophical differences of approaches to diabetes management in the elderly population but rather to discuss and suggest a generalized glucose-lowering approach focused on the one constant standard in managing diabetes in the long-term care (LTC) setting. That is, above all else, to improve or maintain quality-of-life while minimizing risks for both hyper- and hypoglycemia. Glycemic goals for some older adults need to be relaxed to avoid hypoglycemia; however, hyperglycemia leading to symptoms or risk of acute hyperglycemic complications should be avoided in all residents.[1,2] This effectively translates into keeping glucose levels under the threshold for hyperglycemic symptoms or <180–200 mg/dl. Doing so not only improves quality of life by avoiding symptoms of hyperglycemia but also reduces the risks associated with hyperglycemia, such as dehydration, poor wound healing, frequent urination, weight loss, etc., and thus improve outcomes.

DOI: 10.2337/9781580404730.10

KNOWING WHEN A CHANGE IS NEEDED

One of the most difficult aspects of managing diabetes medications within the LTC setting is to know when therapy changes should be made and taking definitive action. For example, when an elderly resident whose diabetes is managed with oral therapy enters the hospital, the oral therapies often are discontinued, and the resident is placed on insulin regardless of how well their glucose has been controlled. This medication change is done because most residents enter the hospital for acute problems that may require more aggressive or flexible glucose-lowering therapy because of stress-induced hyperglycemia or a significant decrease in appetite. When the resident is discharged, however, oral therapies may or may not be reinstated regardless of how well the resident's glucose was controlled before admission. If the resident were discharged to a short-stay facility for services, such as physical therapy, there may not be any change made to the diabetes therapies even if the resident were being given doses of sliding-scale insulin (SSI) for episodes of hyperglycemia. This type of scenario often takes place when hospitalists and short-stay facility prescribers believe that because diabetes is a long-term condition; their intervention would have little to no impact on overall glucose control. Therefore, these prescribers think the diabetes is best managed by the resident's primary health care provider upon discharge. Unfortunately, this approach often misses an opportunity to improve the resident's glucose control, which could directly improve the resident's recovery time and quality of life as well as decrease the risk of acute complications that could cause a readmission to the hospital.

Protocol-Driven Decision Process

Assessing the need for a therapy change can be based on simple principles. First, is the resident experiencing episodes of either hyper- or hypoglycemia? Second, is the resident's A1C outside acceptable limits? If the answer is yes to either of these questions, then a change in therapy is warranted.

An A1C value within an acceptable range should not be used as the sole criteria for appropriateness of current therapy. For example, an 80-year-old resident with a multitude of comorbid conditions may have an A1C value of 7.2%, which places him or her well within an acceptable A1C range for a younger individual. However, this resident may be experiencing episodes of severe hyper- and hypoglycemia that may or may not be documented. If fluctuations are suspected but not documented, an increase in blood glucose testing is needed, especially at suspected times of hyper- or hypoglycemia to determine whether wide fluctuations in glucose are occurring.

Another principle that can be used to assess the need for diabetes therapy change is to conduct a drug utilization review. Using this approach would not only identify a need for a diabetes therapy change in an individual resident, but also could identify facility or staff issues that should be addressed with education. The best example of this would be a facility that frequently is utilizing glucagon. Glucagon is indicated for the treatment of severe hypoglycemia in cases in which the person with diabetes is unconscious or cannot be treated with oral options (e.g., glucose tablets, gel, fruit juice, or milk). If an individual frequently requires glucagon to treat hypoglycemia, this is a clear indication for the need of a therapy change to stabilize blood glucose levels. If on the other hand, multiple residents are being given glucagon to treat hypoglycemia, it is possible the treatment approach is too aggressive or that the glucagon is being used inappropriately. In this case, the treatment approach could be considered a medication error that needs to be addressed.

Another common indicator for potential need of therapy change to improve glucose control would be the prolonged use of SSI or correction insulin doses. In this case, glucose levels are allowed to reach hyperglycemic levels and then are treated after the fact. This approach to therapy causes wide fluctuations in glucose levels placing the resident at significant risk for both severe hyper- and hypoglycemia complications. The American Medical Directors Association's (AMDA) Diabetes Clinical Practice Recommendations encourages discontinuation of SSI within 1 week of admission. Additionally, as of 2012, SSI therapy was included on the American Geriatrics Society (AGS) Beers criteria and now is considered inappropriate therapy for the elderly.[3]

A PRACTICAL APPROACH TO DIABETES THERAPY SELECTION FOR THE SNF RESIDENT

Once a resident has been identified as being in need of a therapy change to improve their glucose control, whether it is to decrease episodes of hyper- or hypoglycemia or simply to stabilize glucose levels, the question becomes which therapy is best. When treating diabetes in the LTC setting it always is best to keep it simple and standardized (KISS). Doing so helps to streamline the process across the continuum of care and across multiple prescribers. Improving glucose control using a science-based standardized process helps to stabilize glucose levels and improves the quality of life for the resident and their caregivers by decreasing the burden of care. A standardized process also can reduce the need for calls to prescribers to address wide glucose fluctuations associated with SSI use. Using a standardized protocol-driven system similar to those used in hospitals also can help decrease the risk of medication errors because of misinterpretation of orders associated with different approaches to managing diabetes, and can improve efficiency.[4] Although the process can be standardized, the goals of therapy still should be individualized to allow for resident-specific variability.

The first step is to choose the best medication or combination of medications that will minimize risk while attaining desired effects. To do so, realistic attainable therapeutic goals need to be determined that will provide for blood glucose levels below the threshold for hyperglycemia, will minimize the risk of hypoglycemia, and at the same time, will not cause increased burden on staff. Although this sounds like a monumental task in the frail elderly, it need not be. At a most basic level, it translates into simply maintaining glucose levels <180–200 mg/dl. Doing so would reduce A1C levels to <8%, which often is deemed acceptable according to the American Diabetes Association (ADA)–recommended framework for glucose targets in older adults.[5] Looser A1C targets may be considered as recommended by the ADA framework for considering glycemic targets (see Table 5.1). Targets that are too high, however, may expose residents to acute risks from glycosuria, dehydration, and hyperosmolar hyperglycemic state if hypergly-cemia is persistent. All of which increase demands on staff, diminish the resident's quality of life, and increase the risk for poor outcomes and readmissions to the hospital.

The second step requires a basic understanding of what to expect from any given class of glucose-lowering agents in terms of A1C (Table 10.1), and apply-ing this to the basic recommendations set forth in currently available algorithms for therapy selection in the management of type 2 diabetes (T2D). As a rule, algorithms recommend the initiation of insulin therapy if glucose targets are not met with the use of three or fewer noninsulin medications.[6,7] Because medications should be reviewed upon admission and throughout a resident's stay, a need for change would be identified whenever a resident is currently on three or more noninsulin glucose-lowering agents and is not meeting recommended A1C or glucose targets. In this case, the resident should be started on physiologic insulin replacement. The AMDA also recommends consideration of insulin therapy if a resident's blood glucose is persistently >180 mg/dl regardless of noninsulin therapies.[8]

For those residents currently receiving fewer than three noninsulin glucose-lowering agents, an assessment can be made as to the need for insulin, based on the resident's current A1C and the desired target A1C. The prescriber would then determine the desired A1C lowering required to reach goal and choose the agent or agents (keeping the total number of agents less than three) that would provide the desired A1C lowering effect without duplicating the mechanism of action

Table 10.1 Average A1C Lowering and Glucose Affected

Therapy class	Average A1C-lowering effect	Most affected blood glucose
Metformin[1]	1–2%	Fasting
Sulfonylureas[2]	1–2%	Fasting and PPG (high risk of hypoglycemia)
Thiazolidinedione[3]	0.5–1.4%	Fasting and PPG
DPP-4 Inhibitor[4]	0.5–0.8%	PPG and fasting
GLP-1 Agonist[4]	0.5–1.6%	PPG and fasting
SGLT2 inhibitor[5]	0.7–1.0%	PPG and fasting
Meglitinides, phenylalanine derivatives[2]	1–1.5%	PPG (risk of hypoglycemia)
α-Glycosidase inhibitor[6]	0.5–0.8%	PPG

[1]Suppress hepatic glucose production; [2]Insulin secretagogue; [3]Peroxisome proliferator–activated receptor (PPAR) activation; [4]Incretin system; [5]Glucose reuptake inhibitor; [6]Inhibit carbohydrate digestion in stomach.

Note: DPP-4 = dipeptidyl peptidase IV; GLP-1 = glucagon-like polypeptide 1; PPG = postprandial plasma glucose; SGLT2 = sodium-dependent glucose transporter two.

or using a contraindicated therapy. For example, a resident currently has been prescribed a thiazolidinedione and a sulfonylurea because metformin had been discontinued due to severe gastric side effects or liver impairment. In this case, the resident's A1C is 9.8%, with the desired target A1C of <8%. An A1C reduction of at least 1.8% is needed with the therapy choices limited to a glucagon-like polypeptide 1 (GLP-1) agonist, meglitinides, or a sodium-dependent glucose transporter two (SGLT2) inhibitor. Use of meglitinides, however, would be contraindicated because of duplication of the current therapy with the sulfonylurea, because both medications are insulin secretagogues. The SGLT2 inhibitor would at best yield a 1% decrease, and the GLP-1 agonist would at best bring the A1C down to only 8.2%. Therefore, the only option that would bring the A1C <8% would be insulin therapy (see Table 10.1; see also Figure 10.1).

Monitoring for Effectiveness

Although all glucose-lowering agents will reduce a resident's A1C, they do so by varying amounts, by different mechanisms of action, and by affecting daily finger-stick results to different degrees at different times. The A1C is only a marker of overall glucose control and should not be used as the only measure of evaluating effectiveness of therapy

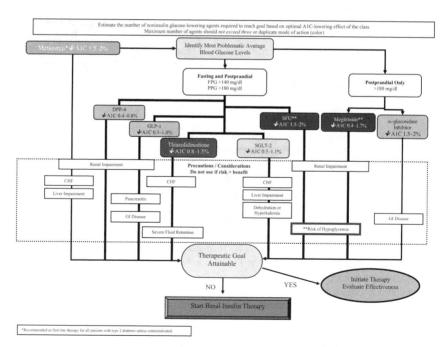

Figure 10.1 Targeted T2D Therapies Decision Tree.

Evaluating the effectiveness of any given therapy depends on monitoring those blood glucose levels most affected by the therapies being used. Doing so enables prescribers to adjust or add therapy to target out-of-target glucose levels. For example, metformin's primary effect is to reduce hepatic glucose production. Therefore, therapy effectiveness should be determined by evaluating fasting blood glucose control. Conversely, meglitinides primarily affect postprandial glucose levels, and therefore postmeal blood glucose levels need to be monitored to evaluate the effectiveness. Other agents affect both and would require measurements of multiple glucose levels to determine effectiveness (Table 10.1).

Avoiding hypoglycemia is a primary and often-overwhelming concern when treating the elderly, yet only three therapies present a risk of hypoglycemia. They are sulfonylureas, meglitinides and insulin. As a rule, sulfonylureas (as a class) present the most significant risk of hypoglycemia in the elderly because of their excessive use and persistent stimulation of insulin secretion from the pancreas. In other words, these agents place the resident at risk for hypoglycemia during times when lower amounts of insulin production are required, such as during the night. Yet nocturnal blood glucose testing is seldom ordered. Serious thought should be given to using such high-risk therapy when lower risk alternatives are available. On the basis of the Beers criteria,[3] glyburide is no longer recommended for use in the elderly, and many prescribers are avoiding the use of sulfonylureas entirely. Regardless of the therapies chosen, glucose monitoring should be targeted to evaluate therapeutic effects as well as hypoglycemic risk time, if warranted by the therapy used, but once glucose levels have been stabilized and maintained within an appropriate target range, the number of finger-sticks may be reduced. If glucose levels do not stabilize and repeated episodes of hyper- or hypoglycemia continue to occur, these occurrences should be considered to be an indication for therapy adjustment or change.

When It Is Time To Go to Insulin

Having determined that a resident's blood glucose levels can no longer be controlled using noninsulin therapy, the next step is to add insulin. Unfortunately, traditional insulin such as neutral protamine Hagedorn (NPH) and regular insulin, and their less-than-ideal peaks and durations of action, have made us leery of hypoglycemia. Take for example the entrenched behavior of having or providing a snack at bedtime. This "diabetes rule" first came about as a result of the use of sulfonylurea-type medications causing nocturnal hypoglycemia and then by the use of insulin, such as NPH, that often had peak activity occurring during the night, or at times when food consumption did not occur, and thus insulin requirements are less. Fortunately, options now are available with minimal risk of nocturnal hypoglycemia. Residents with diabetes, however, often are being given snacks that increase the blood glucose before they go to sleep, whether they need them or not. Needing snacks, it should be pointed out, is usually an indication to change therapy to avoid the hypoglycemia the snacks are intended to treat.

Appropriate insulin therapy starts with understanding normal insulin physiology. Simply put, the body produces a given amount of insulin each day, ~50% of which provides the baseline amount of insulin the body needs to maintain euglycemia during the fasting state. Because the amount of basal insulin produced is relatively constant, we easily can mimic the effect by using insulin that is relatively peakless, such as insulin glargine or insulin detemir.

Adding basal insulin and titrating to its most effective dose improves glucose control by providing for the body's basic insulin requirements during the fasting state and is independent of food consumption. It should be given regardless of the resident's eating. This is why most hospitals now utilize basal insulin over traditional regular, NPH, or premix insulin. Even in instances in which a resident requires doses of SSI, when basal insulin is added and titrated until fasting blood glucose is stabilized to target levels, the need for SSI doses diminishes, especially when residents are not eating.

Mealtime insulin requirements on the other hand vary from meal to meal depending on how a resident eats. Physiologic insulin production at meals is glucose mediated so the pancreas produces exactly the amount of insulin needed to handle the glucose increase associated with the amount of carbohydrate consumed and digested. To mimic this meal-associated insulin response, and further reduce or eliminate SSI insulin use, some fundamental changes are needed in current beliefs about dosing insulin at meals. The following may be helpful in changing beliefs:

1. A dose of rapid-acting insulin given for a meal is for the *meal*. It is needed to handle the subsequent carbohydrate-induced rise in blood glucose regardless of the blood glucose level before the meal.

2. Blood glucose levels taken before the meal should be used to determine whether a correction dose of insulin is needed to bring blood glucose levels back into target range. This correction (plus or minus) then is added to the meal insulin dose.

   For example: a resident is prescribed 5 units of rapid-acting insulin daily at lunch, but today the blood glucose reading before lunch is elevated, and the prescriber has indicated the resident should be given 2 additional units. In this case, the meal dose is still 5 units and the correction dose is 2 units, for a total of 7 units given.

3. If corrections are required routinely at any given meal or at bedtime, the preceding meal's prescribed insulin dose needs to be adjusted (revised) by the number of units on average required for the correction. Making these adjustments ultimately leads to more accurate dosing of rapid-acting insulin at meals and fewer corrections being required overall, which has an added benefit of possibly reducing the number of finger-sticks required if blood glucose levels stabilize.

4. Administering rapid-acting insulin doses *after* the meal is preferable when consumption is unpredictable. This allows for adjustments to the dose based on consumption, rather than giving the dose before a meal and risking hypoglycemia if the resident does not eat, or not giving insulin and waiting until blood glucose levels become hyperglycemic to give SSI doses.

Optimal glucose control without hypoglycemia requires insulin therapy that mimics normal physiology as closely as possible. To choose the right insulin, there needs to be a basic understanding of the advantages and disadvantages of each form of insulin with respect to its onset of action, peak, and duration of activity.

In other words, when the peaks in activity and duration of action do not match the physiologic need, the result will be wide fluctuations in glucose, both high and low.

The use of basal insulin with little to no peaking effect and more steady-state activity allows us to appropriately match physiologic insulin requirements during the fasting state and has made initiation of insulin therapy in the resident T2D a relatively straight-forward process. This lack of peaking activity means that basal insulin has little to no effect on meals and can be given regardless of whether or not the resident eats with no significant risk for hypoglycemia compared with NPH predecessors.

On the other hand, rapid-acting insulin can be used to focus peaks of glucose-lowering activity when they are needed most. That is, preventing glucose levels from raising because of meals with much more predictable responses. Rapid-acting insulin dosing also offers greater flexibility than traditional regular insulin in that its rapid onset and relatively short duration of action makes it ideal for use at meals (see Table 10.2).

Table 10.2 Properties of Insulin

	Onset	Duration	Glucose change
Physiologic endogenous meal response	Immediate*	1–3 hours*	<40 mg/dl
Injected insulin given at start of meal			
Rapid-acting insulin	5–10 minutes	Most active in first 3 hours	Individualized response
Regular given at meal	30–90 minutes	≥6 hours	Initial hyperglycemia due to digestion with delayed insulin response followed by high risk of hypoglycemia 3–6 hours after meal
Physiologic endogenous basal (fasting state)	Continuous	Relative steady state (less nocturnal)	None
Glargine	Steady state	Steady state	Minimal
Detemir	3–5 hours	Dose dependent 5.7–23 hours	Minimal once titrated
NPH	2–4 hours; peak 4–10 hours	10–18 hours	Unpredictable glucose lowering effect, high risk of hypoglycemia

Note: NPH = neutral protamine Hagedorn.

*Depending on carbohydrate content of the meal.

Insulin glulisine and insulin lispro have the advantage of being indicated for dosing after meals, which gives an additional option of withholding the mealtime insulin dose if the resident does not eat or adjusting the dose based on actual carbohydrate consumption. Because the onset of action of rapid-acting insulin is within minutes and its duration of action on average is only 3–4 hours, this type of insulin more closely matches normal digestion time even when given after the meal is consumed. Unfortunately, the rapid onset and short duration of action also means rapid-acting insulin is not medication-pass friendly. Administering a dose of rapid-acting insulin during a premeal medication pass, when the food has not arrived or the resident has not started to eat, is an invitation for severe hypoglycemia. Rapid-acting insulin needs to be considered prandial insulin, always given with a meal to handle the rise in glucose associated with a meal. The exception to this rule would be when a dose of rapid-acting insulin is needed to correct an out-of-target blood glucose reading. Correction doses of rapid-acting insulin can be added to the prandial dose to bring an occasional high-premeal reading back down to target or these doses may be given by themselves at other times when a previous dose of rapid-acting insulin is past its duration of action, such as at bedtime. However, extreme caution should be used giving correction insulin at bedtime as this insulin will be peaking during the night, when the resident is sleeping. Corrections given at bedtime should only provide enough units of rapid-acting insulin to bring blood glucose levels down to <180 mg/dl, thus eliminating the hyperglycemia with minimal risk of hypoglycemia during the night.

Routine use of correction doses, however, is an indication that the previous dose of rapid-acting insulin needs to be adjusted so the need for correction doses is reduced or eliminated (Figure 10.2).

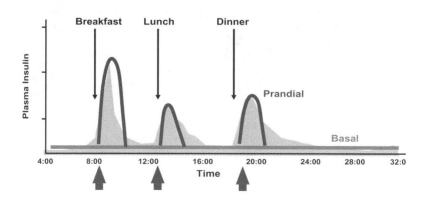

Figure 10.2 Insulin Dosing Profile Superimposed on Endogenous Insulin Profile (Shaded Area).

Source: Adapted from White JR Jr, et al. *Postgraduate Medicine* 2003;113:30–36.

Starting Insulin in the Resident with T2D

An appropriate protocol can help eliminate most of the barriers to utilizing a new insulin therapy approach. Protocols help streamline the order process across prescribers, provide for timely titration without unnecessary phone calls to prescribers, allow for more dosing flexibility, which can minimize both hyper- and hypoglycemic episodes, and most importantly, improve glucose control in accordance with current standards of care. Understanding the basics of initiating physiologic insulin therapy will make adoption of new insulin protocols easier.

Unlike conventional insulin therapies, starting physiologic insulin in the resident with T2D can be accomplished using a straight-forward stepwise approach. This simply involves adding basal insulin to the current noninsulin therapy, titrating to goal, and then starting mealtime rapid-acting insulin if needed. Before discussing titration, it is important to be familiar with the differences between the two basal insulin currently available.

Key Issues Comparing Insulins Glargine and Detemir

	Insulin glargine	Insulin detemir
Dosing	Once daily	1–2 times per day.
Duration of action	24 hour	5.7–23 hours (dose dependent).
Mode of action	Precipitates upon injection with slow release over 24 hours	Highly protein bound to albumin.

Insulin detemir and insulin glargine and new biosimilar insulin should not be considered equivalent and therefore interchangeable dose per dose. Insulin detemir for example is highly protein bound with a dose-dependent duration of action and therefore may require more than once-daily dosing as well as a significantly larger number of units per daily than insulin glargine.[9]

Adding basal insulin and then titrating to its most effective dose improves glucose control by providing for the body's insulin requirements during the fasting state, which is for the most part independent of food consumption. This is why most hospitals now utilize basal insulin over traditional regular, NPH, or premixed insulin. Even in those instances in which a resident requires doses of rapid-acting insulin to correct for episodic hyperglycemia (sliding scale) when basal insulin is added and titrated appropriately, the blood glucose tends to stabilize and the need for sliding correction doses diminishes, especially when residents are not eating.

Starting Basal. Several methods of titration have been suggested for basal insulin. Each has distinct advantages and disadvantages that should be assessed before determining which protocol to use. The ADA and the European Association for the Study of Diabetes (EASD) suggest starting with 10 units and increasing the dose by 2 units every third day until fasting blood glucose levels are <100 mg/ dl. Hospitals often start physiologic insulin by estimating total insulin requirements using a weight-based calculation of 0.4–1 units/kilogram (u/kg) depending on patient type and current blood glucose levels. Half of the calculated daily requirement is given as basal insulin and the other half is given as rapid-acting insulin distributed across meals if the patient is eating. Adjustments to the doses then are made on a daily basis, using large unit adjustments to improve control quickly. Many prescribers in LTC feel these types of titrations are too aggressive for the frail elderly, especially targeting fasting blood glucose <100 mg/dl. The American Medical Directors Association recommends the following in their Diabetes Clinical Practice Recommendations for Long-Term Care.

Key Issues General AMDA Recommendations

Option 1

- Give 10 units of basal insulin once daily.
- Titrate q (every) third day or weekly until fasting blood glucose is in the target range.
- Add rapid-acting insulin before meals based on need.

Option 2

- Give 10 units of basal once daily.
- Titrate up q third day or weekly until bedtime and fasting glucose are about equal (regardless of level).
- Then add rapid-acting insulin at evening meal.
- Titrate until bedtime glucose is in the target range.
- Then add rapid-acting insulin at breakfast and lunch if needed.

Physiologic basal insulin represents ~50% of the total daily insulin requirement. The other 50% is in the form of insulin produced to handle prandial glucose increases associated with normal total daily carbohydrate intake. Because physiologic basal insulin production is a relatively steady state regardless of whether or not the resident is fasting, doses of injected-basal insulin should be given regardless of eating status. Basal insulin should *not* be expected to cover peaks in glucose associated with meals because glucose levels rise quickly after consumption of carbohydrates, and insulin administered to cover these glucose elevations should have a limited duration, which basal insulin does not provide. During the titration process for basal insulin, adjustments are based on fasting blood glucose levels, mealtime glucose increases are not considered. For example, if a resident is experiencing significant hyperglycemia after meals, they might have significant hyperglycemia at bedtime and subsequently through to morning. If the basal insulin dose is increased enough to reduce bedtime hyperglycemic blood glucose to target by morning (an 8-hour time period), at meals the resident still will experience episodes of hyperglycemia; however, the resident also may have significant risk of hypoglycemia because of the excess basal insulin continually reducing blood glucose over time when meals are only intermittent.

One way to avoid over titration of insulin glargine is to monitor bedtime and fasting blood glucose levels during the basal titration period. Titration should stop and the current dose should be maintained when fasting blood glucose levels reach goal *or* when bedtime blood glucose is approximately equal to the fasting blood glucose, regardless of the level. Basal insulin when dosed correctly should *maintain* blood glucose during the fasting state (overnight) through suppression of hepatic glucose production. Therefore, when bedtime blood glucose levels are approximately equal to fasting blood glucose levels, the basal dose being administered would appear to be appropriate. If glucose levels at bedtime and fasting are equal to but not at goal, this is an indication the resident may need mealtime insulin doses. Initiating mealtime insulin then will improve bedtime glucose levels and the same basal insulin dose should now maintain the better bedtime blood glucose levels through the night. Figures 10.3 and 10.4 provide a simplified order for this process, using insulin glargine (Figure 10.3) and insulin detemir (Figure 10.4), respectively.

If insulin detemir is used, blood glucose testing also should include a pre-evening meal blood glucose test to evaluate the need for an additional dose of insulin detemir in the morning to provide full basal coverage. If so, both doses should be titrated until bedtime and fasting glucose levels stabilize. If readings are approximately equal to but above goal, the addition of rapid-acting insulin at meals should be considered (Figure 10.5).

Incorporating the principles of physiologic insulin therapy into prescribing may appear to be challenging, given the need for resident-specific insulin dosing, and the wide range of prescribing currently seen in LTC. Protocols and orders that are both standardized and yet flexible enough allow to for prescriber preferences are essential. Adjustments of mealtime doses can be done on a dose-per-dose basis if the process is simple, consistent, and resident specific and if it is based on the physiologic needs of the resident. This includes adjustments of doses for carbohydrate consumption as well as out of target glucose levels. Because the use of SSI is now considered inappropriate therapy and carbohydrate counting is considered to be too complicated, the question becomes how can meal-to-meal dose adjustments be made safely? Doing so involves three basic principles:

1. A dose of insulin should be prescribed for each meal based on the average prescribed carbohydrate for that meal and not just the blood glucose before the meal.
2. A resident's insulin sensitivity must be determined to allow for the dose to be adjusted when glucose levels are out of target.
3. A simplified protocol must be provided to allow for dose adjustments based on the amount of food consumed. This requires dosing of the prandial insulin *after* the meal rather than before.

All three principles can be incorporated easily into a single order (Figure 10.6). First, the prescribed dose of rapid-acting insulin at each meal should follow physiologic principles. If glargine is used as the basal insulin, then the total daily insulin dose (TDD) of rapid-acting insulin should be approximately equal to the glargine dose with the distribution of the rapid-acting insulin equal to the

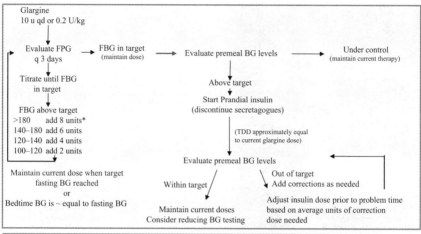

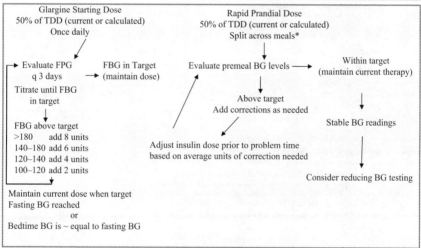

*May be given after meals and withheld if NPO
Note: This titration algorithm was not developed for frail elderly or for residents in LTC.
Starting weight based total daily dose (TDD) insulin requirements:
- 0.3 u/kg (0.14 u/lb.) body wt. for underweight or very physically active
- 0.5 u/kg (0.23 u/lb.) body wt. for normal wt. minimal physical activity
- 0.8 u/kg (0.36 u/lb.) body wt. for obese, minimally physical activity

Source: Adapted from Leahy JL, Cefalu WF, Eds. *Insulin Therapy.* New York, NY, Marcel Dekker, Inc., 2002.

Figure 10.3 Starting Glargine Insulin Therapy in LTC.

percentage of carbohydrate distribution across meals. For example, if a resident requires 30 units of insulin glargine per day, the resident should require ~30 units of rapid-acting insulin per day as well. The prescribed distribution is shown in Table 10.3.

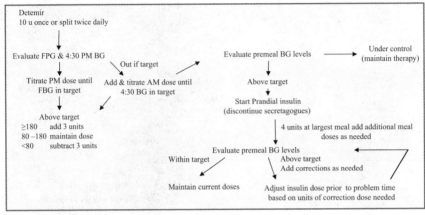

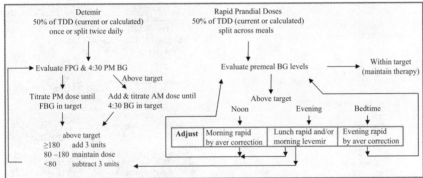

Note: Starting weight–based total daily dose (TDD) insulin requirements:
- 0.3 u/kg (0.14 u/lb.) body wt. for underweight or very physically active
- 0.5 u/kg (0.23 u/lb.) body wt. for normal wt. minimal physical activity
- 0.8 u/kg (0.36 u/lb.) body wt. for obese, minimally physical activity

Source: Adapted from Leahy JL, Cefalu WF, Eds. *Insulin Therapy.* New York, NY, Marcel Dekker, Inc., 2002.

Figure 10.4 Starting Detemir Insulin Therapy in LTC.

Insulin detemir may require a higher dose to maintain the same A1C reduction as insulin glargine. For this reason the 50:50 rule of basal versus meal insulin may not be applicable if insulin detemir has been prescribed, and dosage and administration adjustments always should be considered when switching between any basal insulin. To avoid the potential risk of hypoglycemia associated with too large a dose of rapid-acting insulin being used at meals, prandial insulin can be started with a low dose starting with the largest meal of the day and then titrate up based on response. Additional doses then would be added to the other meals as needed. The other option is to do a weight-based calculation of the resident's insulin requirements and then give 50% of the calculated TDD as rapid-acting insulin, distributed across the meals (Table 10.3).

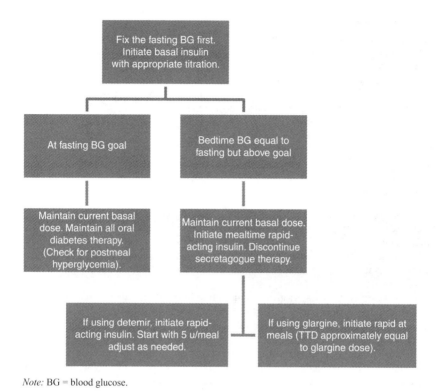

Note: BG = blood glucose.

Figure 10.5 Steps in Initiating Basal Insulin.

Table 10.3 Example of Distribution of Daily Carbohydrate Intake, Prescription

Meal	Percent of daily carbohydrate in meal plan	Insulin dose
Breakfast	30%	10 units (30% of TDD of rapid-acting insulin)
Lunch	40%	15 units (40% of TDD of rapid-acting insulin)
Supper	20%	5 units (20% of TDD of rapid-acting insulin)
Large snacks	10%	3 units (10% of TDD of rapid-acting insulin)*

Note: If snacks require <3 units of insulin, insulin doses may be omitted if glucose levels do not increase significantly. TDD = total daily dose.

*In general, correction insulin should not be given at bedtime, because of the potential for hypoglycemia during the night. If bedtime glucose is elevated and still high the next morning, correction insulin may be added to the prebreakfast dose.

When glucose levels are occasionally *not* in target, then supplemental doses of rapid-acting insulin are required to bring the glucose level back under control as quickly as possible, regardless of the cause. Supplemental dosing involves estimating corrective doses based on the resident's individual insulin sensitivities. To determine the resident's insulin sensitivity, simply determine their current TDD of insulin and divide this into 1,500. For example, a resident using 50 units/ day of insulin would have a calculated insulin sensitivity of 30 (1,500 / 50 = 30). This means they should require 1 extra unit of rapid-acting insulin for every 30 mg/ dl their blood glucose is above target. If their glucose levels were below target, then withholding 1 unit from the prescribed dose should allow the blood glucose to raise 30 mg/dl. Dose adjustment charts based on insulin sensitivities that are similar to traditional SSI dosing charts can make adding correction doses to the prescribed dose easy to incorporate (Figure 10.6).

Sliding-Scale Insulin (SSI) Versus Correction Insulin. The use of SSI dosing has been discouraged by AMDA, ADA, American Association of Clinical Endocrinologists (AACE), and AGS for some time. Yet one study indicated that 84% of residents entering a facility from an acute hospital setting on SSI, remain on it for the duration of their stay in SNFs and >50% of all residents using insulin have sliding-scale orders.[10]

Although SSI has been around since insulin was discovered, it has never had the science to support its use. In fact, data overwhelmingly support no improvement in glucose control, longer hospital stays, and increased risk of hypoglycemia with its use.[11] For these reasons, SSI is now included on the AGS Beers list and is considered inappropriate therapy for the elderly.[12] It can be argued that any dose of insulin that is based on a blood glucose level is simply a sliding scale, regardless of what you call it. How insulin corrections are used actually determines whether or not the dose should be considered sliding scale. If a dose of insulin is always and only dependent on blood glucose readings, then you are using a sliding scale. If on the other hand, the prescribed doses of rapid-acting insulin given for meals are occasionally supplemented or decreased to bring blood glucose readings back

☐ Low dose correction algorithm (patients/residents requiring less than 40 units of insulin/day)		☐ Medium-dose correction algorithm (patients/residents requiring 40 – 80 units of insulin/day)	
Pre-meal glucose (mg/dl)	**Additional insulin (units)**	**Pre-meal Glucose (mg/dl)**	**Additional insulin (units)**
150 – 199	1	150 – 199	1
200 – 249	2	200 – 249	3
250 – 299	3	250 – 299	5
300 – 349	4	300 – 349	7
Greater than 349	5	Greater than 349	8
☐ High-dose correction algorithm (patients/residents requiring 40 units of insulin/day)		☐ Individual correction algorithm	
Pre-meal glucose (mg/dl)	**Additional insulin (units)**	**Pre-meal glucose (mg/dl)**	**Additional insulin (units)**
150 – 199	2	150 – 199	
200 – 249	4	200 – 249	
250 – 299	7	250 – 299	
300 – 349	10	300 – 349	
Greater than 349	12	Greater than 349	

Figure 10.6 Correction Insulin Algorithms.

into a given target range, this is a correction. When corrections continually are being made to prescribed doses of insulin at meals over extended periods of time without a valid reason, this practice could be considered a sliding scale. Use of sliding-scale insulin is no longer considered an acceptable practice, and dose reductions with eventual discontinuation should begin as soon as possible to reduce the potential risk of an inappropriate therapy F-Tag during survey.[13]

There are, and always will be, circumstances in which it is necessary and valid to give correction doses of insulin to bring blood glucose levels back into the target range. These include infections, short-term or high-dose tapering steroid therapy, and consumption of high-calorie foods not part of the meal plan. Because all of these situations are temporary in nature, you would not want to make permanent adjustments to fixed doses of insulin. At some point, the condition will resolve and insulin requirements will decrease, thus leading to increased risk for hypoglycemia. When correction doses are needed routinely without a definitive temporary cause, the prescribed mealtime dose for the preceding meal should be adjusted by the average correction being used to stabilize the glucose fluctuations and eliminate the need for routine corrections.

Last, adjusting prandial insulin doses based on carbohydrate consumption can be somewhat more challenging, because it will require some changes in protocol for both dosing insulin after meals and for documenting consumption. In this case, consumption records should indicate the percentage of carbohydrate consumed from the meal rather than the percentage of the total meal consumed. Although some hospitals and a few LTC facilities have moved to a carbohydrate-counting protocol to determine prandial insulin doses, this still is considered too complicated for the average SNF.

Use of traditional documentation of total meal consumption to adjust insulin doses can result in less accurate insulin dosing, leading to glucose fluctuations, because the dose of rapid-acting insulin required for a meal is affected minimally by the amount of protein and nonstarch vegetables consumed. Ideally, the chart should indicate how the resident is eating in terms of carbohydrate compared with protein and vegetables. In addition to more detailed documentation forms, an in-service presentation and training by the facility's dietitian or a certified diabetes educator on carbohydrate recognition is recommended for anyone involved in documenting consumption or dosing insulin.

It is important to make the adjustment protocol practical by using a simple algorithm for adjusting the prescribed mealtime insulin dose based on consumption. This can be accomplished using protocols as shown in Table 10.4.

An example of a documentation system is shown in Figure 10.7.

1. Blood Glucose
   Blood glucose reading
   (may be documented by any qualified staff member before the meal).
2. Correction Dose
   Insulin dose adjustment needed to bring glucose back to target (+ or –)
   (determined by medication nurse when injection is given).
   (Current BG – Target BG) ÷ Correction Factor,
   or dose from a chart provided by the prescriber.

Table 10.4 Mealtime Insulin Based on Percentage of Carbohydrate Consumed

Approximate percent of meal carbohydrate consumed	Prescribe meal dose adjustment
100%	Give full prescribed dose
75%	Give 75% of prescribed dose
50%	Give 50% of prescribe dose
25%	Give 25% of prescribed dose
<25%	Hold dose

3. Percentage of Carbohydrate Consumed
   Amount of carbohydrate for meal consumed
   (determined and documented by staff member documenting consumption).
   Should be documented as >75%, 50%, < 25%.
4. Meal Dose
   Insulin dose needed for percentage of meal's carbohydrates consumed
   (determined by medication nurse when injection is given).
   Documented as follows:

   a. >75% = full prescribed dose,
   b. 50% = half of prescribed dose,
   c. <25% = withhold prescribed dose.

5. Total Dose
   Insulin dose given to resident
   (documented by medication nurse at the time of injection).
   (Meal dose ± any correction required.)

After a few days or at the end of the week, the prescriber can take this single document and quickly assess the resident's eating, insulin dosing, and blood glucose control. He or she then should be able to quickly determine the average correction insulin dose being given per meal and adjust the previous meal's prescribed dose by the average correction being used. For example, if over a week's time, an average of 2 extra units of insulin is needed at lunch because glucose levels are consistently above goal, then the breakfast prescribed dose of insulin should be increased by 2 units. Once blood glucose levels are stabilized and corrections are no longer needed, blood glucose testing may be able to be reduced to twice daily (morning and supper one day, lunch and bedtime the next). This testing reduction is possible because the prandial doses of insulin are for the meal, not the blood glucose and because corrections are not required, and insulin doses need not be adjusted, other than based on consumption that is independent of premeal glucose levels.

In addition to providing for dosage adjustments for consumption and blood glucose levels, this type of protocol also makes transition away from sliding-scale dosing possible after a relatively short period of time as is recommended by

Glucose/Insulin Dose Tracking Form

Patient _____ **WEEK Starting** ___ / ___ / ___ **Correction Factor** **1 unit per** _____ **mg/dl**

Carbohydrate/meal: B _____ **L** _____ **D** _____

DAY	Fasting Prescribed Insulin Dose ___				Lunch Prescribed Insulin Dose ___				Dinner Prescribed Insulin Dose ___				Bedtime	
	BG	% Carb Consumed	Meal Dose	Correction Dose	BG	% Carb Consumed	Meal Dose	Correction Dose	BG	% Carb Consumed	Meal Dose	Correction Dose	BG	Correction Dose
SUN														
MON														
TUE														
WED														
THU														
FRI														
SAT														
Average														

Note: BG = blood glucose.

Figure 10.7 Example Documentation System to Record Insulin Given and Percent of Carbohydrate Eaten.

AMDA. Use of insulin pen devices (discussed earlier in Chapters 5 and 9) rather than traditional vials and syringes also may help to improve efficiency, decrease nursing time, and potentially reduce dosing errors. Unlike vials, however, the rule for any medication pen device is *one pen, one resident*. A single pen should *never* be used for multiple residents.

Physiologic insulin therapies should not be considered too complicated or time consuming to implement. They initially do require more insulin dose adjusting by nursing staff and standardized orders that allow it. Using a physiologic approach to insulin, however, should be seen as a win-win situation because of the following:

- It improves quality of life for the resident.
- It improves adherence to established clinical recommendations and it improves quality indicators such as dehydration associated with hyperglycemia.
- It decreases weight loss and improves healing, all of which are a focus in the State Operations Manual.
- It provides more predictability and decreases episodes of both hyper- and hypoglycemia requiring extensive nursing time or readmission to acute care hospitals and reduces the need for phone calls to prescribers.

REFERENCES

1. U.S. Census Bureau. Available at http://www.census.gov/acs/www/. Accessed 13 February 2014.
2. American Diabetes Association: Standards of medical care for residents with diabetes. *Diabetes Care* 2014;37(Suppl 1):S14–S80.
3. American Geriatrics Society. Available at www.americangeriatrics.org/files/documents/beers/2012BeersCriteria_JAGS.pdf. Accessed 13 February 2014.
4. Yu CH, Sun XH, Nisenbaum R, Halapy H. Insulin order sets improve glycemic control and processes of care. *Am J Med.* 2012 Sep;125(9):922–928.e4.
5. Kirkman MS, et al. Diabetes in older adults. *Diabetes Care* 2012;35:2650–2664.
6. Inzucchi, SE, et. Al. Management of hyperglycemia in type 2 diabetes: A patient-centered approach: position statement of the American Diabetes Association (ADA) and the European Association for the Study of Diabetes (EASD). *Diabetes Care* 2012;35:1364–1379.
7. Bergenstal RM, Buse JB, et al. Management of hyperglycaemia in type 2 diabetes: a patient-centered approach. Position statement of the American Diabetes Association (ADA) and the European Association for the Study of Diabetes (EASD). *Diabetologia* 2012;55:1577–1596.
8. American Medical Directors Association. *Diabetes management in the long-term care setting clinical practice guideline.* Columbia, MD: AMD 2008, revised 2010.
9. Rosenstock, J, et al. A randomised, 52-week, treat-to-target trial comparing insulin detemir with insulin glargine when administered as add-on to glucose-lowering drugs in insulin-naive people with type 2 diabetes. *Diabetologia* 2008;51:408–416.

10. Pandya N, Thompson S, Sambamoorthi U. The prevalence and persistence of sliding scale insulin use among newly admitted elderly nursing home residents with diabetes mellitus. *Journal of the American Medical Directors Association* 2008;9(9):663–669.
11. MacMillan DR. The fallacy of insulin adjustment by the sliding scale. *Journal of the Kentucky Medical Association* 1970;68:577–579.
12. Fick D, Semla T, Beizer J,et al. American Geriatrics Society Updated Beers Criteria for Potentially Inappropriate medication use in older adults. Journal of the American Geriatrics Society 2012;doi, 10.1111/j.1532-5415.
13. Centers for Medicare and Medicaid Services. State operations manual: Appendix PP: Guidance to surveyors for long term care facilities. Available at https://www.cms.gov/Medicare/Provider-Enrollment-and-Certification/GuidanceforLawsAndRegulations/Downloads/som107ap_pp_guidelines_ltcf.pdf. Accessed 13 February 2014.

11

Monitoring

Linda B. Haas, PhC, RN, CDE

INTRODUCTION

M anagement of diabetes in long-term care (LTC) settings is usually complex.[1-3] To help ensure that these complex residents receive optimal diabetes care, careful monitoring is essential. This monitoring includes parameters such as glycemic control, blood pressure, kidney function, and lower extremity status. In addition, nutrition, hydration, and cognition status should be monitored. For this monitoring to be most effective, documentation of the observations and findings is vital so that residents' progress or deterioration can be tracked and interventions can be implemented in a timely manner. Documentation is critical to facilitate continuity of care and to help ensure residents' safety during transitions, such as admission, transfers to and from acute hospitals or the emergency room (ER), transfers within the LTC facility, change of providers, shift changes, and discharge from the LTC facility. Nutrition therapy in older adults and foot care are covered in Chapters 7 and 12, respectively; thus, this chapter will not deal with these aspects of long-term care. This chapter will address methods to monitor glycemic control, blood pressure, hydration, kidney function, and cognition, and review the importance of monitoring residents during transitions.

Glycemic Control

Once glycemic targets are determined (see Chapter 5), attainment of and deviations from these targets can be assessed using capillary blood glucose monitoring (CBGM) and A1C. CBGM enables staff and residents, if the residents are able and willing, to identify glycemic patterns. When using handheld monitors for CBGM, it is critical to use single-use, disposable finger-puncture devices (gauge 30 to prevent tissue damage) or for each resident to have his or her own personal device to prevent the spread of bloodborne illnesses, such as hepatitis.[4-6] Several factors can influence the accuracy of CBGM. These factors include high altitude, hematocrit, pH level, high oxygen level (such as seen in residents using oxygen therapy), sugars (such as may be in dialysates), hypertriglyceridemia, and acetaminophen.[7] Some handheld glucose monitors allow testing on sites other than the fingertip, called alternate site testing (AST). Using AST may be helpful for residents who are having frequent CBGM or who would prefer that their fingertips not be punctured so often. When using AST, however, there are several cautions of which to be aware. AST is accurate when blood glucose levels are stable, such as in the morning and before meals. AST is *not* accurate when blood glucose levels are changing, such as after eating and exercise. The fingertip and the pad of the palm nearest the thumb are the most accurate sites to use after eating and exercise. In addition, AST *never* should be used to assess for hypoglycemia; only the fingertip should be used if hypoglycemia is suspected.[8,9]

Frequency of CBGM. CBGM is used to identify blood glucose readings out of range, as well as glycemic patterns, to evaluate the medication regimen. Unfortunately, no data indicate the optimal frequency of CBGM in the LTC setting. *The Guide for Management of Diabetes in LTC*, however, does offer several practical suggestions.[10] This guide recommends standing orders for CBGM or a protocol based on each resident's diabetes treatment. This type of protocol can be individualized as indicated. The guide suggests the following for CBGM frequency:[10]

1. First week of admission:

   ■ Residents treated with insulin—CBGM four times daily, before meals and at bedtime
   ■ Residents treated with oral medicines (or noninsulin injections)—CBGM two times daily (vary times before meals and at bedtime)

2. Ongoing testing once stabilized, as ordered by clinician:

   ■ Residents treated with insulin—test two times daily (vary times before meals and at bedtime
   ■ Residents treated with oral medicines (or noninsulin injections)—test two times weekly (vary times before meals and at bedtime)

3. Increase CBGM during illness, surgery, high stress, or when staff detects a sudden change in the resident's condition

Furthermore, the frequency can be determined by residents' glycemic goals and response to treatment.

Use of CBGM Data. A major purpose of CBGM is to allow providers to identify residents' glycemic patterns. To identify glycemic patterns, legible documentation of the results is imperative. A frequent practice in LTC is to put 1 month of data on a single page. Although this practice may save space, it makes pattern identification difficult. CBGM results should be documented in a manner that facilitates glycemic pattern recognition. Chapter 2, Figure 2.1 gives an example of a form for 2-week documentation of CBGM, which facilitates pattern recognition. In addition to legible documentation of CBGM results, Figure 2.1 also has space for insulin doses, so that all staff caring for a resident treated with insulin can easily and quickly see the type and amount of insulin a resident has received and when it was given. (See also Figure 10.7.) This type of documentation allows staff to see the resident's response to the insulin. In addition, this documentation facilitates identification by the provider that a resident may be getting too many supplemental insulin doses and enables easier recognition that the baseline insulin dose may need to be changed. Documentation of CBGM also allows for identification of glucose levels out of the target range, so that action can be taken quickly and troubleshooting as to the possible causes can be initiated without delay. CBGM is a useful tool to help ensure resident safety, but it needs to be done at appropriate times, not done unnecessarily and, importantly, be documented in a way that allows this tool to be used by all staff in a timely manner.

Value of Capillary Blood Glucose Monitoring (CBGM)

- Guides therapeutic decisions
- Dependent on legibility
- Most valuable if documentation of CBGM combined with documentation of insulin is provided

---

Long-term glycemic control usually is monitored with the A1C test. Although no data support how frequently this test should be done in LTC, the recommendations of the California Healthcare Foundation/American Geriatrics Society Guidelines for Care seem reasonable.[11] These guidelines suggest that elders whose glycemic targets are not being met should have their A1Cs measured every 6 months or more frequently as indicated. Elders whose A1Cs have been stable for several years can have their A1Cs measured annually.

Blood Pressure Monitoring

Monitoring a resident's blood pressure can give staff information on the effectiveness of that resident's blood pressure medications as well as that resident's fluid status. There are scant data to indicate how often residents' blood pressure should be monitored. One study showed that residents with hypertension achieved acceptable blood pressure control, and readings were taken on an average of every 14 days (range 2–31 days).[12] Staff should keep in mind that residents with coronary artery disease have shown higher mortality rates at the low, as well as the high, blood pressure ranges.[13] Thus, if a resident's systolic blood pressure is <120 mmHg or diastolic blood pressure is <70 mmHg, more frequent blood pressure monitoring may be indicated.

If a resident seems dehydrated (see the following section) or becomes dizzy when standing up, orthostatic blood pressure monitoring is indicated. Up to 70% of the institutionalized elderly may have orthostatic hypotension.[14] Thus, monitoring this very common condition seems prudent and may help prevent falls and other comorbidities. Orthostatic hypotension is defined as a persistent reduction of systolic blood pressure at least 20 mmHg or diastolic blood pressure of 10 mmHg, within 3 minutes of standing or head-up tilt to at least 60 degrees on a tilt table.[14] There is an aging-associated impairment of the baroreflex, which normally helps maintain blood pressure with position change. In addition, residents with autonomic dysfunction, which is common in diabetes, may experience orthostatic hypotension after excessive nocturia or after meals.[15] Residents with orthostatic hypotension should sit before they stand, stand slowly, and hold on to a secure object when going from sitting to standing, and they should stand for a few moments before walking. Residents with orthostatic hypotension will benefit from using assistive devices for standing and walking.

Hydration

Hydration is an important factor to monitor, particularly for the frail elderly with diabetes. Dehydration occurs frequently and is a form of fluid–electrolyte imbalance. Dehydration is a serious condition in LTC facilities and can have many contributing causes, including decreased thirst sensation and lean body mass, and the functional renal decline associated with aging.[15] In addition, factors such as hot and humid weather, diarrhea, vomiting, and fever can contribute to dehydration. Functional factors, such as immobility, dysphagia, visual impairment, and incontinence also can cause dehydration.[16] In residents with diabetes, the osmotic diuresis related to hyperglycemia can cause dehydration, which in turn can lead to worsening hyperglycemia and even to a hyperosmolar hyperglycemic state, which can be fatal. Several estimates can be used to assess adequate fluid intake; a common one is 100 ml/kg for the first 10 kg, 50 ml/kg for the next 10 kg, and 15 ml/kg for any remaining kilograms.[17]

To estimate adequate hydration[17]

- 100 ml/kg for the first 10 kg
- 50 ml/kg for the next 10 kg
- 15 ml/kg for any remaining kilograms

Thus a resident who weighs 70 kg (154 lb) should consume ~1,065 ml (at least 1 quart [4 cups]) of fluid each day. Assessment for dehydration includes monitoring for skin tenting, concentrated urine, oliguria, sunken eyes, orthostatic hypotension, tachycardia, constipation, weight loss, and mental confusion.[16] The Illinois Council on Long Term Care has suggested a proactive approach to prevent dehydration in LTC residents.[18] The measures include routine monitoring for signs of dehydration and of residents' fluid consumption, with documentation of fluid intake in nursing notes. An accurate intake and output form also is helpful to monitor fluid status. Other suggested measures from the Illinois Council include the following:[18]

- Keep a list of residents at high risk for dehydration at strategic locations as a staff reminder for fluid monitoring.
- Establish hydration protocols to be used when fluid and electrolyte status is threatened.
- Schedule fluid administration at least three times a day between meals.
- Note residents' preferences for types and temperature of fluids.
- Leave easily accessible, filled, fresh water pitchers and glasses at the bedside. Supply straws and special glasses as indicated.
- Offer a full glass of water with medications; review medications to assess effect on hydration (e.g., diuretics).

■ Use a positive approach when offering fluids, rather than just asking if the resident wants fluids. For example, staff can say "here is your juice (or water)" or "would you like water or juice" instead of "would you like some water?"

Other measures to prevent or treat dehydration and subsequent orthostatic hypotension include exercising in a horizontal position, such as swimming or bed exercises (moving the feet up and down to activate the gastrocnemius [calf] muscle). Fitted elastic support hose or compression stockings may help increase venous return to the heart. To be effective, however, support hose or stockings must be worn all day.[15]

Some facility issues may contribute to residents' dehydration.[16] These include inadequate staffing, attitudes and beliefs of staff, inadequate positioning of cognitively and functionally impaired residents to facilitate safe drinking (i.e., not sitting them up), inadequate staff knowledge, and inadequate or incomplete documentation of food and fluid intake. As with estimating carbohydrate intake, LTC staff may benefit from education on the importance of hydration, how to identify at-risk residents, ways to estimate and encourage hydration, and correct documentation of fluid intake.

Kidney Status

Residents with diabetes are at high risk for chronic kidney disease (CKD), particularly if they have hypertension. In addition to diabetes and hypertension, other risk factors for CKD include age; obesity; family history; and African American, American Indian, and Hispanic ethnicity.[19]

Kidney function usually is monitored using the estimated glomerular filtration rate (eGFR) test and urine albumin. The eGFR is the preferred test for screening and monitoring kidney function.[20] Urine protein, however, also should be monitored as albuminuria (urine protein by dipstick trace positive or positive) has been associated with severe hypoglycemia in people with type 2 diabetes (T2D).[21] Table 11.1 was developed by the National Kidney Foundation to delineate CKD progression.[22]

Table 11.1 Classification of CKD by the National Kidney Foundation's Kidney Disease Quality Initiative

Stage	Description	GFR (ml/minute/1.73 m²)
1	Kidney damage with normal or increased GFR	>90
2	Kidney damage with mildly decreased GFR	60–90
3	Moderately decreased GFR	30–59
4	Severely decreased GFR	15–29
5	Kidney failure	<15 (dialysis)

Reprinted with permission from the National Kidney Foundation: NKF KDOQI Guidelines. Available from www.kidney.org/professionals/kdoqi/guidelines_ckd/p4_class_g1.htm. Accessed 18 March 2014.

If a resident has CKD, glycemic control to the resident's individualized target is very important, as is treating hypertension to target. There is evidence that treatment of hypertension in people with diabetes with an angiotensin-converting enzyme (ACE) inhibitor or angiotensin receptor blocker (ARB) may slow the progression of CKD,[20] particularly in people with Stages 1–3 CKD.[19] Residents treated with these medications should have kidney function and serum creatinine monitored within 1–2 weeks of starting therapy, every time the dose is increased, and then annually.[11] If further blood pressure treatment is indicated to reach goals, or if a resident has congestive heart failure, β-blockers are effective in reducing mortality.[19] Because the elderly may have poor tolerance for lowering blood pressure, antihypertensive medications should be introduced gradually to avoid complications. It is recommended to lower systolic blood pressure by 20 mmHg. If this lowering is tolerated, then the antihypertensive medication dose may be increased and the resident should be monitored. Glycemic and blood pressure control should be achieved with the least amount of risk to the resident (i.e., hypoglycemia and hypotension). In addition to hypertension treatment, people with Stages 1–3 CKD may benefit from treatment with statins, if they have dyslipidemia.[19]

Cognition

Cognitive impairment is an issue with many LTC residents and is more prevalent is residents with diabetes.[23] The causes of the increased cognitive impairment in residents with T2D are multifactorial and may be related to white matter abnormalities[24] and may progress more rapidly than in residents without diabetes.[25] The decreased cognition in diabetes can be manifested as decreased word and information processing speed, word recall, and executive functioning.[26] Executive function is the cognitive ability that enables other abilities and behaviors and is involved in goal-directed behavior. Importantly, both hyperglycemia[11] and hypoglycemia[27] can be associated with decreased cognition. Thus, prevention, recognition, and adequate treatment of these conditions may lessen or resolve the decreased cognition. In addition, cognitive impairment is associated with an increased incidence of severe hypoglycemia.[28] Thus, any resident who exhibits new or worsening decreased cognition should have their blood glucose levels monitored more closely, particularly those whose diabetes is being treated with insulin.

Cognitive impairment increases with increasing age, and cognitively impaired elders frequently have multiple other conditions.[29] Thus, it is reasonable to screen all residents with diabetes for cognitive impairment on admission, at least yearly thereafter, and with any change in their clinical status. Several tools can be used to screen for cognitive impairment.[30] A quick and easy tool is the Mini Mental State Examination (MMSE), which has questions about attention, orientation, memory, calculation, and language. The MMSE, however, has few questions related to executive function, which often is impaired in the elderly with diabetes. Other screening tools are the clock-drawing test and the clock-in-a box test. Several simple tools are available for screening older adults for cognitive dysfunction, functional status, and fall risk.[31] Because high and low blood glucose levels can be associated with fairly sudden changes in cognition, if there is a sudden change in cognition, blood glucose levels should be checked and treated if low, or diabetes medication should be adjusted if glucose levels are high Thus, any resident who exhibits new or worsening cognitive impairment should have their blood glucose levels monitored more closely.

Strategies for working with cognitively impaired residents with diabetes are the same as the strategies used for all cognitively impaired residents, except that monitoring for high and low blood glucose levels should be done more frequently. Address the cognitively impaired resident by name, identify yourself, and explain why you are there. It is helpful to use lay terminology when referring to what you are doing or going to do. For example, cognitively impaired residents may respond better to being told that their blood sugar is being tested versus being told that their blood glucose levels are being monitored. In addition, signals (cues) can aid memory and verbal analogies may be helpful. Use short sentences and focus on one thing at a time. In addition, cognitively impaired residents usually need more time to process what is happening. All regimens, including those for diabetes, should be as simple as possible. Glycemic targets should be geared toward preventing hyper- and hypoglycemia.

TRANSITIONS OF CARE

LTC residents are at high risk for adverse events during transitions of care and need particularly careful monitoring at these times. Transitions of care include initial admission to the facility, transfers within the LTC facility, for example, from one level of care to another, provider changes, transfers to and from acute care hospitals and ERs, and discharge from the facility to home or another facility.[32] Accurate and complete information transfer regarding the course of treatment, health status, and medications will help these transitions. Transitions can increase hospital readmissions and duplication of services, which causes unnecessary increased use of resources. In addition, these transitions are a major cause of medication errors. Often during transitions, it is difficult to identify the responsible provider, which causes a dilemma for "hands-on" staff. Information being transferred or received should be monitored for accuracy and completeness, and any inaccuracies or incompleteness identified should be remedied as soon as possible. Transitional care is defined as actions that ensure coordination and continuity of care and is based on a comprehensive care plan.[32]

When newly admitted residents have diagnosed diabetes, the current meal plan, activity level, medications, previous self-care education, self-care abilities, laboratory tests (including A1C), lipids, kidney function, hydration status, and previous episodes of hypoglycemia (including symptoms and ability to self-recognize and self- treat) should be identified. These parameters should be monitored over time to identify changes in the resident's status promptly and any need for regimen adaptions and changes.

On admission, all residents without identified diabetes should be screened to identify undiagnosed diabetes. In this way, residents may be newly diagnosed with diabetes when admitted to the LTC facility. It is important that these residents also are monitored closely as they are at high risk for complications of diabetes, particularly lower extremity complications requiring surgery, such as gangrene, debridement, and amputation.[33]

LTC residents are at high risk for unplanned readmissions to acute care hospitals within 30 days of discharge from these hospitals. One reason for this readmission is medication changes that are made upon admission to the acute-care hospital or on discharge, without notification of LTC staff.[32] Another issue is the lack of communication regarding course of treatment and response to treatment in the acute-care setting, as well as completed and pending laboratory tests.[34] Both the facility that is transitioning the resident and the facility that is receiving the resident should validate the transfer, identify discrepancies, and intervene in a timely manner. For residents with diabetes, continuance of sliding-scale insulin after admission or transfer back to the LTC facility is a long-standing problem.[35] The American Medical Directors Association (AMDA) recommends that sliding-scale insulin dosing be reviewed 1 week after admission to an LTC facility or when readmitted from an acute-care setting and be converted to basal or bolus insulin therapy (see Chapters 5 and 10). Accurate and complete written communication should also flow from LTC facilities to other institutions and ERs.

Continuity of Care

The need to monitor continuity of care is particularly acute when residents are admitted or transferred. The AMDA has several sample admission and transfer forms available for download.[36] *Transitions of Care in the Long-Term Care Continuum* is available for download free of charge from this site. Staff turnover is another issue that affects the continuity-of-care needs of these residents. LTC staff turnover is high, particularly in hands-on caregivers, so that continuity of care is affected adversely.[37] Systems, thorough documentation, and good staff communication, can help make up for this high turnover and help meet the needs of residents with diabetes. It is important to include the residents and their families in the communication loop.

CONCLUSION

Residents with diabetes in LTC facilities often have many comorbidities and present challenges to staff at all levels to provide appropriate and safe care. The structured environment of the LTC facility, however, provides an opportunity for careful monitoring and to facilitate monitoring of the many aspects of diabetes care.[38] This monitoring includes the same parameters as for all residents, and in addition, adds parameters specific to diabetes, such as glycemic control, particularly high and low blood glucose levels. In addition, because of their diabetes, carbohydrates and fluids must be monitored carefully. Documentation is a critical part of monitoring and can facilitate communication between and among staff to ensure residents' safety and prevent duplication of services and, thus, wasted resources. Many tools are available that can assist monitoring of these residents and facilitate communication among staff and in transfers. Several of these tools are online, are delineated in this book, and usually can be downloaded and used without cost.

REFERENCES

1. Gadsby R, Barker P, Sinclair AJ. People living with diabetes resident in nursing homes—assessing levels of disability and nursing needs. *Diabetic Medicine* 2011;28:778–780.
2. Van Rensbergen G, Nawrot T. Medical conditions of nursing home admissions. *BMC Geriatrics* 2010;10:46. doi: 10.1186/1471-2318-10-46
3. Travis SS, Buchanan RJ, Wang S, Kim M. Analyses of nursing home residents with diabetes at admission. *Journal of the American Medical Directors Association* 2004;5:320–327.
4. Centers for Disease Control and Prevention. Infection prevention during blood glucose monitoring and insulin administration. In Atlanta, GA, Centers for Disease Control and Prevention, 2012, p. 1–8.
5. Duffell EF, Milne LM, Seng C, Young Y, Xavier S, King S, Shukla H, Ijaz S, Ramsay M. Five hepatitis B outbreaks in care home in the UK associated with deficiencies in infection control practice in blood glucose monitoring. *Epidemiology and Infection* 2011;139:327–335.
6. Thompson ND, Barry V, Alelis K, Cui DP, Joseph F. Evaluation of the potential for bloodborne pathogen transmission associated with diabetes care practices in nursing homes and assisted living facilities, Pinellas County. *Journal of the American Geriatrics Society* 2010;58:914–918.
7. Lajara R, Magwire ML. Accuracy considerations for self-monitoring of blood glucose: Practical tools for primary care physicians. *Practical Diabetology* 2013;32:6–10,19–23.
8. Ellison JM, Stegmann JM, Colner SL, Michael RH, Sharma MK, Ervin KR, Horwitz DL. Rapid changes in postprandial blood glucose produce concentration differences at finger, forearm, and thigh sampling sites. *Diabetes Care* 2002;25:961–964.
9. Peled N, Wong D, Gwalani SL. Comparison of glucose levels in capillary blood samples obtained from a variety of sites. *Diabetes Technology and Therapeutics* 2002;4:35–44.
10. Nettles A, Laurel R. Managing diabetes in the resident. In *Diabetes management in long-term care facilities: A practical guide.* 6th edition. Nettles A, Laurel R (Eds). MN, Minnesota Department of Health, 2011, p. 35. Available at http://www.ltcdiabetesguide.org. Accessed 30 June 2013.
11. California Health Care Foundation/American Geriatric Society Panel on Improving Care for Elders with Diabetes, Guidelines for improving the care of the older person with diabetes mellitus. *Journal of the American Geriatrics Society* 2003;51:S265–S280.
12. Tsuyuki RT, McLean DL, McAlister F. Management of hypertension in elderly long-term care residents. *Canadian Journal of Cardiology* 2008;24:912–914.
13. Denardo SJ, Gong Y, Nichols WW, Messerti FH, Bavry AA, Cooper-DeHoff RM, Handberg E, Champion A, Pepine CJ. Blood pressure and outcomes in the very old hypertensive coronary artery disease patients: An INVEST substudy. *American Journal of Medicine* 2010;123:719–726.
14. Freeman R, Wieling W, Axelrod FB, Benditt DG, Benarroch E, Biaggioni I, Cheshire WP, Chelimsky T, Cortelli P, Gibbons CH, Goldstein DS,

Hainsworth R, Hilz MJ, Jacob G, Kaufmann H, Jordan J, Lipsitz LA, Levine BD, Low PA, Mathias C, Raj SR, Robertson D, Sandroni P, Schatz I, Schondoroff R, Stewart JM, van Dijk JG. Consensus statement of the definition of orthostatic hypotension, neurally mediated syncope and the postural tachycardia syndrome. *Clinical Autonomic Research* 2011;21:69–72.

15. Sclater A, Alagiakrishnan K. Orthostatic hypotension: A primary care primer for assessment and treatment. *Geriatrics* 2004;59:22–27.

16. Garcia ME. Dehydration of the elderly in nursing homes. In *Nutrition noteworthy*. Los Angeles, CA, University of California–Los Angeles, 2001, p. 1–6.

17. Gasper P. Water intake of nursing home residents. *Journal of Gerontological Nursing* 1999;25:23–29.

18. Illinois Council on Long Term Care, Family Resource Center. IL: Illinois Council on Long Term Care, 2012. Available at http://www.nursinghome. org/fam/fam_018.html. Accessed 20 July 2012.

19. Fink HA, Ishani A, Taylor BC, Greer NL, MacDonald R, Rossini D, Sadiq S, Lankireddy S, Kane RI, Wilt TJ. Chronic kidney disease stages 1–3: Screening, monitoring, and treatment. Comparative effectiveness, Review No. 37. Agency for Healthcare Research and Quality. Rockville, MD, Minnesota Evidence-based Practice Center, 2012. Available at www.effectivehealthcare. ahrq.gov/reports/final.cfm. Accessed 16 October 2012.

20. Solini A, Ferrannini E. Pathophysiology, prevention and management of chronic kidney disease in the hypertensive patient with diabetes mellitus. *Journal of Clinical Hypertension* 2011;13:252–257.

21. Yun J-S, Ko SH, Ko SH, Song K-H, Ahn Y-B, Yoon K-H, Park Y-M, Ko SH. Presence of macroalbuminuria predicts severe hypoglycemia in patients with type 2 diabetes: A 10-year follow-up study. *Diabetes Care* 2013;36:1283–1289.

22. Eknoyab G, Levin NW. Executive summary. In *NKF Kidney Disease Outcomes and Quality Initiative: Clinical practice guidelines for chronic kidney disease: Evaluation, classification and stratification.* Eknoyab G, Levin NW (Eds). New York, NY, National Kidney Foundation, 2002. p. 12. Available at https:// www.kidney.org/professionals/kdoqi/pdf/ckd_evaluation_classification_ stratification.pdf. Accessed 10 February 2014.

23. Zeyfang A, Watson JD. Perspectives on diabetes care in old age: A focus on frailty. In *Diabetes in old age.* 3rd ed. Sinclair AJ, Ed. London, England, John Wiley & Sons, 2009, p. 193–194.

24. Reijmer YD, Brundel M, de Bresser J, Kappelle LJ, Leemsns A, Biessels GJ. Microsomal white matter abnormalities and cognitive function in type 2 diabetes. *Diabetes Care* 2013;36:137–144.

25. Ravona-Springer R, Luo X, Schmeidler J, Wysocki M, Lesser G, Rapp M, Dahlman K, Grossman H, Haroutunian V, Beeri MS. Diabetes is associated with increased rate of cognitive decline in questionably demented elderly. *Dementia and Geriatric Cognitive Disorders* 2010;29:68–74.

26. Spauwen PJJ, Kohler S, Verhey FRJ, Stehouwer CDA, van Boxtel MPJ. Effect of type 2 diabetes on 12-year cognitive change: Results from the Maastricht aging study. *Diabetes Care* 2012;36:1554–1561.

27. Lekarcyk JA, Himmel L, Munshi MN. Blood glucose monitoring and underlying question of hypoglycemia are both essential to preventing hypoglycemia in nursing home residents. *Diabetes Spectrum* 2013;31:28–30.
28. Punthakee Z, Miller M, Launer L, ACCORD Group of Investigators; ACCORD-MIND Investigators. Poor cognitive function and risk of severe hypoglycemia in type 2 diabetes: Post hoc epidemiologic analysis of the ACCORD trial. *Diabetes Care* 2012;35:787–793.
29. Cigolle CT, Langa KM, Kabeto MU, Tian Z, Blaum CS. Geriatric conditions and disability: The health and retirement study. *Annals of Internal Medicine* 2007;147:156–164.
30. Munshi MN, Grande L, Hayes M, Ayres D, Suhi E, Capelson R, Lin S, Milberg W, Weinger K. Cognitive dysfunction is associated with poor diabetes control in older adults. *Diabetes Care* 2006;29:1794–1799.
31. Society of Hospital Medicine. Clinical toolbox for geriatric care. Available at www.hospitalmedicine.org/geriresource/toolbox/determine.htm. Accessed 30 June 2013.
32. Association of American Medical Directors. *Transitions of Care in the Long-Term Care Continuum Clinical Practice Guideline.* Columbia, MD, American Medical Directors Association, 2010.
33. Bethel MA, Sloan FA, Belsky D, Feinglos MN. Longitudinal incidence and prevalence of adverse outcomes of diabetes mellitus in elderly patients. *Archives of Internal Medicine* 2007;167:921–927.
34. Were MC, Li X, Kesterson J. Adequacy of hospital discharge summaries in documenting test with pending results and outpatient follow-up providers. *Journal of General Internal Medicine* 2009;24:1002–1006.
35. Pandya N, Thompson S, Sambamoorthi U. The prevalence and persistence of sliding scale insulin use among newly admitted elderly nursing home residents with diabetes mellitus. *Journal of the American Medical Directors Association* 2008;9:663–669.
36. American Medical Directors Association. Clinical practice guidelines in the long term care setting. Available at www.amda.com/tools/guidelines.cfm. Accessed 3 July 2014.
37. Donoghue C. Nursing home staff turnover and retention; An analysis of national level data. *Journal of Applied Gerontology* 2010;29:89–106.
38. Quinn CC, Gruber-Baldini AL, Port CL, Conrad M, Stuart B, Hebel R, Zimmerman S, Burton L, Zuckerman IH, Fahlman C, Magazziner J. The role of nursing home admission and dementia status on care for diabetes mellitus. *Journal of the American Geriatrics Society* 2009;57:1628–1633.

12

Foot Care in Long-Term Care

Jeffrey M. Robbins, DPM*

INTRODUCTION

As our population ages and more baby boomers reach retirement age, the number of residents in nursing homes and assisted-living facilities will increase dramatically. This increase will create an increasing need for health care providers to deal with the pedal manifestations of common chronic conditions present in this patient cohort. The principles of the patient-centered medical home require a new paradigm in how we manage this challenging population and these principles can apply to long-term care (LTC). This new paradigm may be especially true for residents with diabetes and other chronic degenerative diseases. The principles of the patient-centered medical home and how they may apply to LTC include the following:

1. Each patient has an ongoing relationship with a personal provider.
2. The patient's personal provider leads the health care team that takes collective responsibility for ongoing care for each patient.
3. The health care team arranges for all of the care needs for the patient during several stages of life: acute care, chronic care, preventive services, and end-of-life care.
4. Care is coordinated and integrated with the entire health care system.
5. There is an emphasis on quality and safety; evidence-based practice and clinical decision-support tools are used to guide decision making.
6. Enhanced access to care is available through systems changes.

Although most people would prefer to live in their own homes, in some cases, medical and psychosocial needs can no longer be met in the private home. Assisted care and LTC facilities provide a safe environment where health care demands can be met on a more consistent basis.[1] This chapter will focus on how to manage the foot health care needs of the patient with diabetes in an LTC facility or assisted-living environment.

Defining Foot Health in Residents with Diabetes

It is important to determine the level of risk for foot wounds, ulcers, and amputations in residents with diabetes. This determination usually is accomplished with an initial foot screening followed by a more in-depth physical examination. This examination should complement the full geriatric assessment, which helps to define the severity of systemic conditions (diabetes, heart disease, and

---

*Opinions expressed in the article are those of the author and do not reflect official positions or policies of the Department of Veterans Affairs.

DOI: 10.2337/9781580404730.12

cognitive dysfunction) and the psychosocial issues facing the patient and family. Several factors can lead to foot problems or compromise existing conditions, including the following:

1. Degree of ambulation
2. Balance
3. Limitation of activity
4. Previous institutionalizations
5. Episodes of social segregation
6. Previous care, including that of foot problems or conditions
7. Emotional adjustment to disease and current life situation
8. Multiple medications and drug interactions
9. The potential of previous neglect and abuse
10. Activities of daily living

Basic Foot Screening

An initial foot screening should be done as part of the admission assessment by the primary care provider or designee to determine the resident's foot risk and how soon a higher level examination should be conducted by a podiatrist. The initial foot screening includes palpation of pedal pulses, testing for protection sensation, and inspection for foot deformities A four-point foot risk scoring system can be used.[2] In this system, 0 represents low risk and 3 signifies the highest possible risk status.

Foot Risk Score 0: Normal Risk

Residents in this normal risk category have diabetes but few other risk factors. They have no evidence of decreased circulation and sensation or foot deformities.

Foot Risk Score 1: Low Risk

The resident in this low-risk category has diabetes and some evidence of vascular compromise, barely palpable or nonpalpable pulses and foot deformity or minor foot infection.[3,4] This resident should be followed up with a more in-depth physical examination to determine the extent of the vascular compromise, if any, and to address any treatable or preventable factors.

Foot Risk Score 2: Moderate Risk

Residents in this moderate-risk category demonstrate sensory loss and one or more of the following: diminished circulation, foot deformity, or minor foot infection. The 5.07 monofilament testing device is a validated instrument that is simple and convenient and readily available to test for protective sensation. The monofilament is pressed against the foot at a number of sites just hard enough to bend the wire. With the residents' eyes closed, they should be able to feel the monofilament. If they cannot, they most likely have a loss of protective sensation (see Figure 12.1).

Residents at moderate risk should be followed-up with a more in-depth physical examination to determine the extent of the vascular compromise, if any, and to address any treatable or preventable factors.

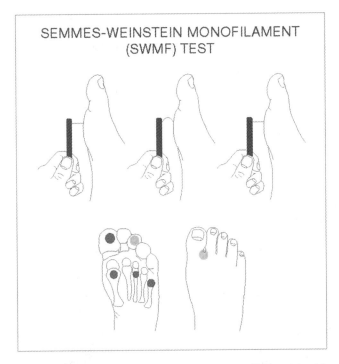

Figure 12.1 How and where to do a 10-gram monofilament test to evaluate protective sensation.

Source: American Diabetes Association. *Foot examination pocket chart.*

Foot Risk Score 3: High Risk

Patients in this high-risk category demonstrate both sensory loss and diminished circulation with foot deformity. The following conditions by themselves are considered high risk:

1. Prior history of foot ulcer or amputation
2. Severe peripheral vascular disease
3. Charcot foot or neuroarthropathy
4. End-stage renal disease

FOOT INSPECTION

The following areas of the foot should be inspected and reported in the basic foot screening:

1. Skin color: The skin can appear normal, or it could be red, white, or mottled. Abnormal coloration may be a sign of vascular compromise. Other discolorations, moles, or areas that are red may indicate the beginning of a wound, especially if it is over a bony prominence.

2. Skin texture: The skin should be smooth and well hydrated. Skin that is thin, excessively dry, flakey, or cracked may indicate simple dry skin, vascular compromise, or possibly a fungal infection. All wounds and ulcerations should be addressed immediately with a consultation to the podiatrist.
3. Edema: Swelling in the feet and ankles should be observed and documented. Edema can be a sign of venous, lymphatic, or other vascular disease, as well as a sign of some types of heart disease.

Key Issues Method to Quantify Edema

The usual method to quantify edema is a 1–7 scale, with each scale number representing 2 millimeter of depth. For example, pressing a finger on the edema for 5 seconds and revealing a 4-millimeter pit would represent a +2 pitting edema.

4. Calluses: Any calluses that appear on the foot should be documented. Calluses can be extremely painful and may cause falls because of balance issues as the resident tries to avoid painful ambulation. Calluses also may cover or mask an ulcer (see Nails).
5. Nails: One of the most common problems in the elderly is hypertrophic nails, which can appear thickened or discolored (yellow, green, brown, or even black) and also may indicate a fungal infection.[2] Excessively thickened nails can cause tissues under the nails to ulcerate, often without the residents' knowledge. This is especially true in residents with neuropathy.
6. Deformities: Hammer toes, bunion deformities, and other bony prominences should be documented as they can be a source of joint pain and discomfort.

Key Issues Plantar Fat Pad Thickness

A reduction in the thickness of the plantar fat pad is a common finding of aging. This can lead to increased discomfort at bony prominences, such as the metatarsal heads, and can lead to calluses or skin breakdown in some cases.

Preventive Foot Care

Once the resident's foot risk level has been determined, a management plan should be instituted. The intensity of the interventions should be based on the severity of the risk. At a minimum, patients in all risk categories should have their feet inspected daily, should have their feet washed daily, and should not walk barefoot. It is also important to define the type of LTC environment. With the changes in health care models, including the patient-centered medical home, more patients will receive assistance in their current homes. They may live in a multigenerational family setting, an independent living environment, an assisted-living center, or a skilled nursing facility. An assessment of the physical abilities of each patient in these settings will help to establish what they can do for themselves and what must be done for them. All levels of care providers can be trained to perform basic foot inspections.

STRATEGIES FOR FOOT CARE FOR EACH FOOT RISK CATEGORY

Basic Foot Care for All Risk Groups

The following strategies for basic foot care apply to all risk groups:

1. Inspect feet daily. Look for marks, discolorations, or any signs of skin breakdown. Make sure to look at the foot in all six planes: dorsal, plantar, lateral, medial, anterior, and posterior (see Figure 12.2).
2. Wash feet daily. Wash and dry between the toes, making sure to pat the feet dry rather than rub. This helps to avoid any towel abrasions for sensitive skin.
3. If feet are excessively dry, use an emollient daily or more often if need. Any excess emollient between the toes should be wiped away.
4. If feet are excessively wet (sweaty), use a daily antifungal foot powder on the foot and in the shoe to reduce perspiration. Use of acrylic socks will help "wick" away moisture from the skin.
5. Do not soak feet. Washing the feet daily is not the same as soaking the feet.[5] Although in some circumstances the provider or podiatrist may recommend foot soaks, it should never be attempted without specific orders. There are two reasons not to routinely soak the feet. First, the foot in diabetes is less able to transfer heat. Because of this inability, even water temperatures under 100°F can cause a burn with the potential loss of tissue. The second reason is that a foot soak can exacerbate an existing infection by allowing water to enter the deep spaces of the foot through the wound and carry pathogens to deeper tissues.
6. Do not allow the resident to walk barefoot. Use slippers or step-in shoes, ensuring that the footwear does not predispose the resident to falling. If the resident does wear slippers, do not allow the resident to walk in slippers for prolonged periods of time as slippers are not strong enough nor supportive enough for walking.
7. Do not cut or trim calluses. This procedure should be done by someone trained to debride hyperkeratotic (thickened) tissue. It is not uncommon to find a wound or ulcer under a painful callus, which requires professional wound care.[6] In addition, in the resident with diabetes, a small nick or cut can quickly degenerate into a major infection.

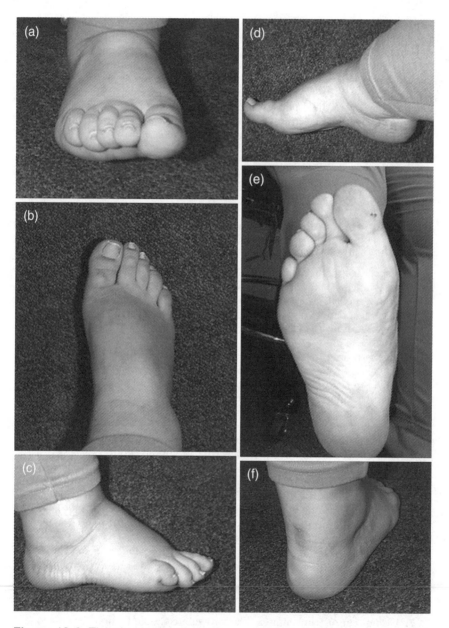

Figure 12.2 The six planes of a foot examination: (a) anterior, (b) dorsal, (c) lateral, (d) medial, (e) plantar, and (f) posterior.

8. Provide appropriate nail care.

  a. Foot risk groups 0 and 1 (normal and low risk): When nails are *normal* color (nails should be translucent and the nail bed should appear flesh colored through the nail) and size, they may be cut carefully by most caregivers. Before trimming, the nails can be softened by placing a washcloth soaked in lukewarm water over the toes for a few minutes before cutting. Normal nails should be cut straight across or follow the shape of the toe. Never cut into a nail groove. Use an emery board (not a nail file) to smooth the edges so there are no sharp or rough edges after clipping the nails.
  b. Foot risk groups 2 and 3 (moderate and high risk) and if the nails are *abnormal*, hypertrophic, or discolored, consult the podiatrist or licensed foot care specialist for proper care.
  c. If a resident in any risk category has ingrown toenails, consult a podiatrist or licensed foot care specialist for proper care.

Shoes and Foot Wear

The shoe serves two essential functions. The first function is to protect feet from environmental factors and the second is to provide proper support to allow effective ambulation. With aging, there is a loss of muscle strength, balance, and the ability to feel (sensory) and to determine where our feet are (proprioception). This is especially true for residents with diabetes, as their disease process will hasten the appearance and severity of these factors associated with aging. Shoes for this patient cohort must be customized for the individual needs of each resident. The basic principles that apply include the following:

1. Most communities have shoe stores that specialize in hard-to-fit sizes or geriatric patients. Seek out a store that advertises employing a certified shoe fitter, called a pedorthist.
2. Shop for shoes late in the day or early evening when the feet are as swollen as they are going to be.
3. Ensure that both feet are measured when shopping for shoes. Feet should be measured for both width and length.
4. Ensure that the shoe fits properly in both width and length. A general guideline is to allow for 0.20–0.25 inches from the longest toe to the front of the shoe.
5. Shoes should not be expected to "stretch" to fit properly. Shoes should be snug but not tight.
6. Make sure the shoe is made out of materials that breathe, such leather or canvas. Avoid plastic shoes, as they are occlusive and do not allow for the proper transfer of heat and moisture.
7. If an orthotic device is needed for pressure relief inside the shoe, make sure the shoe has removable inserts to accommodate the orthosis to prevent undue pressure on other parts of the foot.
8. Slippers should be used only for inside the facility and only for short walks from room to room. Slippers are not cushioned enough or

supportive enough to be used for walking on hard surfaces or for any length of time. Slippers are not designed for weight-bearing activities and residents should be encouraged to use other types of footwear that are easy to get on and off (clog type, slip-on sneakers, etc.)

9. In cases in which foot deformities cannot be accommodated in commercially available shoes, a custom-molded shoe may be necessary. These shoes are made from plaster casts taken of the patient's feet and constructed by a laboratory that specializes in custom shoes. It is essential that a podiatrist or pedorthist ensure that the custom-molded shoe fits properly after it is constructed. These shoes commonly require repeated adjustments before they fit properly.[2,7,8]

10. Clean socks should be worn daily and should be made out of materials that wick moisture away from the body. Materials such as acrylics in combination with other natural fibers are suggested. Additionally, many socks for at-risk feet provide extra padding for the toes and heels. Patients with vascular problems should avoid socks that restrict flow unless used purposefully for lower leg edema, as appropriate.

CONCLUSION

Providing foot care in the aging population in general, and for those in LTC facilities in particular, is a significant challenge. As we age, we tend to lose our ability to provide even the most basic self–foot care, such as foot inspection and nail trimming. In addition, the current health care system does not support payments for this basic foot care in many geriatric populations despite the risk associated with improper foot care.[9] As such, this role increasingly will fall on family, nursing, and other health care providers at the patient's expense. It is essential that preventive foot care be provided to avoid serious and sometimes limb-threatening complications.

REFERENCES

1. Hefland AE. Institutional podiatric care: administration and organization. In *Public Health and Podiatric Medicine: Principles and Practice*. 2nd ed. Helfand AE (Ed).Washington, DC, American Public Health Association Press, 2006
2. Veterans Health Administration. VHA directive 2012-020: Prevention of amputations in veterans everywhere program. Available at www.va.gov/vhapublications/ViewPublication.asp?pub_ID=2778. Accessed 15 January 2014.
3. Knutson D, Yeager B. Physical examination. In *The Aging Foot*. Gabel LL, Haines DJ, Papp KK (Eds). Columbus, OH, U.S. Department of Health and Human Services, Public Health Service, Health Resources and Services Administrations, Bureau of Health Professions, Division of Medicine, The Ohio State University, Department of Family Medicine, 2004, p. 1–12.
4. Hefland AE. Improving early recognition of foot problems in the long-term care resident. In *Foot Health Training Guide for Long-term Care Personnel*. Helfand AE, Ed. Baltimore, MD, Health Professions Press, Inc., 2007, p. 15–26.

5. Hefland AE. Improving early recognition of foot problems in the long-term care resident: Clinical Podogeriatric Assessment. In *Foot Health Training Guide for Long-term Care Personnel.* Helfand AE, Ed. Baltimore, MD, Health Professions Press, Inc., 2007, p. 15–26.

6. Hefland AE. A guide to foot care for older adults. In *Foot Health Training Guide for Long-term Care Personnel.* Helfand AE, Ed. Baltimore, MD, Health Professions Press, Inc., 2007, p. 105–120.

7. Yeager B. Primary prevention. In *The Aging Foot.* Gabel LL, Haines DJ, Papp KK, Eds. Columbus, OH, U.S. Department of Health and Human Services, Public Health Service, Health Resources and Services Administrations, Bureau of Health Professions, Division of Medicine, The Ohio State University, Department of Family Medicine, 2004, p. 1–9.

8. Yeager B. Common pedal manifestations. In *The Aging Foot.* Gabel LL, Haines DJ, Papp KK, Eds. Columbus, OH, U.S. Department of Health and Human Services, Public Health Service, Health Resources and Services Administrations, Bureau of Health Professions, Division of Medicine, The Ohio State University, Department of Family Medicine, 2004, p. 1–16.

9. Hefland AE. Basic Consideration for geriatric footwear. In *Foot Health Training Guide for Long-term Care Personnel.* Helfand AE, Ed. Baltimore, MD, Health Professions Press, Inc., 2007, p. 95–104.

13

Visual Impairment in Older Adults

Ann S. Williams, PhD, RN

INTRODUCTION

Visual impairment commonly co-occurs with diabetes, especially among older adults. In 2011, 4 million adults with diabetes, or about 19.1% of the 20.9 million people with diagnosed diabetes, reported having trouble seeing, even with their glasses or contact lenses on.[1] Among people with diabetes age ≥45 years, the prevalence is even higher, estimated at 20%. Although nearly half of those with visual impairment and diabetes report diabetic retinopathy as the cause of their vision loss, other causes also are common, notably cataracts, glaucoma, and age-related macular degeneration (see Table 13.1).[2] Furthermore, people with existing vision loss from earlier in life can and do develop diabetes as they age. In fact, evidence exists that older adults with vision loss have higher rates of physical inactivity and diabetes than those without vision loss.[3]

Among older adults, rates of visual impairment are reported at even higher rates in long-term care (LTC) facilities than in community-dwelling populations.[4-7] West et al. suggested several reasons for this, including a high overall frequency of eye disease among the elderly; a high rate of admission to LTC facilities of people with visual impairment because of difficulties remaining independent; and lack of access to vision care, resulting in problems ranging from outdated eyeglass prescriptions to untreated new eye disease.[4]

Vision loss with diabetes has profound effects on quality of life. This combination of conditions has been linked to increased risk of falling,[8-10] fractures,[11] ophthalmic infections and emergencies,[12] and both clinical depression and anxiety.[13-17] Such negative physical and psychological sequelae are not inevitable, however. Providing adequate vision care and visual rehabilitation (use of low-vision and nonvisual tools and techniques) can greatly diminish the physical and psychosocial problems associated with vision loss.[18-20]

This chapter covers basic information about the disease process, effects on vision, and treatments for the most common causes of visual loss in older adults with diabetes: cataracts, diabetic retinopathy, glaucoma, and macular degeneration. The chapter also includes a brief overview of visual rehabilitation services and an overview of the tools and techniques for independent diabetes self-management by people with visual impairment or blindness.

DOI: 10.2337/9781580404730.13

Table 13.1 Common Causes of Visual Impairment

Condition	Disease process	Effects on vision	Treatments
Age-Related Macular Degeneration (ARMD)	All types: The macula is damaged. Dry ARMD is most common and less severe, and may occur in one or both eyes. The macula thins and dries out, distorting vision. Yellow deposits (*drusen*) may form in the macula. Stages are early (no vision loss), intermediate (some vision loss), and advanced (blurred spot in central vision).	Progresses slowly, causing blurred vision, eventually loss of central vision.	No proven treatment exists. The Age-Related Eye Disease Study (AREDS) showed that a high-dose combination of Vitamins C and E with β-carotene, zinc and copper slows progression from intermediate to advanced ARMD. The doses are higher than in any multivitamin and have shown no effect in preventing ARMD.
	Wet ARMD is caused by an overgrowth of new blood, weak vessels that leak blood and fluid.	Initially, straight lines appear wavy, progressing quickly to blurred central vision.	Can be treated with laser surgery, photodynamic therapy (an injected medication activated by shining light into the eyes), and injections into the eyes. These treatments do not cure ARMD but can slow its progression and preserve sight.
Cataract	Clouding of the lens of the eye, which can become thicker, cloudy, and yellow as a person ages. Usually happens slowly, over a period of years.	Vision becomes blurred and indistinct, especially in low-light situations. Loss can be so gradual that the person may not notice it in earlier stages. Other possible symptoms: glare sensitivity, double vision ("ghost images"), and loss of sensitivity to colors.	For early cataracts: good lighting, antiglare sunglasses, magnifiers, high contrast, and elimination of sources of glare. For most cataracts that interfere with daily living, surgical removal of the clouded lens and replacement with an intraocular, clear plastic lens is recommended. (Thick glasses are no longer needed with intraocular lenses.)

Diabetic retinopathy, macular edema, retinal bleeding, and retinal detachment	In early stages, swelling and blockages of the tiny blood vessel in the retina prevent a good blood supply. Fluid may leak out into the macula, causing swelling, or macular edema, and blurring the central vision. In later stages, more blockages develop, some areas of the retina die off. Many new blood vessels grow in the retina. They are fragile and break easily, causing bleeding into the retina and the vitreous gel. With extensive damage and scarring, the retina can pull away from the back of the eye, causing retinal detachment.	In the early stages, vision is not affected. In the later stages, the person may have blurring, spots floating around the field of vision ("floaters"), and areas missing in the visual field. Because the brain fills in what it thinks was there, people with missing portions of the visual field may not know they are not seeing certain areas; careful testing of the vision may be necessary to identify this type of loss. Bleeding into the vitreous gel blocks light from reaching the retina, causing total blindness. Retinal detachment can cause a sudden loss of vision.	Intensive management of diabetes is vital to all efforts to treat diabetic retinopathy and prevent its progression. For macular edema: laser surgery or injections into the eyes. May not improve vision, but can prevent further loss by stopping growth of blood vessels. For blood in the vitreous gel: vitrectomy, i.e., surgery to remove bloody fluid and replace it with a clear fluid. For detached retina: surgical reattachment; to be successful this must be done soon after detachment.
Glaucoma	Any of a group of diseases that damage the optic nerve through fluid pressure within the eye.	In early stages, vision is normal and there is no pain. If pressure is measured, it may be high.	Regular screening at routine eye exams, through measuring pressure in the eye; visual acuity and fields; and a dilated eye exam to see the optic nerve. Early detection allows for treatment in early stages and preservation of vision.

(Continued)

Table 13.1 Common Causes of Visual Impairment (Continued)

Condition	Disease process	Effects on vision	Treatments
	Most common types are open-angle glaucoma (the fluid in the eye drains, but too slowly) and angle-closure glaucoma (the fluid does not drain). Both cause increased fluid pressure in the eye. Low-tension or normal-tension glaucoma causes damage even though the fluid pressure is normal.	Later, peripheral vision gradually decreases. A person may miss seeing things on either side of the normal visual field. Eventually, the person sees as if looking through a tunnel. Angle-closure glaucoma can develop suddenly, with severe pain, nausea, redness of the eye, and blurred vision. This is a medical emergency, and must be treated immediately.	High-risk groups: African American >40 years, everyone >60 years, especially Mexican Americans, and anyone with a family history of glaucoma. Most common treatment: topical eye medication, administered through eyedrops, usually several times a day (prostaglandins, β-blockers, adrenergics, carbonic anhydrase inhibitors, or cholinergics). Less commonly, laser or conventional surgery may be used.

Sources: National Eye Institute. Eye health information, 2013. Available at www.nei.nih.gov/health/. Accessed 7 February 2014; Houde SC, Huff MH. Age-related vision loss in older adults. A challenge for gerontological nurses. *Journal of Gerontological Nursing* 2003;29(4):25–33; Rosenberg EA, Sperazza LC. The visually impaired patient. *American Family Physician* 2008;77(10):1431–1436; Tumosa N. Eye disease and the older diabetic. *Clinics in Geriatric Medicine* 2008;24(3):515–527, vii; Watkinson S. Visual impairment in older people: the nurse's role. *Nursing Standards* 2005;19(17):45–52; quiz 4–5; Young JS. Age-related eye diseases: a review of current treatment and recommendations for low-vision aids. *Home Healthcare Nursing* 2008;26(8):464–471; quiz 72–73; Jackson GR, Owsley C. Visual dysfunction, neurodegenerative diseases, and aging. *Neurologic Clinics* 2003;21(3):709–728; American Foundation for the Blind. Your eye condition, 2013. Available at www.visionaware.org/section.aspx?FolderID=6. Accessed 7 February 2014.

VISUAL LOSS IN OLDER ADULTS

Definitions of Vision and Visual Loss

The following standard definitions are used to describe vision and visual loss:[21,22]

Visual acuity: A clinical measure of the eye's ability to distinguish detail. It usually is expressed as a fraction that describes how well the person can read a line of print on a Snellen chart (the typical eye chart with the letter "E" at the top.) A person with 20/40 vision can read a line of print at 20 feet what a typical person can see at 40 feet.

Visual field: A clinical measure of the entire area that an eye can see when the eye is directed forward. It usually is expressed in degrees of vision.

Normal vision: Visual acuity between 20/12.5 and 20/25, and a visual field of 160 degrees.

Visual impairment: A general term indicating a loss of vision that affects how a person can function. It includes low vision, legal blindness, and total blindness.

Low vision: Functionally, a loss of vision that makes it difficult for the individual to complete daily activities that are usual for that person, such as reading, cooking, walking outside, or recognizing faces. Clinically, this includes any level of visual acuity between 20/70 and 20/200. It also may include factors not usually measured, such as decreased contrast sensitivity, increased glare sensitivity, and difficulty with light or dark adaptation. People with this level of vision still can see many things and often can use large print, magnifiers, special lighting, and other adaptive aids to accomplish whatever they want or need to do.

Mild low vision: Visual acuity between 20/30 and 20/60.

Moderate low vision: Visual acuity in the best eye of 20/70 to 20/200

Severe low vision: Visual acuity between 20/200 and 20/400.

Profound low vision: Visual acuity between 20/500 and 20/1,000.

Legal blindness: Visual acuity in the best eye of ≤20/200, with the best possible correction; or a visual field of ≤20 degrees. With this level of vision, a person still may have some sight that is helpful in daily living, such as seeing areas of light and dark. Vision, however, is quite limited. People with legal blindness usually need to rely on their nonvisual senses to accomplish everyday tasks.

Total blindness, or no light perception: An inability to see anything with either eye.

Parts of the Eye

The major parts of the eye are as follows:[23]

Cornea: The clear outer layer, located at the front of the eye; a part of the eye's focusing system.

Iris: The colored part of the eye, which adjusts the size of the pupil to regulate the amount of light entering the eye.

Pupil: The dark opening in the middle of the iris, the area where light enters the eye. As the iris adjusts its size, it can grow larger or smaller to allow more or less light to enter.

Lens: A clear disc behind the iris that helps to focus an image formed by the light entering the eye onto the retina, so the person can see clearly.

Vitreous gel: A clear fluid that fills the eye. Light travels through the vitreous gel to reach the retina.

Retina: The light-sensitive area at the back of the eye, the retina converts the images formed by light into electrical impulses, or visual messages, which are carried by nerves to the brain.

Macula: A small, very light-sensitive area in the center of the retina. The macula contains the fovea.

Fovea: The center of the retina, responsible for clear and detailed central vision.

Optic nerve: A bundle of >1 million nerve fibers responsible for carrying visual messages from the retina to the brain, where those messages are interpreted (Figure 13.1).

Common Causes of Visual Loss

The most common causes of visual loss are age-related macular degeneration, cataracts, diabetic retinopathy, and glaucoma. A description of the disease process, its effects on vision, and treatments for each of these can be found in Table 13.1.

There are many other additional causes of visual impairment common among older adults, including dry eye syndrome, visual neuropathy, stroke, trauma, and vision loss from any cause earlier in life. In addition, evidence is accumulating that there may be some loss of contrast sensitivity, producing functional visual impairment, associated with Alzheimer's disease and other neurodegenerative disorders.

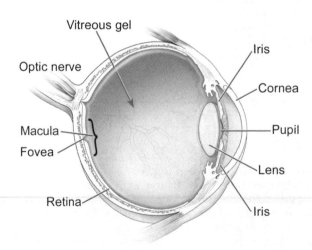

Figure 13.1 Eye diagram showing the macula and fovea (black and white).
Source: National Eye Institute. Diagram of the eye, 2013. Available at www.nei.nih.gov/health/eyediagram/index.asp. Accessed 19 March 2013.

What Does Visual Loss Look Like?

The photos in Figure 13.2 give you an idea of what it looks like when a person has visual impairment from the most common causes.[24] A video that shows a simulation of various types of visual impairment can be found on the Vision Aware website.[25]

VISUAL REHABILITATION

Available Services

Visual rehabilitation services can include a wide variety of specialized training and counseling services that can help people who have vision loss continue to perform everyday activities independently. Vision rehabilitation professionals include the following:[19,26]

- **Low-vision therapist:** Helps people to use any remaining vision as effectively as possible. These therapists can recommend special

(a)

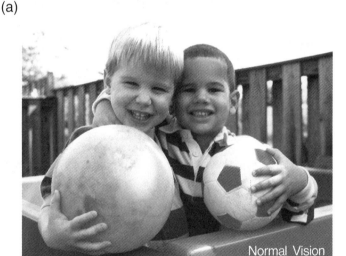

Normal Vision

Figure 13.2 (a) Normal vision. (b) A scene as it might be viewed by a person with glaucoma. (c) A scene as it might be viewed by a person with cataract. (d) A scene as it might be viewed by a person with diabetic retinopathy. (e) A scene as it might be viewed by a person with age-related macular degeneration. (f) A scene as it might be viewed by a person with myopia (nearsightedness). (g) A scene as it might be viewed by a person with retinitis pigmentosa.

Source: National Eye Institute. Eye disease simulations, 2009. Available at www.nei.nih.gov/health/examples. Accessed 19 March 2013.

(b)

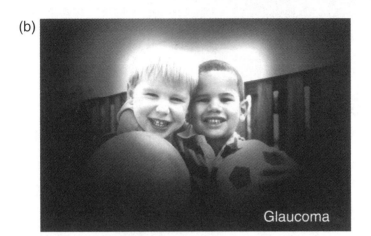

Glaucoma

(c)

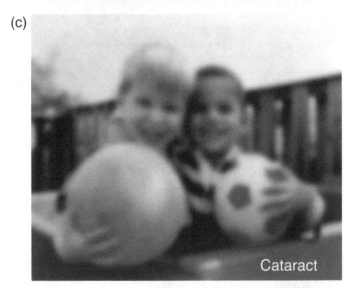

Cataract

(d)

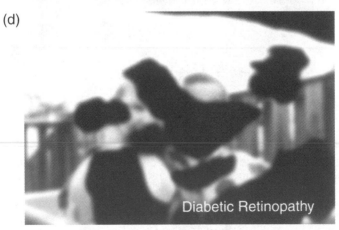

Diabetic Retinopathy

Figure 13.2 (Continued)

(e)

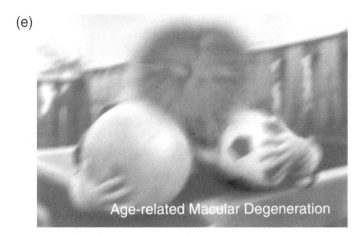

Age-related Macular Degeneration

(f)

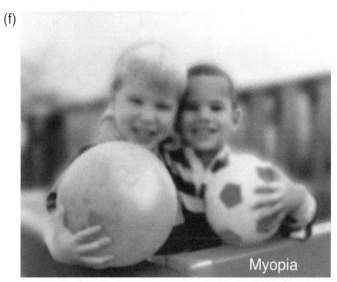

Myopia

(g)

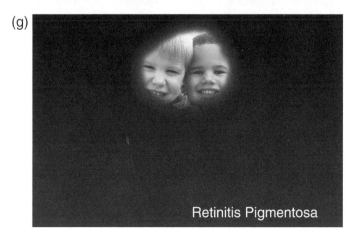

Retinitis Pigmentosa

Figure 13.2 (Continued)

techniques, optical devices, optimal lighting, or electronic devices. Their work is highly individualized, taking into consideration the individual's eye condition, functional vision, and the visual tasks they wish to do.

- **Occupational therapists (OTs):** Help people with disabilities, including visual impairment, to learn ways they can safely and effectively do every-day activities that are important to them, such as caring for themselves and their families or working and volunteering. Some OTs specialize in low-vision services.
- **Vision rehabilitation therapist:** Helps people with visual impairment to use nonvisual techniques (or any remaining vision) to safely and effectively do everyday tasks like cooking, grooming, cleaning, reading, handling money, using a computer, and enjoying recreation and leisure activities.
- **Orientation and mobility specialist:** Helps people learn travel skills, or how to move through the environment safely, effectively, and inde-pendently, for example, by using a white cane. This includes both under-standing exactly where one is (orientation) and knowing how to move through that environment (mobility).

In an LTC setting, visual rehabilitation professionals can provide consulta-tion, and sometimes teaching, to help residents in a variety of ways. Examples of helpful services they might provide include recommending a particular type of lighting to help a resident function effectively in her room; suggesting fonts and types of paper to enable a resident with low vision to read necessary informa-tion independently; teaching a resident with new blindness how to use nonvisual techniques for bathing, dressing, and feeding her- or himself; helping a resident with visual impairment find a way to continue a favorite leisure activity, such as reading, knitting, or playing cards; or teaching a resident with new vision loss how to safely and independently make her or his way from the bedroom to the bathroom, activity room, and dining room. An OT consultation would be particu-larly appropriate for a resident who had impairments in both vision and manual dexterity, such as a person with both age-related macular degeneration and rheu-matoid arthritis or stroke.

Locating Visual Rehabilitation Services

Both public and private agencies provide visual rehabilitation services. These include the following:

- **State vocational rehabilitation services:** Every state in the U.S. offers visual rehabilitation and orientation and mobility services for people with visual disabilities. Most include low-vision services and many include special services for seniors.
- **The Veterans Health Administration (VHA):** The VHA offers com-prehensive visual rehabilitation services for veterans who qualify. Because the visual rehabilitation services offered to veterans are of high quality and often include the purchase of equipment that may not be funded by state or private agencies, it is highly recommended that veterans with

visual impairment explore their eligibility for these services. To learn more about eligibility, see the Military Benefits website.[27]

- **Private blindness agencies and low-vision clinics:** Many areas, especially large cities, have private agencies that provide a variety of visual rehabilitation and low-vision services. Some offer comprehensive services, while others offer only specific services. Most private agencies work collaboratively with any publically funded programs in the area.
- **National Library Service for the Blind and Physically Handicapped (NLS):** Although not truly a rehabilitation program, the NLS of the Library of Congress is an important publically funded service offering Braille and audio reading materials to any U.S. resident who cannot read standard text because of visual or other disabilities. NLS materials are sent without any charge through the U.S. mail. Both books and periodicals are available. Anyone who qualifies for NLS recorded audio materials is entitled to receive a special player for those materials free of charge. As of this writing, the NLS is in a transition period, transferring the entire collection from audiocassettes to a digital format. New users of the NLS currently are receiving the new digital recorders. For more information about the NLS, see the Library of Congress website.[28]

To locate services available in a particular area or to find specific visual rehabilitation services for a particular need, refer to the comprehensive online directory maintained by the AFB.[29]

Low-Vision Aids

A wide variety of special devices, or low-vision aids, are available to help people manage daily life with low vision. These include the following:

- **Optical magnifiers:** Magnifiers can be handheld and can come with a small light that points to the magnified area. They also can come on a stand, with a flexible neck and a clamp to attach the magnifier to a table or as a hands-free magnifier that hangs around the neck.
- **Telescopic glasses or monoculars:** Can help a person to see objects more clearly at a distance, such as faces of people who are across a room, or a television.
- **Tinted glasses, or glare shields:** Can help reduce glare and therefore improve functional vision for people who have an eye condition that causes a problem with glare, such as cataract or diabetic retinopathy.
- **Video magnifiers or closed-circuit televisions:** These devices project a video image on a screen, allowing magnification without the distortion that limits the usefulness of optical magnifiers. They mainly are used for reading, although they can be used for other visual tasks. These devices are available both as handheld video magnifiers and for use on a table or desk, with a standard television or computer screen. Handheld magnifiers allow up to 20× magnification, and those attached to a screen allow 30–60× magnification. In addition, most allow the user to change the color of the image, for example, from black print on a white background

to white print on a blue or black background. This feature can greatly improve functional vision for people who are bothered by glare.

■ **Nonoptical devices:** Many nonoptical devices can make life easier for people with visual impairment. For example, a person with low vision may use a large-print calendar; large-print address book; writing pens that makes a thick, dark line; and a telephone with large print number keys. A person who is blind may appreciate having a talking watch, talking personal weight scale, and playing cards marked in both Braille and print to enable her to play card games with sighted friends. These and other similar items may be recommended by visual rehabilitation professionals and are available through specialty catalogues and some local stores that carry low-vision products. For a list of companies that carry many low-vision items, see the AFB website.[30]

DIABETES SELF-MANAGEMENT FOR PEOPLE WITH VISUAL IMPAIRMENT

Although many residents in LTC need some assistance performing diabetes self-management tasks, such as blood glucose monitoring or organizing and administering medications, individuals who live in assisted living can do much of their diabetes self-management themselves. In rehabilitation settings, the expectation is that the person will learn to manage as independently as possible in preparation for returning home. In the LTC facility, however, the resident may have limited capacity for true self-management.

Visual impairment itself is not a contraindication to independent diabetes self-management. In the community, many people who have diabetes and visual impairment manage all their own routine diabetes self-management by themselves. In fact, many individuals with low vision and total blindness succeed with complex self-management tasks, such as using an insulin pump. To accomplish independent diabetes self-management, however, people with visual impairment need specialized knowledge of low-vision or nonvisual tools and techniques for diabetes care. Fortunately, the knowledge and skills needed are not difficult to master.

Table 13.2 contains a list of the American Association of Diabetes Educators 7 (AADE7) Self-Care Behaviors, which are the essential self-management behaviors for everyone who has diabetes. For each behavior, the table summarizes the needs for low-vision or nonvisual tools and techniques for independent self-management and resources or professional referrals to help an individual meet those needs. This table contains only a summary; for more complete information about tools and techniques, see "Diabetes and Vision Loss: A Guide to Caring for Yourself When You Have Vision Loss" on the AFB website.[31]

Diabetes educators may be available to assist residents or staff in the LTC facility. The AADE has a position statement affirming that all diabetes educators have a responsibility to provide diabetes education for people with disabilities in ways that allow them to achieve similar behavioral goals as people without current disabilities. In other words, if a diabetes educator teaches insulin injections, or blood glucose monitoring, or problem solving to persons without disabilities,

Table 13.2 Low-Vision and Nonvisual Tools and Techniques for the AADE7 Self-Care Behaviors

Self-care behavior	Low-vision or nonvisual needs	Resources and professional referrals
Healthy eating	Nutrition information in low-vision or nonvisual formats: large print, audio recording, Braille, or digital formats; or simple, large pictures.	Referral to a dietitian, preferably a certified diabetes educator. Some resources for diabetes information in accessible formats can be found on the AFB's "Your Diabetes 411 Page."[a]
	Low-vision or nonvisual food measurement.	Nested measuring cups, talking food scale, simple estimation using hands and area on a plate.
Being active	Physical activities adapted for visual impairment.	Can do almost anything with adaptations: chair exercises, tai chi, walking, swimming, golfing, tandem bicycle riding, and competitive sports.[b,c] Visual rehabilitation professionals can advise on adaptations.
	Special precautions for exercise safety, considering all long-term medical conditions, especially those affecting eyes, heart, and feet.	Consult with physician before increasing activity. Possible referral to a physical therapist or to cardiac rehabilitation.
Monitoring	Large-print or talking equipment for measuring blood glucose, weight, blood pressure, and body temperature.	A diabetes educator can help a person choose an appropriate blood glucose meter and learn to use it. A visual rehabilitation professional can advise where to purchase other talking health care equipment.
Taking medication	A system to label, recognize, and organize medications.	Use large print, Braille, tactile, or talking labeling systems. Share "Guidelines for Prescription Labeling" with the pharmacist.[d]
	If using insulin, a low-vision or nonvisual system for measuring insulin: syringe magnifier, insulin pens, or tactile insulin measurement devices.	A diabetes educator can teach low-vision or nonvisual insulin measurement.
Problem solving	A low-vision or nonvisual method for keeping records of blood glucose, food, exercise, and laboratory results.	A vision rehabilitation professional can advise on appropriate large-print, computerized, audio-recorded, or Braille recordkeeping.

(Continued)

Table 13.2 Low-Vision and Nonvisual Tools and Techniques for the AADE7 Self-Care Behaviors (Continued)

Self-care behavior	Low-vision or nonvisual needs	Resources and professional referrals
	Information in accessible formats about techniques for diabetes self-management and self-management in unusual situations.	Resources for diabetes information in accessible formats can be found on AFB's "Your Diabetes 411 Page."[a]
Healthy coping	Adjustment to chronic disease and disability; treatment of depression or anxiety; stress management.	Mental health professionals; support groups; guided imagery; prayer, meditation, or yoga instruction; books about emotional wellness.
Reducing risks	Information about reducing long-term risks.	Resources for diabetes information in accessible formats can be found on AFB's "Your Diabetes 411 Page."[a]
	Nonvisual foot care.	Can be taught by a diabetes educator.

Note:
a. American Foundation for the Blind. Diabetes and vision loss: Your diabetes 411 page. Available at http://www.afb.org/info/living-with-vision-loss/eye-conditions/diabetes-and-vision-loss/your-diabetes-411-page-connecting-to-available-info/1235. Accessed 7 February 2014.
b. Vision Aware. How can I manage my diabetes? 2013. Available at www.visionaware.org/section.aspx?FolderID=6&SectionID=111&DocumentID=5709. Accessed 7 February 2014.
c. American Foundation for the Blind. Diabetes and vision loss: Being active, 2013. Available at www.afb.org/section.aspx?FolderID=2&SectionID=93&TopicID=409&SubTopicID=300&DocumentID=4230. Accessed 7 February 2014.
d. American Society of Consultant Pharmacists Foundation, American Foundation for the Blind. Guidelines for prescription labeling and consumer medication information for people with vision loss, 2008. Available at www.afb.org/Section.asp?SectionID=3&TopicID=329&DocumentID=4064. Accessed 7 February 2014.

Sources: American Foundation for the Blind. A guide to living with diabetes and vision loss, 2013. Available at www.afb.org/seniorsite.asp?SectionID=63&TopicID=396. Accessed 19 March 2013; Vision Aware. How can I manage my diabetes? 2013. Available at www.visionaware.org/section.aspx?FolderID=6&SectionID=111&DocumentID=5709. Accessed 19 March 2013.

she or he also must provide such services to people with disabilities, including visual impairment. Therefore, if a person with visual impairment and diabetes in LTC is undergoing rehabilitation with the expectation of returning to independent living in the community, a diabetes educator should be involved to ensure that the person is able to perform all necessary diabetes self-management skills. To see whether a diabetes educator is available in your area, visit the AADE website.[32]

Recommendations for Long-Term Care Facilities

LTC facilities can improve the quality of life for people with diabetes and visual impairment by implementing the following recommendations:

1. Find out how visual rehabilitation services are provided in the local area. Contact both public and private agencies that provide these services to learn exactly what is available and how to make referrals. Keep this information where it is readily available.
2. Know how to make referrals for talking books and ensure that all residents who qualify are offered this service.
3. Consider the lighting throughout the building. Because different eye conditions may require different types of lighting, having flexible options is desirable. For example, bright, scattered overhead lighting may be best for some people, whereas a direct beam of light from a lamp is better for others.
4. For residents with low vision, work with a low-vision specialist to determine the type of light that will enable each person to function best, and consider this in making room assignments. For example, some people with low vision would benefit from a room that faces direct sunlight during the day; others may function worse in such placement if the glare from direct sunlight diminishes their function.
5. Prevent avoidable visual impairment and maximize useful vision. Ensure that all residents have regular professional eye care to screen for and treat eye diseases and to ensure that their prescription lenses (glasses or contact lenses) meet their current refraction needs.
6. When a resident has visual impairment, find out whether that person has received visual rehabilitation. If not, make a referral, and be sure that the person is offered all appropriate options. Note that visual rehabilitation is provided outside the health care system through state rehabilitation services. Each state in the U.S. has such services, and they are listed on the AFB resource list.[29]
7. If a person is expected to return to independent living at home, ensure that a diabetes educator is included on the rehabilitation team.

CONCLUSION

Visual impairment is very common in LTC residents and often contributes to their admission. Careful follow-up is necessary in order to try to prevent further visual deterioration. Fortunately, there are many resources available to visually impaired residents, including specialized staff, programs, visual aids, and government assistance.

REFERENCES

1. Center for Disease Control and Prevention. Diabetes data and trends, 2013. Available at http://apps.nccd.cdc.gov/DDTSTRS/default.aspx. Accessed 9 February 2014.
2. Congdon N, O'Colmain B, Klaver CC, Klein R, Munoz B, Friedman DS, et al. Causes and prevalence of visual impairment among adults in the United States. *Archives of Ophthalmology* 2004;122(4):477–485.

3. Jones GC, Crews JE, Danielson ML. Health risk profile for older adults with blindness: An application of the International Classification of Functioning, Disability, and Health framework. *Ophthalmic Epidemiology* 2010;17(6):400–410.

4. West SK, Friedman D, Munoz B, Roche KB, Park W, Deremeik J, et al. A randomized trial of visual impairment interventions for nursing home residents: study design, baseline characteristics and visual loss. *Ophthalmic Epidemiology* 2003;10(3):193–209.

5. Brezin AP, Lafuma A, Fagnani F, Mesbah M, Berdeaux G. Prevalence and burden of self-reported blindness and low vision for individuals living in institutions: a nationwide survey. *Health Quality Life Outcomes* 2005;3:27.

6. Mitchell P, Hayes P, Wang JJ. Visual impairment in nursing home residents: The Blue Mountains Eye Study. *Medical Journal of Australia* 1997;166(2):73–76.

7. Tielsch JM, Javitt JC, Coleman A, Katz J, Sommer A. The prevalence of blindness and visual impairment among nursing home residents in Baltimore. *New England Journal of Medicine* 1995;332(18):1205–1209.

8. Klein BE, Moss SE, Klein R, Lee KE, Cruickshanks KJ. Associations of visual function with physical outcomes and limitations 5 years later in an older population: The Beaver Dam eye study. *Ophthalmology* 2003;110(4):644–650.

9. Schwartz AV, Vittinghoff E, Sellmeyer DE, Feingold KR, de Rekeneire N, Strotmeyer ES, et al. Diabetes-related complications, glycemic control, and falls in older adults. *Diabetes Care* 2008;31(3):391–396.

10. Strotmeyer ES, Cauley JA, Schwartz AV, Nevitt MC, Resnick HE, Bauer DC, et al. Nontraumatic fracture risk with diabetes mellitus and impaired fasting glucose in older white and black adults: the health, aging, and body composition study. *Archive of Internal Medicine* 2005;165(14):1612–1617.

11. Ivers RQ, Cumming RG, Mitchell P, Peduto AJ. Diabetes and risk of fracture: The Blue Mountains eye study. *Diabetes Care* 2001;24(7):1198–1203.

12. Wipf JE, Paauw DS. Ophthalmologic emergencies in the patient with diabetes. *Endocrinology and Metabolism Clinics of North America* 2000;29(4):813–829.

13. Cox DJ, Kiernan BD, Schroeder DB, Cowley M. Psychosocial sequelae of visual loss in diabetes. *Diabetes Educator* 1998;24(4):481–484.

14. Roy MS, Roy A, Affouf M. Depression is a risk factor for poor glycemic control and retinopathy in African-Americans with type 1 diabetes. *Psychosomatic Medicine* 2007;69(6):537–542.

15. Lamoureux EL, Fenwick E, Moore K, Klaic M, Borschmann K, Hill K. Impact of the severity of distance and near-vision impairment on depression and vision-specific quality of life in older people living in residential care. *Investigative Ophthalmology and Visual Science* 2009;50(9):4103–4109.

16. Rees G, Tee HW, Marella M, Fenwick E, Dirani M, Lamoureux EL. Vision-specific distress and depressive symptoms in people with vision impairment. *Investigative Ophthalmology and Visual Science* 2011;51(6):2891–2896.

17. Varma R, Wu J, Chong K, Azen SP, Hays RD. Impact of severity and bilaterality of visual impairment on health-related quality of life. *Ophthalmology* 2006;113(10):1846–1853.

18. Williams AS, Ponchillia SV. Psychosocial sequelae of visual loss in diabetes. *Diabetes Educator* 1998;24(6):675–676.

19. American Foundation for the Blind. AFB senior site, 2013. Available at www. afb.org/seniorsitehome.asp. Accessed 7 February 2014.
20. National Federation of the Blind. Information packet for seniors, 2013. Available at https://nfb.org/info-packet-seniors. Accessed 7 February 2014.
21. American Foundation for the Blind. Key definitions of statistical terms, 2008. Available at www.afb.org/Section.asp?SectionID=15&DocumentID=1280. Accessed 7 February 2014.
22. American Optometric Association. Low vision, 2013. Available at www.aoa. org/x5240.xml. Accessed 7 February 2014.
23. National Eye Institute. Diagram of the eye, 2013. Available at www.nei.nih. gov/health/eyediagram/index.asp. Accessed 7 February 2014.
24. National Eye Institute. Eye disease simulations, 2009. Available at www.nei. nih.gov/health/examples. Accessed 7 February 2014.
25. Vision Aware. Vision simulation video, 2013. Available at http://www.vision-aware.org/section.aspx?FolderID=6&SectionID=116&DocumentID=3393. Accessed 7 February 2014.
26. Association for the Education and Rehabilitation of the Blind and Visually Impaired. Who are vision professionals? 2014. Available at www.aerbvi.org/ modules.php?name=News&file=article&sid=1219. Accessed 7 February 2014
27. Military Benefits. VA Health Care: Blindness Rehabilitation. Available at www.military.com/benefits/veterans-health-care/blindness-rehabilitation. Accessed 7 February 2014.
28. Library of Congress. That all may read... The national library service for the blind and physically handicapped. Available at www.loc.gov/nls/index.html. Accessed 6 February 2014.
29. American Foundation for the Blind. Comprehensive online directory. Available at www.afb.org/services.asp. Accessed 7 February 2014.
30. American Foundation for the Blind. Sources of specialty products. Available at www.afb.org/results.asp?OrganizationcodeId=76. Accessed 7 February 2014.
31. American Foundation for the Blind. A guide to living with diabetes and vision loss, 2013. Available at www.afb.org/seniorsite.asp?SectionID=63&TopicID=396. Accessed 7 February 2014.
32. National Eye Institute. Eye health information, 2013. Available at www.nei. nih.gov/health/. Accessed 7 February 2014.

14

Cardiovascular Disease in the Older Adult with Diabetes

Laurie Quinn, PhD, RN, APN, CDE, FAAN

INTRODUCTION

Although diabetes has increased dramatically in all age-groups throughout the past two decades; diabetes remains a disease of aging. Approximately 11.3% of U.S. residents >20 years of age have diabetes.[1] This number increases to 26.9% among those ≥65 years of age.[1] People with diabetes have heart disease death rates about two to four times higher than those without diabetes.[1] In 2004, heart disease was noted on 68% of diabetes-related death certificates among people aged ≥65 years.[1] The risk for stroke is two to four times higher among people with diabetes than those without diabetes. In 2004, stroke was noted on 16% of diabetes-related death certificates among people age ≥65 years.[1]

The current epidemic of diabetes and the aging of the U.S. population have contributed to the growing number of older adults with diabetes. The estimated prevalence of diabetes in nursing homes increased from 16.3 to 23.4% from 1995 to 2004, and the most commonly reported diabetes-related comorbidity was cardiovascular disease (CVD).[2] Evidence-based guidelines for the primary and secondary prevention of CVD among adults have been developed but with few age-related modifications. Therefore, their application to the treatment of older adults with *CVD and diabetes*, especially those residing in long-term care (LTC) facilities, is challenging. This chapter focuses on evidence-based treatment of the primary factors (e.g., dyslipidemias and hypertension) leading to primary and secondary CVD events in older adults with diabetes, discussing recommendations (if available) for those residing in LTC facilities.

LIPID DISORDERS IN ADULTS

The American College of Cardiology/American Heart Association Guideline on the Treatment of Blood Cholesterol to Reduce Atherosclerotic Cardiovascular Risk in Adults (Adult Treatment Panel IV [ATP IV]) was released in November 2013.3 This evidence-based treatment guideline was designed to reduce atherosclerotic cardiovascular disease (ASCVD) in adults and replace the existing ATP III criteria.[4]

The ATP IV expert panel found insufficient evidence to support the continued use of specific low-density lipoprotein cholesterol (LDL-C) and/or non–high-density lipoprotein cholesterol (non-HDL-C) treatment targets. Therefore, in ATP-IV, no recommendations are provided for specific

DOI: 10.2337/9781580404730.14

LDL-C or non–HDL-C targets for primary or secondary prevention of ASCVD. Instead, there is an ASCVD risk assessment based on Pooled Cohort Equations (PCEs) using data from five NIH Heart, Lung, and Blood Institute (NHLBI)-sponsored longitudinal population-based cohorts of African American and non-Hispanic white adults.4 Such equations estimate risk for first occurrence nonfatal myocardial infarction, coronary heart disease (CHD) death, or fatal or nonfatal stroke on the basis of age, sex, race, smoking status, total cholesterol level, HDL-C level, systolic blood pressure (treated or untreated), and diabetes.3 These PCEs are used to estimate 10-year ASCVD risk to guide the treatment regimen, particularly statin treatment.4 Downloadable applications to calculate the 10-year risk for ASCVD risk are available to assist the health-care provider in determining treatment strategies.5

Lifestyle modifications (e.g., adherence to a healthy diet, maintaining a healthy weight, regular exercise, optimal control of blood pressure and diabetes, avoidance of tobacco products) are recommended for all adults to decrease risk for ASCVD.6 Healthy lifestyle behaviors are recommended alone or in concert with cholesterol-lowering drugs. Central to the ATP IV treatment guidelines is the use of statin therapy in individuals, where the benefits of ASCVD reduction outweigh the risk of adverse events associated with statin use. The four major statin benefit groups include 1) individuals with clinical ASCVD, 2) individuals with primary elevations of LDL-C ≥190 mg/dl, 3) individuals with diabetes aged 40–75 years with LDL-C 70–189 mg/dl without clinical ASCVD, and 4) individuals without clinical ASCVD or diabetes with LDL-C 70–189 mg/dl and an estimated 10-year ASCVD risk ≥7.5%.6

The appropriate intensity of statin therapy is based on ASCVD risk and potential for adverse effects. The ATP IV panel classifies statin treatment as high-, moderate-, and low-intensity therapy (Table 14.1).6

The evidence supporting the major recommendations of ATP IV are extensively detailed in the ATP IV report.6 The NHLBI grade for the strength of the recommendations is presented in Table 14.2.

Table 14.1 Intensities of Statin Therapy under ATP IV

Classification	LDL-C Decrease (%)	Example
High intensity	≥50	atorvastatin 40–80 mg daily rosuvastatin 20–40 mg daily
Moderate intensity	30 to <50	simvastatin 20–40 mg daily pravastatin 40–80 mg daily
Low intensity	<30	simvastatin 10 mg daily pravastatin 10–20 mg daily

Table 14.2 ATP IV Recommendation Grades

Grade	Classification	Description
A	Strong recommendation	This suggests that there is a high certainty that the benefit (balance between risks and benefits of treatment) is substantial.
B	Moderate recommendation	This suggests that there is a moderate certainty from evidence that the overall benefit is moderate to substantial. In addition, there is high certainty that the overall benefit is moderate.
C	Weak recommendation	There is some moderate certainty based on evidence that there is a small overall benefit.
D	Recommendation against	There is at least moderate certainty based on evidence that there is no overall benefit and that the risk of the intervention outweighs the benefits.
E	Expert opinion	The net benefit is not clear and may be related to a variety of factors (e.g., insufficient evidence, unclear evidence, conflicting evidence); however the Work Group (i.e., the ATP panel) thought that a recommendation should be made. This is an area for future research.
N	No recommendation for or against	The net benefit is not clear and may be related to a variety of factors (e.g., insufficient evidence, unclear evidence, conflicting evidence); however the Work Group (i.e., the ATP panel) thought that no recommendation should be made. This is an area for future research.

Major Recommendations for the Treatment of Blood Cholesterol to Reduce ASCVD Risk in Adults

Target Cholesterol Goals[6]

■ There are no recommendations provided for treatments designed to address specific LDL-C or non–HDL-C targets for primary or secondary prevention of ASCVD (Grade = N).

Secondary Prevention[6]

■ High-intensity statin therapy should be initiated or continued as first-line therapy in adults ≤75 years of age with clinical ASCVD. Clinical ASCVD risk includes acute coronary syndromes, history of myocardial infarction (MI), stable or unstable angina; coronary or other arterial revascularization, stroke, trans-ischemic attack (TIA), or peripheral arterial disease assumed to be of atherosclerotic origin (Grade = A).

■ There are individuals in whom high-intensity statins are indicated, but statin use is contraindicated. In addition, there are individuals who are predisposed to adverse events from statins (e.g., those with myopathy). Moderate-intensity statins should be used (if tolerated) in these individuals (Grade = A).

■ Individuals >75 years of age with clinical ASCVD can be evaluated in terms of ASCVD risk-reduction benefits, adverse effects, and drug-drug interactions. Additionally, patient preferences should be considered in initiating or continuing moderate- or high-intensity statin use (Grade = E).

Primary Prevention in Individuals ≥21 Years of Age with LDL-C ≥190 mg/dl[6]

■ Individuals with LDL ≥190 mg/dl or triglycerides ≥500 mg/dl should be evaluated for secondary causes of hyperlipidemia (Grade = B).

■ Individuals with a *primary untreated* LDL-C ≥190 mg/dl should be treated with statins regardless of their estimated 10-year ASCVD risk. In this group, high-intensity statin therapy should be used unless contraindicated. For those who are unable to tolerate high-intensity statin therapy, the maximum tolerated statin dose should be used (Grade = B).

■ In individuals with *primary untreated* LDL-C ≥190 mg/dl, statin therapy can reasonably be intensified to achieve at least a 50% reduction in LDL-C (Grade = E).

■ In individuals aged ≥21 years with a *primary untreated* LDL-C ≥190 mg/dl, after maximum intensity of statin therapy is achieved, a non-statin drug may be considered to further lower LDL-C (Grade = E).

Primary Prevention in Individuals with Diabetes and with LDL-C 70–189 mg/dl[6]

■ In this group (individuals with diabetes and with LDL-C 70–189 mg/dl), aged 40–75 years, moderate-intensity statin therapy should be initiated or continued (Grade = A).

■ In this group, high-intensity statin therapy is reasonable for adults 40–75 years of age who have an estimated 10-year ASCVD risk of ≥7.5% (Grade = E).

■ In this group, aged <40 or >75 years, it is reasonable to evaluate potential for ASCVD benefits and adverse effects of statins, drug-drug interactions, and consideration of patient preferences when deciding to initiate, continue, or intensify statin therapy (Grade = E).

Primary Prevention in Individuals without Diabetes and with LDL-C 70–189 mg/dl[6]

■ In this group of individuals (without diabetes and with LDL-C 70–189 mg/dl) without clinical ASCVD, the PCEs should be used to estimate 10-year ASCVD risk and to guide initiation of statin therapy for the primary prevention of ASCVD (Grade = B).

■ In this group of individuals without *clinical* ASCVD, aged 40–75 years, with an estimated 10-year ASCVD risk of ≥7.5%, moderate- to high-intensity statins should be initiated (Grade = A).

■ In this group of individuals without *clinical* ASCVD, it is reasonable to offer treatment with moderate-intensity statin to those 40–75 years of age with an estimated 10-year ASCVD risk of 5 to <7.5% (Grade = C).

- In this group of individuals without *clinical* ASCVD, it is reasonable to discuss potential for ASCVD risk-reduction benefits and adverse effects, drug-drug interactions, and patient preferences prior to initiating statin therapy (Grade = E).
- In adults with LDL-C <190 mg/dl who are not identified as part of a statin benefit group or for whom a treatment decision is uncertain after risk assessment, one may consider additional factors to make an informed decision about statin treatment. Statin therapy for primary prevention only may be considered after evaluating potential for ASCVD risk-reduction benefits, adverse effects, drug-drug interactions, and patient preferences (Grade = E).

Heart Failure and Hemodialysis[6]

- The APT IV Panel makes no recommendations regarding beginning or discontinuing statin therapy in patients with New York Heart Association (NYHA) class II–IV ischemic systolic heart failure or in patients who are on maintenance hemodialysis (Grade = N).

Members of the American Diabetes Association's (ADA) Professional Practice Committee plan to review the ATP-IV guidelines as they relate to patients with diabetes and prediabetes.[7] A thorough assessment of these recommendations could not be completed for publication of the ADA's 2014 Standards of Care,[8] but will be addressed in publication of the 2015 Standards of Care. Therefore, the remainder of the recommendations presented in this chapter for *lipid management in adults with diabetes* are based on existing guidelines.[8] In addition, the ATP IV guidelines identify individuals for whom existing available data do not support statin therapy and no recommendations can be made.[9] Because no ATP IV recommendations could be made on adults aged ≥75 years unless clinical ASCVD disease was present, the recommendations in this chapter for older adults with diabetes are based on existing guidelines.

Lipid Management in Older Adults

Older adults are heterogeneous with respect to their clinical and functional status. The *younger* old generally are categorized as those ages 65–79 years, whereas the *older* old generally are classified as >80 years old. High-serum LDL-C and low HDL-C are predictive of primary and secondary CVD risk among older adults.[10] There remains controversy, however, as to whether target lipid goals and treatment modalities are the same for *younger* and *older* elderly adults. This controversy is due, in part, to the exclusion of *older* elderly participants from clinical research trials. Regardless, statin therapy remains a first-line pharmacological treatment in LDL-C reduction among older adults. Some of the evidence supporting the use of statins is described in the following paragraphs.

A meta-analysis of data from nine randomized clinical trials (RCT) examined the relationship between all-cause mortality and statin use in 19,569 older adults (65-82 years of age) with CHD.[11] The results of the meta-analysis concluded that the pooled rates of all-cause mortality were 15.6% with statins and 18.7% with placebo. Additionally, the use of statins was associated with a relative risk reduction in all-cause mortality of 22% over 5 years; a reduction in CHD mortality by 30%; nonfatal MI by 26%; need for revascularization by 30%; and stroke by 25%.[11] Unfortunately, the *oldest old* were poorly represented in this meta-analysis; only the Prospective Study of Pravastatin in the Elderly at Risk (PROSPER) trial included subjects beyond 80 years of age.[12]

The Cholesterol Treatment Trialists' Collaboration (CTT) was a systematic prospective meta-analysis of statin treatment in 90,056 adults enrolled in 14 RCTs.[13] Results of this meta-analysis indicated that LDL-C reductions in those patients older than 65 years of age were associated with a 19% reduction in the risk of major CVD events; these results were similar to those in individuals under 65 years of age. In the same meta-analysis, the CTT studied the effects of statin therapy among the 18,686 adults with diabetes (1,466 with type 1 diabetes [T1D] and 17,220 with type 2 diabetes [T2D]) and noted a 21% decrease in major CVD events per 40-mg/dl reduction in serum LDL-C. The decrease in major vascular events was similar among diabetes subjects with preexisting vascular disease and those with no such history. There was no evidence that the relative effects of statin therapy differed by diabetes type (T1D or T2D), sex, age (<65 years or >65 years), SBP or diastolic blood pressure (DBP), smoking, BMI, renal function, predicted annual risk of a major vascular event, or the baseline lipid profile.

The Heart Protection Study (HPS)[14] and the PROSPER study[12] were RCTs that included older adults with diabetes. The HPS included both middle-aged and older adults (ages 40–80 years); 28% of the participants were 70 years of age or older. The PROSPER study included only older adults (ages 70–82 years). In the HPS, 5963 adults *with* diabetes and 14,573 *without* diabetes and occlusive arterial disease were randomly allocated to receive 40 mg simvastatin daily or placebo. In the analysis of the subjects with diabetes, lowering LDL-C by 40 mg/dl reduced the risk of major vascular events by about 25% during 5 years of treatment. There were similar proportional reductions in risk among people *with* or *without* diabetes regardless of age (<65 years or ≥65 years), sex, vascular disease, or lipid levels.

The PROSPER trial enrolled 5,804 older adults with a history of, or risk factors for, vascular disease to 40 mg/day pravastatin or placebo.[12] Over a period of 3.2 years, pravastatin reduced the primary endpoint (a composite of coronary death, nonfatal MI, and fatal or nonfatal stroke) by ~15%. There were 623 subjects in the diabetes cohort randomized to placebo (n = 320) or pravastatin (n = 303). Unfortunately, the number of individuals with diabetes was too small to permit accurate interpretation of the treatment effect.

The Collaborative AtoRvastatin Diabetes Study (CARDS) was an RCT designed for primary prevention of CVD in those with T2D.[15] The primary objective of the CARDS trial was to investigate whether treatment with atorvastatin (10 mg/day) reduced the incidence of major CVD events in adults with T2D compared with placebo. The study participants included individuals ages 40–75 years with LDL-C ≤160 mg/dl, fasting triglycerides ≤600 mg/dl, and at least one additional risk factor (hypertension, retinopathy, microalbuminuria or macroalbuminuria, or current smoking) but no history of CHD, stroke, or severe peripheral vascular disease. Twelve percent of the subjects in the CARDS trial were ≥70 years of age. The group treated with atorvastatin 10 mg/day had on average a 26% (54-mg/dl) reduction in total cholesterol and a 40% (46-mg/dl) reduction in LDL-C. The average reduction in triglyceride levels was 19% (35 mg/dl), with a 1% (0.77-mg/dl) increase in HDL-C levels compared with placebo. The relative risk reduction in the primary endpoint of first acute CHD event (including fatal and nonfatal MI, unstable angina, acute CHD death, resuscitated cardiac arrest), coronary revascularization procedures, or stroke (fatal or nonfatal) was reduced by 37% with atorvastatin 10 mg/day compared with placebo. Stroke was reduced by 48%; however, the 27% reduction in all-cause mortality was not statistically significant.

Fibrates have been shown to be beneficial in improving the lipid profile in people with T2D, especially those with low HDL-C and high triglycerides. Trials of fibrate therapy that included diabetes subgroups were the *primary prevention* Helsinki Heart Study (HHS)[16] and the *secondary prevention* Veterans Affairs HDL Intervention Trial (VA-HIT).[17] In the HHS, the lipid-lowering effects of simvastatin and gemfibrozil were examined in 96 men with T2D. The simvastatin group received 10–40 mg/day in progressive increases over 24 months, whereas the gemfibrozil group received 1,200 mg/day throughout the 24 months. Simvastatin was most effective in reducing LDL-C and total cholesterol, whereas gemfibrozil was most effective in increasing HDL-C and decreasing triglyceride levels. In the VA-HIT, participants were randomized to either 1,200 mg/day gemfibrozil or placebo and followed for an average of 5 years. Seventy-seven percent of the participants in the VA-HIT were >60 years of age. In a subanalysis of 627 subjects with diabetes, there was a 24% reduction in CHD among those treated with gemfibrozil.

Guidelines for Lipid Management in Adults with Diabetes

The American Diabetes Association (ADA) developed, based on the ATP III criteria, the following guidelines for the treatment of lipid disorders in people with diabetes.[8]

- Lifestyle modifications are recommended to improve the lipid profile of individuals with diabetes. These modifications should focus on decreasing saturated fats, *trans* fats, and cholesterol intake. In addition, intake of n–3 fatty acids, viscous fiber, and plant stanols or sterols should be increased; weight loss (if indicated) should be encouraged; and physical activity should be increased.
- Regardless of the baseline lipid levels, statin medications should be added to lifestyle modifications for diabetes patients with overt CVD and those without overt CVD who are >40 years old with one or more of the other CVD risk factors.
- In patients with who are at lower risk than described (e.g., those who do not have overt CVD and are <40 years old), statin therapy should be considered in addition to lifestyle modifications if LDL cholesterol remains >100 mg/dl, or in those individuals with multiple CVD risk factors.

- In individuals without overt CVD, the primary LDL cholesterol goal is <100 mg/dl.
- In individuals with overt CVD, a lower LDL cholesterol goal of <70 mg/dl may be considered; the use of a high dose of a statin to achieve this goal remains an option.
- If drug-treated individuals do not reach the above targets on maximally tolerated statin therapy, a reduction in LDL cholesterol of about 30–40% from baseline values should be considered an alternative therapeutic goal.
- Serum triglycerides levels <150 mg/dl and HDL cholesterol >40 mg/dl (males) and >50 mg/dl (females) are desirable targets. The preferred strategy, however, is the use of statin medications to achieve LDL cholesterol targets.
- If lipid targets are not reached on maximally tolerated doses of statins, combination therapy using statin medications and other lipid-lowering agents may be considered; however, these have not been shown to provide benefit and are not broadly recommended.

Guidelines for Treatment of Lipid Disorders in Older Adult with Diabetes

The most comprehensive evidence-based guidelines for the treatment of lipid disorders in older adults with T2D were published recently by the European Diabetes Working Party for Older People.[18] The levels of evidence and grades of recommendations for this study are detailed in Tables 14.3 and 14.4, respectively. Their guidelines include the following:

- The 10-year risk of developing symptomatic CVD should be calculated for all individuals who have two or more risk factors to assess the need for primary prevention (Evidence level 1+, Grade of recommendation B).
- In patients with no history of CVD, a statin should be offered to those with an abnormal lipid profile if their 10-year cardiovascular risk is >15% (Evidence level 1–, Grade of recommendation A).
- A statin should be offered to individuals with an abnormal lipid profile who have proven CVD (Evidence level 1+, Grade of recommendation A).
- Consider statin therapy in older subjects with diabetes to reduce the risk of stroke as part of secondary prevention of CVD (Evidence level 2++, Grade of recommendation B).
- A fibrate should be considered in patients with an abnormal lipid profile who have been treated with a statin for at least 6 months but in whom the triglyceride level remains elevated (≥204 mg/dl) (Evidence level 2+, Grade of recommendation C).

Guidelines for Treatment of Lipid Disorders in Older Adults with Diabetes in LTC Facilities

There are no published evidence-based guidelines for lipid management in individuals with diabetes residing in LTC facilities. The general consensus among health care providers is that all residents with diabetes require risk–

Table 14.3 Levels of Evidence

1++	High quality meta-analyses, systematic reviews of RCTs, or RCTs with a very low risk of bias
1+	Well conducted meta-analyses, systematic reviews of RCTs, or RCTs with a low risk of bias
1−	Meta-analyses, systematic reviews of RCTs, or RCTs with a high risk of bias
2++	High-quality systematic reviews of case-control or cohort or studies
	High-quality case-control or cohort studies with a very low risk of confounding, bias, or chance and a high probability that the relationship is causal
2+	Well-conducted case-control or cohort studies with a low risk of confounding, bias, or chance and a moderate probability that the relationship is causal
2−	Case-control or cohort studies with a high risk of confounding, bias, or chance and a significant risk that the relationship is not causal
3	Nonanalytic studies (e.g., case reports, case series)
4	Expert opinion

Note: RCT = randomized clinical trials.

Source: Sinclair AJ, Paolisso G, Castro M, Bourdel-Marchasson I, Gadsby R, Rodriguez Manas L. European Diabetes Working Party for Older People 2011 clinical guidelines for type 2 diabetes mellitus. Executive summary. *Diabetes and Metabolism* 2011;37(Suppl3):S27–S38. Reprinted with permission from the publisher.

Table 14.4 Grades of Recommendation

A	At least one meta-analysis, systematic review, or RCT rated as 1++, and directly applicable to the target population; or
	A systematic review of RCTs or a body of evidence consisting principally of studies rated as 1+, directly applicable to the target population, and demonstrating overall consistency of results
B	A body of evidence including studies rated as 2++, directly applicable to the target population, and demonstrating overall consistency of results; or
	Extrapolated evidence from studies rated as 1++ or 1+
C	A body of evidence including studies rated as 2+, directly applicable to the target population and demonstrating overall consistency of results; or
	Extrapolated evidence from studies rated as 2++
D	Evidence level 3 or 4; or
	Extrapolated evidence from studies rated as 2+

Note: RCT = randomized clinical trials.

Source: Sinclair AJ, Paolisso G, Castro M, Bourdel-Marchasson I, Gadsby R, Rodriguez Manas L. European Diabetes Working Party for Older People 2011 clinical guidelines for type 2 diabetes mellitus. Executive summary. *Diabetes and Metabolism* 2011;37(Suppl3):S27–S38. Reprinted with permission from the publisher.

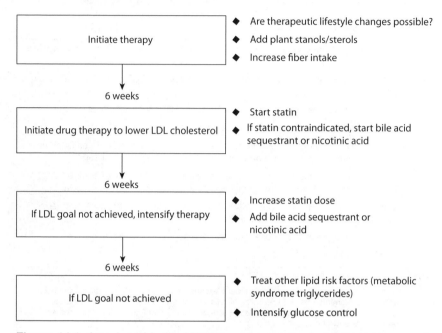

Figure 14.1 American Medical Directors Association's treatment approach for residents in the LTC setting with diabetes, hyperlipidemia, and cardiovascular complications.

Source: Adapted from the National Heart, Lung, and Blood Institute. Third report of the Expert Panel on Detection, Evaluation, and Treatment of High Blood Cholesterol in Adults (Adult Treatment Panel III). Available at http://www. nhlbi.nih.gov/guidelines/cholesterol/index.htm. Accessed 13 February 2014. Reprinted with permission from the publisher.

benefit analysis in terms of potential and current medical therapy, including pharmaceutical therapy for dyslipidemias. The American Medical Directors Association's (AMDA) proposed the following treatment approach for residents in the LTC setting with diabetes, hyperlipidemia, and cardiovascular complications with a fair or better prognosis (Figure 14.1). Caution should be used when prescribing statins or fibrates to frail older adult with diabetes residing in LTC facilities. Many nonfrail residents, however, may benefit from pharmacological treatment of dyslipidemia, particularly in the secondary prevention of CVD.

HYPERTENSION IN ADULTS

Approximately one in three adults in the U.S., or an estimated 68 million people, have hypertension.[1] The public health goal of controlling blood pressure is to reduce morbidity and mortality from CVD and kidney disease. Prevention and management of hypertension among U.S. adults over the past decade has been based on guidelines established by the *Seventh Report of the Joint National Committee on Prevention, Detection, Evaluation, and Treatment of High Blood Pressure* (JNC VII).[19] The primary focus of the JNC VII guidelines is helping individuals to achieve SBP goals because most patients with hypertension reach DBP goals once SBP goals have been attained. In people >50 years old, SBP >140 mmHg is a much more important CVD risk factor than DBP. The risk of developing CVD beginning at a blood pressure of 115/75 mmHg doubles with each increment of 20/10 mmHg. Individuals with a SBP of 120–139 mmHg may benefit from health-promoting lifestyle modifications to prevent CVD.

Blood pressure classification and general management based on JNC VII criteria are presented in Table 14.5. Clinical trials have demonstrated that several pharmacological classes of drugs, including angiotensin-converting enzyme (ACE) inhibitors, angiotensin-receptor blockers (ARB), β-blockers, calcium channel blockers (CCB), and thiazide-type diuretics, reduce the complications of hypertension. The JNC VII report states that thiazide-type diuretics should be used as pharmacological treatment for most patients with uncomplicated hypertension, either alone or combined with drugs from other classes.[19] Certain high-risk conditions are compelling indications for the initial use of antihypertensive drug classes other than thiazide-type diuretics.[19] Most individuals with hypertension will require two or more antihypertensive medications to achieve the target blood pressure goal (<140/90 mmHg, or <140/80 mmHg for patients with diabetes). If blood pressure is >20/10 mmHg above target blood pressure goal, consideration should be given to initiating therapy with two agents, one of which usually should be a thiazide-type diuretic.[19]

Hypertension in Older Adults

The prevalence of hypertension increases with age; ~66.7% of men and 78.5% of women age ≥75 years have hypertension.[1] The clinical management of hypertension in the older adult is complicated by the presence of CVD, specific target organ damage (e.g., kidney disease), and other comorbidities. Additionally, most hypertension trials had upper age limitations or did not present results categorized by age.[20] The results of the Blood Pressure Control in the Very Elderly Trial, which included adults ages 80–105 years, were published recently.[21] This clinical trial demonstrated greater than expected benefits of blood pressure control in this older adult cohort. In particular, there was a 30% reduction in strokes, 64% reduction in heart failure, and 21% reduction in total mortality with blood pressure lowering. As in the management of dyslipidemia in the older adult, information is limited to develop evidence-based guidelines for the management of older adults with hypertension; clinical management is based on consensus and expert opinion.

The recently published ACCF/AHA Consensus Document on Hypertension in the Elderly[20] has provided the most extensive review on the management of hypertension in the older adult. The recommendations are summarized in the following paragraphs.

Table 14.5 Classification and Management of Blood Pressure for Adults[a]

Blood pressure classification	SBP[a] (mmHg)	DBP[a] (mmHg)	Lifestyle modification	Initial drug therapy Without compelling indication	Initial drug therapy With compelling indications[b]
Normal	<120	and <80	Encourage		
Prehypertension	120–139	or 80–89	Yes	No antihypertensive drug indicated.	Drug(s) for compelling indications.[c]
Stage 1 hypertension	140–159	or 90–99	Yes	Thiazide-type diuretics. For most; may consider ACEI, ARB, BB, CCB, or combination.	Drug(s) for the compelling indications.[c] Other antihypertensive drugs (diuretics, ACEI, ARB, BB, CCB) as needed.
Stage 2 hypertension	≥160	or ≥100	Yes	Two-drug combination for most[d] (usually thiazide-type diuretic and ACEI or ARB or BB or CCB).	

Note: ACEI = angiotensin converting enzyme inhibitor; ARB = angiotensin receptor blocker; BB = β-blocker; CCB = calcium channel blocker; DBP = diastolic blood pressure; SBP = systolic blood pressure.

a. Treatment determined by highest blood pressure category.
b. Examples of compelling conditions include heart failure, postmyocardial infarction, diabetes, high CHD risk, recurrent stroke prevention.
c. Treat patients with chronic kidney disease or diabetes to blood pressure goal of <130/80 mmHg.
d. Initial combined therapy should be used cautiously in those at risk for orthostatic hypertension.

Source: Chobanian AV, Bakris GL, Black HR, et al. The Seventh Report of the Joint National Committee on Prevention, Detection, Evaluation, and Treatment of High Blood Pressure: The JNC 7 report. *Journal of the American Medical Association* 2003;289(19):2560–2572. Reprinted with permission from the publisher.

Clinical Assessment, Diagnosis, and Evaluation. The consensus panel supports a targeted approach to the management of the older adults with known or suspected hypertension. Their evaluation includes history and physical examination and laboratory evaluation to *1*) accurately determine blood pressure, *2*) identify treatable or reversible causes of elevated blood pressure, *3*) assess target organ damage, *4*) assess for additional CVD factors and comorbid conditions that may affect prognosis, and *5*) identify factors that may influence adherence to therapy. The consensus panel suggests a more deliberate and focused approach to laboratory testing because there does not appear to be evidence to support routine testing. Their recommendations include *1*) assessment for renal dysfunction (i.e., urinalysis for albuminuria); *2*) blood chemistries, including potassium, creatinine, and estimated glomerular filtration rate; *3*) cholesterol panel (total cholesterol, HDL-C, LDL-C, and triglycerides); *4*) fasting blood glucose and A1C, if indicated; and *5*) electrocardiogram. Additionally, the consensus panel has suggested that in selected older adults, a two-dimensional echocardiogram may be useful to evaluate left ventricular hypertrophy and left ventricle dysfunction that may warrant additional therapy (e.g., ACE inhibitors, β-blockers).

Hypertension Management. Several factors need to be considered in the management of hypertensive older adults. Some important factors include cognitive function; insurance coverage and financial ability; and adverse effects of medications, including cognitive changes related to lower blood pressure values. The clinical trials reviewed by the consensus panel did demonstrate benefits from a blood pressure of <150/80 mmHg; however, the generally recommended blood pressure goal in uncomplicated hypertension in older adults with hypertension is <140/90 mmHg. An SBP goal of <140 mmHg is appropriate for most patients age ≤79 years. These target blood pressures are based on expert opinion rather than on data from RCTs. Whether target blood pressure goals for those age ≥80 years should be the same as for those between 65 and 79 years old is not known. Older adults with mild hypertension may be candidates for nonpharmacological interventions as initial therapy; however, drug therapy may be necessary if unresponsive to nonpharmacological therapy.

Initiation of Drug Treatment. The initial antihypertensive drug should be started at the lowest dose and gradually increased, depending on the blood pressure response, until the maximally tolerated dose is reached. If the blood pressure response is not adequate after reaching a maximally tolerated dose, a second drug from a different class should be added. If there are adverse effects or no therapeutic response from this second medication, a drug from another class should be substituted. If a diuretic is not the initial drug, it usually is prescribed as the second drug. If the antihypertensive response is inadequate after reaching full doses of two classes of drugs, a third drug from another class should be added. When blood pressure is >20/10 mmHg above goals, therapy should be initiated with two antihypertensive drugs. An algorithm for the treatment of hypertension in the older adult is presented in Figure 14.2.

Most important, the pharmacological treatment of hypertensive older adult subjects should be individualized. The consensus panel recommends that before adding new antihypertensive drugs, the possible reasons for the poor blood pressure response should be examined. Older adults often are taking more than six prescription drugs. Therefore, polypharmacy and drug interactions are important concerns. In addition, it is always essential to determine whether individuals are following prescribed therapy recommendations.

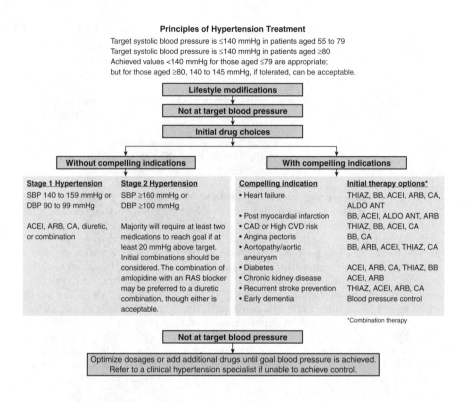

Principles of Hypertension Treatment
Target systolic blood pressure is ≤140 mmHg in patients aged 55 to 79
Target systolic blood pressure is ≤140 mmHg in patients aged ≥80
Achieved values <140 mmHg for those aged ≤79 are appropriate;
but for those aged ≥80, 140 to 145 mmHg, if tolerated, can be acceptable.

Figure 14.2 Algorithm for treatment of hypertension in the elderly.

Note: ACEI = angiotensin converting enzyme inhibitor; ALDO ANT = aldosterone antagonist; ARB = angiotensin receptor blocker; BB = β-blocker; CA = calcium antagonist; CCB = calcium channel blocker; DBP = diastolic blood pressure; SBP = systolic blood pressure, THIAZ = thiazide diuretic .

Source: Aronow WS, Fleg JL, Pepine CJ, et al. ACCF/AHA 2011 expert consensus document on hypertension in the elderly: A report of the American College of Cardiology Foundation Task Force on Clinical Expert Consensus Documents developed in collaboration with the American Academy of Neurology, American Geriatrics Society, American Society for Preventive Cardiology, American Society of Hypertension, American Society of Nephrology, Association of Black Cardiologists, and European Society of Hypertension. *Journal of the American Society of Hypertension* 2011;5:259–352. Reprinted with permission from the publisher.

Guideline for Hypertension Management in Older Adults with Diabetes

The importance of hypertension management in the treatment of those with diabetes cannot be underestimated. In the U.K. Prospective Diabetes Study, tight blood pressure control (mean blood pressure, 144/82 mm/Hg) in individuals with hypertension and T2D was associated with a reduction in the risk of deaths related to diabetes, strokes, microvascular complications related to diabetes, progression of diabetic retinopathy, and deterioration in visual acuity.[22] The European Diabetes Working Party for Older People has published evidence-based guidelines for the treatment of hypertension disorders in older adults with T2D.[18] The authors provided a strong caveat that interventions designed to reduce CVD risk reduction in older adult subjects with diabetes are based on tolerability, clinical factors, disease severity, appropriate blood pressure targets (i.e., those that can be achieved with monotherapy or combination pharmacological therapy), and agreement with the primary care provider. These evidence-based guidelines include the following:

- The threshold for the treatment of hypertension in older adults with T2D should be ≥140/80 mmHg and present for >3 months. Blood pressure should be measured on at least three separate occasions during a period of lifestyle management counseling—for example, behavioral changes, exercise, weight loss, smoking cessation, and nutritional advice (Evidence level 2++, Grade of recommendation B).

- In nonfrail older adult subjects with diabetes (>80 years of age), an acceptable blood pressure in treated patients is an SBP of 140–145 mmHg and a DBP <90 mmHg (Evidence level 1+, Grade of recommendation B).

- For frail older adults with diabetes (e.g., multisystem disease, dementia, caregiver-dependent LTC facility) avoiding heart failure and stroke may be of greater relative importance than microvascular disease, an acceptable blood pressure is <150/90 mmHg (Evidence level 2+, Grade of recommendation C, extrapolated data).

- For older adults with diabetes *without* diabetic renal disease and a sustained blood pressure (≥140/80 mmHg), first-line pharmacological therapies can include the use of ACE inhibitors, ARBs, long-acting CCB, β-blockers, or thiazide diuretics (Evidence level 1+, Grade of recommendation A).

- For older adults with diabetes with microalbuminuria or proteinuria, with a sustained blood pressure (≥140/80 mmHg), pharmacological treatment with an ACE inhibitor or ARBs is recommended (Evidence level 1+, Grade of recommendation B).

- Use of a perindopril (a specific type of an ACE inhibitor)-based regimen in older adults with T2D (with or without hypertension) improves both microvascular and macrovascular outcomes (Evidence level 1+, Grade of recommendation A).

Guidelines for Hypertension Treatment in Older Adults with Diabetes in LTC Facilities

A review of the literature revealed no evidence-based guidelines on the treatment of hypertension in older adults with diabetes residing in LTC facilities. The AMDA has recommended that older adults with diabetes and hypertension who are being treated with ACE inhibitors and residing in an LTC facility have an eGFR monitored regularly and that their medication dose should be adjusted if hyperkalemia develops or if the eGFR is <30 ml/minute/1.73 m^2.[23] Beyond this, there are no other recommendations on hypertensive older adult care among those with diabetes in an LTC setting.

RECOMMENDATIONS TO REDUCE CVD IN OLDER ADULTS WITH DIABETES

Antithrombotics can be used in both the *primary* and *secondary* prevention of CVD in older adults with diabetes. The European Diabetes Working Party for Older People has published evidence-based guidelines on antithrombotic therapy.[18]

- At this time, there is insufficient evidence to routinely recommend low-dose aspirin for older adults with T2D for the *primary* prevention of stroke or CVD mortality (Evidence level 1+, Grade of recommendation A).
- All older adults with T2D, irrespective of baseline CVD risk, should be offered aspirin treatment at a dose of 75–325 mg/d for *secondary* prevention (Evidence level 2++, Grade of recommendation B).

The use of aspirin in older adults with diabetes must be balanced with each individual's clinical condition. There are a number of contraindications to antiplatelet therapy (e.g., active liver disease, allergy, anticoagulation therapy, recent gastrointestinal bleeding, and thrombocytopenia). A review of the literature did not reveal any specific recommendations for residents of LTC settings.

Lifestyle Management for the Prevention of CVD in Adults with Diabetes

Medical nutrition therapy (MNT) is an essential component of diabetes care and is necessary for the primary and secondary prevention of CVD. MNT is designed to provide individual food and meal plans based on assessment, therapy goals, and use of dietary approaches that meet each individual's needs. The overall goals of MNT are to attain and maintain normal blood glucose, blood pressure, and lipid levels; prevent or treat nutrition-related complications (e.g., obesity, dyslipidemia, CVD, hypertension, and nephropathy); improve health through healthy food choices and physical activity; and address individual nutrition needs.[24] ATP III encourages TLC for the primary and secondary prevention of CVD in all adults.[25] TLC recommendations include the following:

- Reduced intake of cholesterol-raising nutrients
- Saturated fats <7% of total calories
- Dietary cholesterol <200 mg/day LDL-lowering therapeutic options
- Plant stanols or sterols (2 grams/day)
- Viscous (soluble) fiber (10–25 grams/day)
- Weight reduction
- Increased physical activity

Lifestyle Management for the Prevention of CVD in Older Adults with Diabetes

The implementation of TLC in older adults with diabetes is highly individualized. Many older adults have changes in taste, vision, or smell that lead to difficulty in food preparation. Significant comorbidities may limit their ability to shop and prepare food. Additionally, older adults may have limited finances that affect their ability to purchase a variety of healthy foods. A change in caloric intake may not be appropriate for all older adults. For example, in frail older adults with diabetes, dietary restriction for lipid lowering is not recommended routinely, as it may cause undernutrition.[23] The European Diabetes Working Party for Older People has provided the following evidence-based guideline for nutrition in the older adult with diabetes.[18]

- Nutritional assessment is recommended for all older adults with diabetes at the time of diagnosis and regularly thereafter. This will allow the identification of resident with undernutrition (Evidence level 2++, Grade of recommendation B).

The goal of this recommendation is to ensure that the older adult with diabetes will have their nutritional status appropriately monitored.

Older adults with diabetes may participate in an individualized exercise plan; however, the frequency and intensity of the training program must be based on each individual's degree of physical fitness. Because there is a strong possibility of underlying CHD in older adults with diabetes, the exercise program must be based on an exercise tolerance test and carefully supervised.[26]

Lifestyle Management for the Prevention of CVD in Older Adults with Diabetes in LTC Facilities

Diabetes UK recently published Good Clinical Practice Guidelines for Care Home Residents with Diabetes.[27] The authors of the guidelines noted that residents of care homes are at nutritional risk. Many of these residents are malnourished and have various degrees of protein energy malnutrition and hypoalbuminuria. Therefore, the guidelines suggest that all adults should be screened for malnutrition on admission to LTC facilities. This recommendation suggests that the health care provider should use caution in the use of nutritional modification as a TLC for lowering CVD risk in LTC residents. A review of the literature did not reveal any other specific recommendations for TLC in residents of LTC settings. At this time, the implementation of TLC in LTC settings is highly individualized based on the individual's clinical status.

CONCLUSION

This chapter has provided a review of medical evidence guiding the management of CVD in older adults with diabetes, including those residing in LTC facilities. The primary targets of review were the treatment of hypertension and dyslipidemia. The recommendations were based largely on ATP III,[25] AMDA,[23]

European Diabetes Working Party for Older People Guidelines,[18] JNC VII,[19] and ACCF/AHA Consensus Document on Hypertension in the Elderly.[20] The two most recent reports[18,20] reflect the growing need for guidance on CVD risk management in older adults with diabetes; however, there is more work to be done. Unfortunately, information on CVD management among residents of LTC settings is not available. Any such information is based on isolated opinions or comments dispersed throughout the literature. In view of the aging population, the further development of guidelines for reducing CVD risk among the older adult (especially those in LTC settings) is warranted.

REFERENCES

1. Centers for Disease Control and Prevention. National diabetes fact sheet: National estimates and general information on diabetes and prediabetes in the United States, 2011. Atlanta, GA, U.S. Department of Health and Human Resources, 2011.
2. Zhang X, Decker FH, Luo H, et al. Trends in the prevalence and comorbidities of diabetes mellitus in nursing home residents in the United States: 1995-2004. *Journal of the American Geriatrics Society* 2010;58(4):724–730.
3. Goff DC Jr, Lloyd-Jones DM, Bennett G, O'Donnell CJ, Coady S, Robinson J, D'Agostino RB Sr, Schwartz JS, Gibbons R, Shero ST, Greenland P, Smith SC Jr, Lackland DT, Sorlie P, Levy D, Stone NJ, Wilson PW. 2013 ACC/AHA Guideline on the Assessment of Cardiovascular Risk: A Report of the American College of Cardiology/American Heart Association Task Force on Practice Guidelines. J Am Coll Cardiol 2013 Nov 12. pii: S0735-1097(13)06031-2. doi: 10.1016/j.jacc.2013.11.005. [Epub ahead of print].
4. Stone NJ, Robinson JG, Lichtenstein AH, Goff Jr DC, Lloyd-Jones DM, Smith Jr SC, Blum C, Schwartz JS; for the 2013 ACC/AHA Cholesterol Guideline Panel. Treatment of blood cholesterol to reduce atherosclerotic cardiovascular disease risk in adults: Synopsis of the 2013 ACC/AHA Cholesterol Guideline. Ann Intern Med 2014 Jan 28. doi: 10.7326/M14-0126. [Epub ahead of print].
5. American Heart Association, American College of Cardiology. 2013 Prevention Guidelines Tools: CV Risk Calculator 2013. Available at https://my.americanheart.org/professional/StatementsGuidelines/PreventionGuidelines/Prevention-Guidelines_UCM_457698_SubHomePage.jsp. Accessed 24 March 2014.
6. Stone NJ, Robinson J, Lichtenstein AH, Bairey Merz CN, Lloyd-Jones DM, Blum CB, McBride P, Eckel RH, Schwartz JS, Goldberg AC, Shero ST, Gordon D, Smith SC Jr, Levy D, Watson K, Wilson PW. 2013 ACC/AHA Guideline on the Treatment of Blood Cholesterol to Reduce Atherosclerotic Cardiovascular Risk in Adults: A Report of the American College of Cardiology/American Heart Association Task Force on Practice Guidelines. J Am Coll Cardiol 2013 Nov 7. pii: S0735-1097(13)06028-2. doi: 10.1016/j.jacc.2013.11.002. [Epub ahead of print].
7. American Diabetes Association. Statement by the American Diabetes Association regarding the American College of Cardiology/American Heart

Association Guideline on the Treatment of Blood Cholesterol to Reduce Atherosclerotic Cardiovascular Risk in Adults. Available at http://www.diabetes.org/newsroom/press-releases/2013/statement-cholesterol-guidelines. html. Accessed 24 March 2014.

8. American Diabetes Association. Standards of medical care in diabetes—2014. *Diabetes Care* 2014;37(Suppl 1):S14–S80.

9. Keaney JF, Curfman GD, Jarcho JA. A pragmatic view of the new cholesterol treatment guidelines. N Engl J Med 2014;370:275–278.

10. Expert Panel on Detection, Evaluation, and Treatment of High Blood Cholesterol in Adults. Executive Summary of the third report of the National Cholesterol Education Program (NCEP) Expert Panel on detection, evaluation, and treatment of high blood cholesterol in adults (Adult Treatment Panel III). *Journal of the American Medical Association* 2001;285(19):2486–2497.

11. Afilalo J, Duque G, Steele R, Jukema JW, de Craen AJ, Eisenberg MJ. Statins for secondary prevention in elderly patients: a hierarchical Bayesian meta-analysis. *Journal* of the *American College* of *Cardiology* 2008;51(1):37–45.

12. Shepherd J, Blauw GJ, Murphy MB, et al. Pravastatin in elderly individuals at risk of vascular disease (PROSPER): A randomised controlled trial. *Lancet* 2002;360(9346):1623–1630.

13. Baigent C, Keech A, Kearney PM, et al. Efficacy and safety of cholesterol-lowering treatment: prospective meta-analysis of data from 90,056 participants in 14 randomised trials of statins. *Lancet* 2005;366(9493):1267–1278.

14. Collins R, Armitage J, Parish S, Sleigh P, Peto R. MRC/BHF Heart Protection Study of cholesterol-lowering with simvastatin in 5963 people with diabetes: A randomised placebo-controlled trial. *Lancet* 2003;361(9374):2005–2016.

15. Colhoun HM, Betteridge DJ, Durrington PN, et al. Primary prevention of cardiovascular disease with atorvastatin in type 2 diabetes in the Collaborative Atorvastatin Diabetes Study (CARDS): Multicentre randomised placebo-controlled trial. *Lancet* 2004;364(9435):685–696.

16. Koskinen P, Manttari M, Manninen V, Huttunen JK, Heinonen OP, Frick MH. Coronary heart disease incidence in NIDDM patients in the Helsinki Heart Study. *Diabetes Care* Jul 1992;15(7):820–825.

17. Rubins HB, Robins SJ, Collins D, et al. Gemfibrozil for the secondary prevention of coronary heart disease in men with low levels of high-density lipoprotein cholesterol. Veterans Affairs High-Density Lipoprotein Cholesterol Intervention Trial Study Group. *New England Journal of Medicine* 1999;341(6):410–418.

18. Sinclair AJ, Paolisso G, Castro M, Bourdel-Marchasson I, Gadsby R, Rodriguez Manas L. European Diabetes Working Party for Older People 2011 clinical guidelines for T2D mellitus. Executive summary. *Diabetes and Metabolism* 2011;37(Suppl3):S27–S38.

19. Chobanian AV, Bakris GL, Black HR, et al. Seventh report of the Joint National Committee on Prevention, Detection, Evaluation, and Treatment of High Blood Pressure. *Hypertension* 2003;42(6):1206–1252.

20. Aronow WS, Fleg JL, Pepine CJ, et al. ACCF/AHA 2011 expert consensus document on hypertension in the elderly: a report of the American College of Cardiology Foundation Task Force on Clinical Expert Consensus Documents developed in collaboration with the American Academy of Neurology,

American Geriatrics Society, American Society for Preventive Cardiology, American Society of Hypertension, American Society of Nephrology, Association of Black Cardiologists, and European Society of Hypertension. *Journal of the American Society of Hypertension* 2011;5(4):259–352.

21. Bulpitt CJ, Beckett NS, Peters R, et al. Blood pressure control in the Hypertension in the Very Elderly Trial (HYVET). *Journal of Human Hypertension* 2012;26(3):157–163.

22. United Kingdom Prospective Diabetes Study. Tight blood pressure control and risk of macrovascular and microvascular complications in type 2 diabetes: UKPDS 38. UK Prospective Diabetes Study Group. *British Medical Journal* 1998;317(7160):703–713.

23. American Medical Directors Association. *Diabetes management in the long-term care setting clinical practice guideline.* Columbia, MD, Author, 2010.

24. Daly A, Powers MA. Medical nutrition therapy. In *Therapy for diabetes mellitus and related disorders.* 5th ed. Lebovitz HE, Ed. Alexandria, VA, American Diabetes Association, 2009, p. 167–178.

25. Pasternak RC. Report of the Adult Treatment Panel III: The 2001 National Cholesterol Education Program guidelines on the detection, evaluation and treatment of elevated cholesterol in adults. *Clinical Cardiology* 2003;21(3):393–398.

26. Halter JB. Diabetes in older adults. In *Therapy for diabetes mellitus and related disorders.* 5th ed. Lebovitz HE, Ed. Alexandria, VA, American Diabetes Association, 2009, p. 362–368.

27. Sinclair AJ. Good clinical practice guidelines for care home residents with diabetes: an executive summary. *Diabetes and Metabolism* 2011;28(7):772–777.

15

Transitions of Care Settings

*Ann Wagle, PhD, RN, NEA-BC**

INTRODUCTION

Care transitions occur when an older adult moves from one setting to another. Community-dwelling older adults who need acute care are admitted to hospital environments. Not infrequently, these same individuals are transferred to skilled long-term care (LTC) nursing facilities for short-term post-acute care before returning to home. Conversely, residents in LTC commonly are transferred to other care settings because of the need of a different level of care or the need to be relocated to another organization or care team. A different level of care may be required as individuals with diabetes are likely to have a history of, or risk for heart disease, cerebrovascular accident (CVA), visual impairment, urinary incontinence, and arthritis.[1] Heart disease and CVA may result in a transfer to acute care, and sequelae of injuries resulting from a fall due to visual impairment, bowel or bladder needs, and immobility or pain resulting from arthritis also may involve a transfer to a higher level of care. Optimal coordination among health care professionals is imperative if these transfers are to achieve the goal of minimal complications and excellent outcomes. Without this coordination, increased hospital readmissions, duplication of services, resource waste, and medication errors may occur.[2–7]

FOUNDATIONAL PRINCIPLES OF CARE

During any transfer among care settings, the risk for insufficient coordination increases regarding aspects of care, such as established individualized routines, particularly when an individual has been a resident in LTC and has established his or her living habits in that setting. In addition, the change and addition of caregivers may result in confusion and increased stress for the individual who is accustomed to a particular LTC setting. Optimal transfer practices can be promoted through principles that are essential to individuals in any setting and are particularly important for individuals with diabetes. For these residents, even small changes in dietary consumption or schedules, activity modification, or alterations in timing of medication administration can result in changes that are life altering.[8] The concepts of individualized care, accountability, communication, documentation, and safety are critical areas affecting transition that merit exploration and emphasis.

---

*Opinions expressed in the article are those of the author and do not reflect official positions or policies of the Department of Veterans Affairs.

DOI: 10.2337/9781580404730.15

233

Individualized Care

Provision of care in LTC through the traditional medical model has been challenged in recent years with the long-awaited implementation of individualization of care. It is no longer acceptable to schedule therapies, daily living, or recreational activities in LTC at the convenience of the organization. Rather, the individual or "resident" determines the daily timetable, which is not limited to 8:00 A.M. to 5:00 P.M. therapies or the "3-Bs" of "Bible, Birthday, and Bingo." Residents should arise, dine, bathe, and attend therapies and other activities each day based on their current wishes, or based on their life patterns as established by the resident or, possibly, a close family member.[9] The resident should be an active participant in his or her plan of care, choosing both the goals of care and the means to achieve those goals. Although this type of individualization of care is also on the horizon of practice in acute-care settings, a resident who currently is transferring from LTC to an acute-care setting may find her- or himself once again in the medical model of care, and thus stripped of her or his ability to contribute to the plan of care because of the acuity of her or his health problem or the change of care setting and caregivers.

Accountability

Another important component of care is that of accountability. In a recent publication, the American Medical Directors Association has recommended the term "discharge" be replaced with that of "transition."[10] The term "discharge" may contribute to a lack of continuity of care because of the implication that the previous care setting is no longer responsible for the individual. The term "transition," however, implies that the responsibility for care continues throughout the transfer process and that clarification of information is an integral part of professional communication. In addition, a competent and compassionate caregiver must be accountable for the transition and the communication of information that surrounds the process. For effective transitions to occur, it is imperative that designated persons on each side of the transition are assigned to each resident with the components of clear feedback and accountability tightly woven into the process for both the sending and receiving care teams. Clear templates for documentation should be devised and revised as needed that verify specific information is conveyed with each transition (see Figure 15.1). Furthermore, subsequent monitoring of transition documentation records is essential to ensure that adequate information is communicated in addition to needed updates of the template on a regular basis.[10]

Communication

Communication continues to be critical in the care and transfer of care for individuals in LTC. Although the implementation of the electronic health record (EHR) has increased the potential for improved communication, the EHR currently is limited to communication within the confines of a particular health system. Communication among health systems does not exist, and in some ways, it is more limited by the inaccessibility of records from one EHR system to

Long-Term Care to Acute Care: Transfer Note

DATE OF NOTE: AUTHOR: EXP COSIGNER:

Current Complaint/Reason for Transfer:

Skin Integrity:

          Location:

Communication Needs:

Behavioral Needs:

A (Antecedent behavior) = Identify situation/conditions that trigger behaviors and
     preventive strategies:
B (Behavior) = Describe problem behaviors frequently presented:
C (Consequence) = Describe interventions known to help manage/control problem behaviors:

Current Pain Level (1–10):

Pain Management:

Safety Needs:
  Fall risk

Special Needs:

NOK Notified of Transfer: Yes/No

Active Inpatient Medications:

HAND-OFF:

          SITUATION
          Name:
          Diagnosis:
          Orientation:
          Activity: Assist Device:
          Suicide Status:
          Nursing Observation: Elopement Risk:

          BACKGROUND
          Pertinent History:
          Allergies:
          Isolation: Yes/No   Type:
          Fall Score:
          Critical Values:
          Code Status:
          Vitals:
          Oxygen: Yes/No   Type/liters:
          Wound: Yes/No   Location:
          Additional Information:

          ASSESSMENT:

          RECOMMENDATION:
Treatments/Interventions:

Figure 15.1 Electronic Template for Documentation.

Diagnostics:
Laboratory

IV site check:

Follow-up needed:

Report given to:

Does the patient/resident have a court-appointed legal guardian?

Is the patient/resident considered to be a danger to self or others?

Has the patient/resident been legally committed?

Does the patient/resident have a history of escape, wandering, or elopement?

Does the patient/resident have mental impairments (either permanent or temporary) that increase their risk of harm to self or others?

Does the patient/resident have physical impairments (either permanent or temporary) that increase their risk of harm to self or others?

SKIN ASSESSMENT:

> Braden Scale (for predicting pressure wound risk):
> Sensory Perception:
> Moisture:
> Activity:
> Mobility:
> Nutrition:
> Friction:
> > Score:

CURRENT SKIN ASSESSMENT
> Skin Color:
> Skin Temperature
> Skin Moisture
> Skin Turgor

SKIN PROBLEMS
> Wound (location, type, description)

INTERVENTIONS

Figure 15.1 (Continued)

another. Until EHRs are universally accessible by health care workers in all segments across health care delivery systems, communication will continue to be compromised.

Kripalani et al. reviewed hospital records and found that numerous components often were missing from discharge summaries, including the responsible hospital physician, main diagnoses, physical findings, medications, follow-up plans, and pending tests.[6] In addition, as much as 25% of discharge letters and summaries never reached the patients' primary caregiver.[6,11] The results of two studies indicated a "packaged discharge," consisting of arranging follow-up appointments, medication reconciliation, patient education and the use of a "transition coach," decreased readmissions and emergency department (ED) visits within 30 days of discharge by 30%, and reduced rehospitalization rates for 6 months, including in populations of individuals >65 years of age with chronic illnesses.[12,13] This type of care coordination is imperative for individuals with diabetes, as stability of insulin or other anti-hyperglycemic agents, along with diet and exercise, must be maintained for optimal outcomes.

Communication must be integrated carefully with documentation and must include the resident's plan of care, pertinent test results, consultant reports, and medication reconciliation. Although the EHR is used widely in many organizations, use of the EHR across organizations is not typical, resulting in a potential for suboptimal communication. In addition, LTC-based care managers once coordinated care across settings, but more recently they are assigned to specific health care organizations, and individuals with several problems may have multiple care managers, thus contributing to the fragmentation of care.[14] Diabetes care and management is complex, and numerous myths exist in the care of diabetes. The individual with diabetes who receives care from numerous health care settings likely will experience miscommunication among health professionals, resulting in a greater potential for misunderstanding of information, and fewer chances to dispel the myths as the illness is explained from a variety of perspectives and in numerous EHRs.

The increased number of care coordinators may be overwhelming to individuals, resulting in a perception of powerlessness related to complex pathophysiology and treatments that are documented poorly across settings. To better explore and understand these communication issues, the Centers for Medicare and Medicaid Services has piloted a tool for use in postacute settings, working to coordinate care and reduce unneeded hospitalizations by improving transitions across settings.[15-17]

Safety

Of primary importance in all care settings is safety of the individual receiving care. The resident and family who are ill-informed about aspects of individualized diabetes care—including planned tests, test results, medication from various sources, and the plan of care—have a greater risk of injury or lack of appropriate implementation of care. A potential problem for the individual with diabetes is that of medication reconciliation. According to the results of one study, 66% of errors related to medication reconciliation happened during transitions of care.[18] During the process of medication reconciliation, medication orders at each point of a resident's care are compared to develop a current, accurate, and comprehensive list of all medications. The medication reconciliation process should be completed each time a resident is admitted or transferred between settings with a goal of reducing complications and poor outcomes that occur from medication errors (see Figure 15.2). This reconciliation is particularly critical for residents with diabetes because of the complex and interrelated nature of the chronic illness. The resident and appropriate family members should be included in the process of medication reconciliation to help ensure that medications are documented thoroughly.

SAMPLE (Patient ID Information)

Medication reconciliation form

List all patient medications prior to assessment, include over-the-counter and alternative medicines (herbals).

Before an outpatient receives any medication as part of their test or procedure, list all of their current home medications looking for allergies, interactions, duplications, or other concerns. A complete reconciliation of medication is required if the patient is to be admitted to the hospital.

Allergies: _____

Information Source:____ Patient   ____ Family   ____ Primary Care Provider

Patient's Pharmacy(s) _____

MAR from _____   ____ Other (specify) _____

____Check here if patient is not currently on any medication.				Last Dose		**Medical Provider Decision:** Continue? Circle One	
Medication Name	Dose	Route	Frequency	Date	Time		
1						Y	N
2						Y	N
3						Y	N
4						Y	N
5						Y	N
6						Y	N
7						Y	N
8						Y	N
9						Y	N
10						Y	N
11						Y	N
12						Y	N
13						Y	N
14						Y	N
15						Y	N

Figure 15.2 Medication Reconciliation Form, Sample 1.

On the lines below, enter orders for new medications that the patient is not currently taking or changes to current regimen.

_____

_____

_____

_____

I have reviewed this list of patient medications and to the best of my knowledge, the additional medications I have ordered will not result in any adverse reaction(s).

Completed by _____ Provider Signature _____ Date/Time _____

            (print name)

Faxed/Given to _____ by _____ Date/Time _____

                 (sign & print name)

Sheet ____ of ____

Figure 15.2 (Continued)

PLANNED AND UNPLANNED TRANSITIONS

Annually, ~2.2 million nursing home residents visit EDs and are 13 times more likely to have been discharged from a hospital within 7 days before the emergent visit. Nearly 50% of these nursing home residents were admitted to the hospital from the ED visit.[19] Although LTC transfers can be planned or unplanned, both require the components of care that include individualized care, accountability, communication, documentation, and safety. A planned transfer from LTC to the acute setting may be due to a scheduled surgical procedure or extensive testing that involves preparation that is outside the scope of LTC. Unplanned transitions may be needed to treat injuries from falls or a sudden or unanticipated change of condition resulting from pneumonia or other illness. In residents with diabetes, unplanned transitions may occur with episodes of hypoglycemia or extreme hyperglycemia. A positive planned transition may occur when an individual improves in the acute-care setting and is ready to return to LTC. Yet another type of planned transition includes end-of-life care decisions or a transition to the home setting, either for a particular event or on a more permanent basis. In each of these transitions, either planned or unplanned, it is critical that the principles of individualized care, accountability, communication, documentation, and safety be maintained.

Physical Needs

The physical needs of an individual with diabetes can be assessed in a variety of methods, including comprehensive physical assessment, diagnostic testing, and monitoring changes in nutrition, hydration, or activity. Although variation occurs among individuals, particular patterns of findings may indicate the need for further evaluation, resulting in a transition to a more acute setting.

The most common lab work for individuals with diabetes is testing blood glucose levels, either with a finger-stick for capillary blood glucose levels or through the venous blood for fasting glucose or A1C levels. Medical thought has evolved regarding ideal levels of blood glucose control for older adults and multiple clinical practice guidelines have been developed.[14,20-24] Detailed information derived from these guidelines can be found in Chapters 4, 5, and 9. Again, the resident should be involved in these decisions regarding personal target levels for blood glucose control with ongoing education and options of care thoroughly explained by the health care team. As transitions occur between health care settings, individualized norms should be communicated carefully among team members, with appropriate documentation to verify preferred blood glucose target values as noted by the health care team, as well as the individual's concerns and preferences. Caregivers should expect that blood glucose values will vary during periods of transition. Insulin doses are likely to be changed, and medications that affect blood glucose levels may be discontinued or added during a hospitalization. In the hospital, blood glucose levels may be checked according to a standardized sick-day management approach. A plan needs to be in place to more closely monitor capillary blood glucose levels until they stabilize during the resident's transition back to his or her LTC environment.

Other types of testing include body systems that have been affected by diabetes or that have the potential for changes due to the disease. These tests include blood pressure, lipid levels, kidney function, liver function, and routine exams for eye health. Careful assessment of skin and feet is important for early intervention of possible risk of skin impairment, and extremities should be evaluated thoroughly for color, temperature, and presence and character of peripheral pulses. Comprehensive information about foot care can be found in Chapter 12. Changes to an individual's "normal" status should be evaluated carefully in the context of current health factors, and specific modifications to the plan of care should be devised with and implemented for that individual. Whatever the individual's baseline, the information should be conveyed explicitly to the caregiver on the receiving end of the transition.

In addition to more typical lab work, the individual with diabetes should be assessed for changes in activity levels. Because physical exercise is related closely to dietary needs and diabetes medication requirements, changes in caloric expenditures can result in hypoglycemia or hyperglycemia. In addition, changes in an individual's routine and general mind-set as noted by consistent and competent staff can help to call attention to physical illnesses, such as pneumonia, constipation, infections, or pressure wounds. Family members are valuable reporters of change in residents' condition. These changes should be well communicated and documented throughout transitions of care.

Cognitive Needs

The challenges of the individual with diabetes can become daunting with the added possibility of cognitive impairments. Confusion resulting from dementia or Alzheimer's disease further complicates the ability of the individual to understand and participate in the care of the already complex illness of diabetes. Of utmost importance in the care of an individual with Alzheimer's disease is the presence of consistent caregivers who know the person and understand that person's behavioral language.[8] The cognitively impaired resident with diabetes may have consistent cues indicating hypoglycemia. Failure to assign consistent caregivers to such a resident may lead to countless unnecessary trips to the ED. Numerous other negative behavioral outcomes can be avoided with the use of knowledgeable and consistent caregivers. Optimal care of individuals with Alzheimer's disease includes limiting caregiving staff to no more than eight individuals.[16] More than eight caregivers often results in confusion for the individual with Alzheimer's disease, and caregivers may have difficulty remembering and documenting the unique preferences of each resident when the number of residents for whom they are responsible increases. Careful and thorough communication with the individual as well as family members is critical when caring for individuals with Alzheimer's disease, because family members may have added concerns as the resident has increased problems with communication and memory.

Some confusion may be reversible if the individual has an infection or inflammatory process that results in delirium. For example, when a resident has a fever, delirium and confusion may result, but this may resolve when the fever is treated and the resident regains his or her former state of health. In these cases, the value of a knowledgeable and consistent caregiver is of utmost importance to recognize differences in cognitive aspects and to report and document these changes appropriately. If possible, the individual may be treated in the LTC setting so caregiver consistency is maintained and the individual's confusion is minimized. If transfer to an acute setting is imperative, family members may be encouraged to stay with the individual to mitigate confusion that may result from the combination of the physical infection as well as a new set of caregivers and the unfamiliarity of the acute-care setting. The idea of consistent caregivers during episodes of delirium may be particularly important given the complexity of treatment related to diabetes and the propensity for changes in blood glucose levels during infections and the accompanying need for closer monitoring of glucose levels during treatment.[25] Proactive treatment often involves recognition of early symptoms of physical infection and inflammation to reduce the potential for confusion resulting from delirium.

Emotional and Social Needs

Most residents with diabetes have family and close friends who serve as formal or informal caregivers and assist with care and some level of decision making. The importance of these family members and close friends should be emphasized, and these individuals should be respected as partners who make valuable contributions to ensure that the resident's preferences are honored in the context of quality and safety.[26] These relationships may be particularly important when the individual in LTC transitions to an acute-care setting, as family and friends who know the resident may serve as a stabilizing entity to support and facilitate consistency of the environment and act as an advocate for the individual in a traditional medical setting. Family involvement, availability, and interest vary widely, however, and persistent communication is needed to potentially engage family members in care and decision making that may present during a transition to and from the acute-care setting, while carefully recognizing the requirements of privacy through Health Insurance Portability and Accountability Act regulations.

Education Needs

Meaningful and continual education is imperative when caring for a resident with diabetes and that responsibility increases when a transition to another care setting takes place. Thorough assessment of the resident and family's current level of knowledge is the first step in conveying additional information that eventually will determine decisions in the plan of care. In addition, the cognitive, affective, and psychomotor domains of learning should be addressed so that the resident and family can develop various perspectives with application and retention of information.

When educating a resident and family about diabetes and the plan of care, a collaborative approach should include the patient and family, medical provider, nurse, dietitian, rehabilitation therapist, certified diabetes educator (if available), and other members of the health care team. The plan of care must include resident preferences to be sustainable in the transition from LTC to acute care and in the return to LTC. Similarly, important factors such as cultural aspects, physical activity patterns, dietary habits, and social cues must be considered.[20,23,27] In this manner, the treatment plan should be one of self-management, and education should address aspects of care that can be understood and supported by the individual and family members.

CONCLUSION

When individuals with diabetes in LTC are transferred to other care settings, careful attention must be given to multiple aspects of care, including individualized care, accountability, communication, documentation, and safety. Whether these transfers are planned or unplanned, coordination of care and comprehensive communication are critical components that must be implemented judiciously to optimize transitions for the individual and family members. Although these areas of care are important for all individuals, strategic consideration must be given to older adults with diabetes to maintain physical, cognitive, and emotional or social health and to prevent major complications and a potential decline in quality of life.

REFERENCES

1. Russell LB, Valiyeva E, Roman SH, et al. Hospitalizations, nursing home admissions, and deaths attributable to diabetes. *Diabetes Care* 2005;28(7):1611–1617.
2. Boockvar K, Fishman E, Kyriacou CK, et al. Adverse events due to discontinuations in drug use and dose changes in patients transferred between acute and long-term care facilities. *Archives of Internal Medicine* 2004;164(5):545–550.
3. Coleman EA. Falling through the cracks: Challenges and opportunities for improving transitional care for persons with continuous complex care needs. *Journal of the American Geriatric Society* 2003;52(5):855–856.
4. Forster AJ, Murff HJ, Peterson JF, et al. The incidence and severity of adverse events affecting patients after discharge from the hospital. *Annals of Internal Medicine* 2003;138(3):161–167.
5. Jencks SF, Williams MV, Coleman EA. Rehospitalizations among patients in the Medicare fee-for-service program. *New England Journal of Medicine* 2009;360(14):1418–1428.
6. Kripalani S, LeFevre F, Phillips CO, et al. Deficits in communications and information transfer between hospital-based and primary care physicians: Implications for patient safety and continuity of care. *Journal of American Medical Association* 2007;297(8):831–341.
7. Sobogal F, Coots-Miyazaki M, Lett JE. Effective care transitions interventions: Improving patient safety and healthcare quality. *CAHQ Journal* 2007(Quarter 2);31(2), 15–19.
8. Crogan NL, Dupler AE. Food choice can improve nursing home resident meal service satisfaction and nutritional status. *Journal of Gerontological Nursing* 2013;39(5):38–45.
9. Mueller C, Burger S, Rader J, Carter D. Nurse Competencies for person-directed care in nursing homes. *Geriatric Nursing* 2013;34:101–104.
10. American Medical Directors Association Public Policy Committee. Improving care transitions between the nursing facility and the acute-care hospital settings [White Papter]. Retrieved from http://amda.com/governance/whitepapers/H10.pdf. Accessed 13 February 2014.
11. Were MC, Li X, Kesterson J, et al. Adequacy of hospital discharge summaries in documenting tests with pending results and outpatient follow-up providers. *Journal of General Internal Medicine* 2009;24(9):1002–1006.
12. Coleman EA, Parry C, Chalmers S, Min SJ. The care transitions interventions: Results of a randomized controlled trial. *Archives of Internal Medicine* 2006;166(17):1822–1828.
13. Jack BW, Chetty VK, Andhony D, et al. A reengineered hospital discharge program to decrease rehospitalization: A randomized trial. *Annals of Internal Medicine* 2009;150(3):178–187.
14. American Medical Directors Association. *Guidelines for diabetes management in the long-term care setting.* Columbia, MD, Author, 2010.
15. Centers for Medicare and Medicare Services (CMS). (2007). MCS-1533-P. Proposed changes to the hospital inpatient prospective payment

systems and fiscal year 2008 rates. Washington, D.C., Federal Register, 2008, vol. 72(85).

16. Centers for Medicare and Medicaid (CMS). Quality Improvement organizations, statement of work. Washington, D.C., U.S. Department of Health and Human Services, Centers for Medicare and Medicaid Services, 2009.

17. RTI International. Post-acute care payment reform demonstration report to Congress supplement—interim report (2011). Centers for Medicare and Medicaid Services' Office of Research, Development, and Information. Retrieved from http://www.cms.gov/Research-Statistics-Data-and-Systems/Statistics-Trends-and-Reports/Reports/downloads/GAGE_PACPRD_RTC_Supp_Materials_May_2011.pdf. Accessed 13 February 2014.

18. U.S. Pharmacopeia. USP patient safety. *CAPSLink* 2005;October. Center for the Advancement of Patient Safety (CAPS). Retrieved from http://www.docstoc.com/docs/52969668/Medication-Errors-Involving-Reconciliation-Failures. Accessed 13 February 2014.

19. Wang HE, Shah MN, Allman RM, Kilgore M. Emergency department visits by nursing home residents in the United States. *Journal of the American Geriatrics Society* 2011;59(10):1864–1872.

20. American Diabetes Association. Standards of medical care in diabetes—2014. *Diabetes Care* 2014;37(Suppl1):S14–S80.

21. Brown AF, Mangione CM, Saliba D, Sarkisian CA, California Healthcare Foundation/American Geriatrics Society Panel on Improving Care for Older Persons with Diabetes. Guidelines for improving the care of the older person with diabetes mellitus. *Journal of the American Geriatric Society* 2003;51(5):S265–S280.

22. Sinclair AJ, Paolisso G, Castro M, Bourdel-Marchasson I, Gadsby R, Rodriguez Mañas L. European Diabetes Working Party for Older People 2011 clinical guidelines for type 2 diabetes mellitus. Executive summary. *Diabetes and Metabolism* 2011;37(Suppl3)(0):S27–S38.

23. Moreno G, Mangione CM, Kimbro L, Vaisberg E, American Geriatrics Society Expert Panel on the Care of Older Adults with Diabetes Mellitus. *Guidelines for improving the care of older adults with diabetes mellitus.* 2nd ed. New York, NY, American Geriatrics Society, 2013.

24. Sinclair A, Dunning T, Colagiuri R, IDF Working Group. International diabetes federation managing older people with type 2 diabetes: Global guideline. 1st ed. Brussels, Belgium, International Diabetes Federation, 2013, p. 1–96.

25. Travis SS, Buchanan RJ, Wang S, Kim M. Analyses of nursing home residents with diabetes at admission. *Journal of the American Medical Directors Association* 2004;5:320–327.

26. Coleman EA, Williams MV. Executing high-quality care transitions: A call to do it right. *Journal of Hospital Medicine* 2007;2(5):287–290.

27. American Diabetes Association. Standards of Medical Care in Diabetes—2013. *Diabetes Care* 2013;36(Suppl1):S11–S66.

16

Where Do We Go from Here?
Conclusions and Recommendations

Sandra Drozdz Burke, PhD, ANP-BC, CDE, FAADE

Specialists in gerontology would agree that the term "older adult" refers to a broad range of ages and a wide spectrum of functional and cognitive abilities. In the same way that geriatrics or gerontology is complex and multifaceted, so too is diabetes in the older adult. The older adult patient or resident with diabetes might be 60, 70, 80, 90, or even 100 years of age. She or he might have new onset or long-standing diabetes. The diabetes could be type 1 (T1D) or type 2 (T2D), and complicated or uncomplicated. The resident might have any number of geriatric syndromes, or none at all. Added to this, the older adult may be living independently or may be a resident of short- or long-term custodial care. This level of heterogeneity in the person, the disease, and the environment adds several layers of complexity to diabetes care and education not found in most other populations. Complicating this image is a profusion of guidelines for the care and management of people with diabetes.

Clinical practice guidelines for diabetes in the older adult are available from various sources, including the American Diabetes Association (ADA), the American Geriatrics Society (AGS), the American Medical Directors Association (AMDA), the U.S. Department of Veterans Affairs/Department of Defense, and the European Diabetes Working Party for Older People.[1-6] Each group recognizes the relative lack of research specific to the care of the older adult population, and there is a real concern about this. We are living in an era of evidence-based medicine and guidelines are designed to serve as a foundation for practice. But let's think about that for a moment. Without research, how can guidelines be established? Data derived from research, particularly from randomized controlled studies, always have been an essential source of information to guide practice. As our population continues to age, discovering solutions for older adults through research continues to be an important objective. But, what do we do while we wait for the results of research studies? What do we do when the research studies do not address the needs of older adults—or subcultures of older adults, such as the long-term care (LTC) population? Is research the only source of evidence? And what, exactly, is evidence-based practice (EBP)?

To engage in EBP, the clinician combines the best and most current evidence about a condition with his or her own clinical judgment and, whenever possible, factors the patient's preferences and values into the decision-making model.[7,8] Research tells us that by engaging in EBP, the clinician is more likely to see consistent outcomes of therapy. "Evidence" comes from many places, including, in some cases, expert or consensus opinion. "Research" refers to many different methods for discovery, not only from randomized controlled trials. Evidence for clinical practice is "graded" or "sorted" and placed into a hierarchy in which

DOI: 10.2337/9781580404730.16

the highest level of evidence is a systematic review (a comprehensive review of research on a particular topic) and the lowest level of evidence is what is known as consensus or expert opinion (see Tables 14.3 and 14.4).[9-11] Thus, it is important for health care providers to recognize that although research is an important source of evidence, it is not the *only* source of evidence. Consensus statements, such as the one jointly published by the ADA and the AGS in 2012[12,13] are developed when experts in the field evaluate and make public what currently is known about a topic. For older adults with diabetes, especially those in LTC settings, much of the current evidence comes from consensus. Consequently, many of the guidelines for clinical care are driven by consensus statements.

COMMON THEMES AMONG GUIDELINES

When it comes to guidelines for the care of the older adult, the conclusions and recommendations from the various groups are similar but not entirely consistent. This makes it difficult for the medical director, the nurse administrator, and the bedside caregiver to know what is best for the resident with diabetes. Recall that EBP involves using the best available evidence in combination with clinician judgment. Familiarity with existing guidelines is an essential element in EBP. Guidelines from the AGS[4,14] are specific to the older adult, whereas guidelines from the ADA are specific to the individual with diabetes. The AMDA guidelines focus on the LTC resident.[3,15] The core recommendations are similar because the clinical experts who wrote the guidelines for their respective organizations are knowledgeable about the clinical recommendations in existence. The astute clinician who reviews recommendations from these three professional groups will recognize a number of common themes.

The first theme to emerge is the importance of individualizing diabetes treatment regimens and management goals. Traditionally, management goals include things such as premeal or postmeal glucose levels, A1C values, blood pressure levels, lipid levels, weight, and BMI. These important aspects of care have been addressed in the chapters on glycemic management (Chapter 5), monitoring (Chapter 11), and cardiovascular disease (Chapter 14). Management goals, however, also should include psychosocial factors, such as quality of life, and behavioral factors, such as those that dictate why or how we choose to consume particular foods or participate in various activities. More information on these essential aspects of care are provided in the chapters on self-care (Chapter 6), nutrition therapy (Chapter 7), and physical activity (Chapter 8). According to most guideline sources to date,[2-6] the actual definition of control will vary according to the particular resident and his or her needs. By definition, the older adult in LTC is more likely to be frail and have multiple comorbid conditions and geriatric syndromes. Whichever guideline is adopted, it is clear that the frail resident will be safer with an A1C goal of ≥8%.[16] Translating the meaning of the A1C to residents is often a little difficult. The plasma (or even capillary) glucose level is more familiar and, therefore, it is an easier number to think about. Residents as well as bedside caregivers might be more comfortable knowing the resident's average glucose level. A conversion calculator is available on the ADA website.[17] Performing a quick conversion when the laboratory results come in will provide clear information about the resident's overall glucose control level. For example when the A1C is 8%, the estimated average glucose (eAG) is 183 mg/dl. This is well above the level associated with hypoglycemia and well below the level associated with symptoms of hyperglycemia. Thinking about abnormally low or excessively high blood glucose levels takes us to the next common theme from practice guidelines: safety.

It is important to know what the resident's goal for glycemic control has been in the weeks and months leading up to admission into the nursing home. Optimal diabetes control in the general population is defined by an A1C level of ≤7%, depending on the individual's characteristics.[18] Some guidelines recommend an even lower target value of ≤6.5% for individuals without coexisting illness or risk of hypoglycemia.[19] As a result, some clinicians advise their patients to work toward achieving values in the near-normal (6%) range. The goal of this level of control is to prevent the development or delay the progression of common chronic complications of persistent hyperglycemia. In the frail elderly resident with diabetes, a common key clinical goal is to keep the individual safe from harm. It is important for clinicians to note that practice guidelines universally point out that hypoglycemia is the limiting factor to achieving normal or near-normal A1C values.[20] Therefore, there is a question of whether or not it is reasonable (and safe) to strive for near-normal glucose levels in an individual who is unlikely to realize the benefit of complication prevention. Take a look at an example: an A1C of 6% translates to an eAG level of 126 mg/dl,[17] which puts the resident at significant risk for hypoglycemia. In those with diabetes, particularly the elderly, hypoglycemia (low blood glucose level, <70 mg/dl) may occur with or without symptoms.[21–23] When the blood glucose level is too low, the resident is at risk for functional problems, such as falling, and may not be able to call for help. In an older adult, hypoglycemia easily can be mistaken for cognitive impairment. Be aware that the resident with hypoglycemia is also at risk for other, even more severe, physiologic problems. In an older adult with comorbid heart disease, low blood glucose can trigger an episode of angina or even precipitate a myocardial infarction.

At the other end of the spectrum, symptomatic hyperglycemia is a serious acute complication. Hyperglycemia, polyuria, polydipsia, and weight loss can affect the resident's sensorium. Progressive hyperglycemia can lead to profound dehydration, the hyperosmolar state, and even death. Thus, while keeping the elder safe from harm can mean keeping the A1C level in a range not lower than 8%, it also means preventing extreme hyperglycemia. The eAG level for an A1C level of 9% is 212 mg/dl. The best upper limits for glucose have yet to be identified, but it is clear that a focus of care should be on preventing symptomatic hyperglycemia.

The chapters on geriatric syndromes and diabetes (Chapter 4), medication management (Chapters 9 and 10), foot care (Chapter 12), visual impairment (Chapter 13), and care transitions (Chapter 15) are all concerned with aspects of safety. As you can see from the perspective of the medical director (Chapter 2) and the nursing home administrator (Chapter 3), diabetes treatment goals, safety, and quality of life are inextricably linked in the LTC setting.

Quality of life is a third common theme among the guidelines. More apparent in the guidelines from the AGS[4,14] than elsewhere is the notion that in the frail elder who has a limited life span, incorporating food or activities that improve the perceived quality of life reduces the burden of living with diabetes for the individual. For example, undernutrition with subsequent weight loss is a common concern affecting LTC residents. Overly restrictive diets are more likely than not to exacerbate the problems of weight loss and failure to thrive. In the area of nutritional management for diabetes in older adults, the evidence fails to support the use of therapeutic, prescribed diets. Chapter 7 makes a strong case for individualized, but liberalized, meal plans for residents of LTC who have diabetes. Clinicians are programmed to think about the importance of weight reduction in the management of T2D, but this may not be appropriate in the nursing home setting. Unplanned weight loss and subsequent failure to thrive are ongoing threats to all LTC residents. Those residents who can exercise some level of control over their daily food intake may be more likely to be satisfied and, perhaps, less likely to skip meals.

Commonalities in Guidelines
- Individualize treatment goals and management strategies
- Safety is critical
- Consider quality of life

THE CHANGING FACE OF DIABETES

One of the most striking observations about diabetes management in the past two decades is how quickly things have changed. Throughout the 20th century, the foundation of diabetes care was the clinical triad of diet, exercise, and medication. Monitoring and patient education were used to support these foundational aspects of care, but a strict approach to care still lingers in many settings, including the nursing home.

It has been 20 years since the results from the landmark Diabetes Control and Complications Trial so clearly demonstrated that improved control of diabetes reduced the risk for or progression of chronic complications in T1D,[24] and it has been nearly that long since the U.K. Progressive Diabetes Study illustrated the effect of improved diabetes control in patients with T2D.[25] These studies and those that have since been published have changed the way we think about diabetes management. We now know that well-controlled diabetes not only prevents or delays complications, we know that early control has long-lasting effects.[26-28] The individual with diabetes has taken center stage now that effective self-management is recognized as the key to success.

THE ROLE OF DIABETES EDUCATION IN LONG-TERM CARE

The role of the diabetes educator in facilitating successful self-management has been established. The focus of diabetes management has moved away from patient compliance with professional "orders" toward empowering the person with diabetes to be an informed, activated partner in care.[29–31] Diet, exercise, medication, and monitoring continue to form the foundation for diabetes management, but the definitions and components of each of these has changed. The American Association of Diabetes Educators (AADE) has translated the foundations of care into seven user-friendly elements. The AADE 7 self-care behaviors incorporate the initial four foundational components as healthy eating, being active, taking medication, and monitoring.[32] Three additional behaviors: healthy coping, problem solving, and reducing risks make up the balance of the AADE 7.[32] For the community-dwelling individual, diabetes care and education is aimed toward empowering the person with diabetes to successfully self-manage his or her condition. Although self-management never is a simple task, the goals for control are defined more easily in the population <60 years of age.

As we have seen throughout this book, diabetes management for the older adult with diabetes who resides in an LTC environment is complicated and not defined consistently. Until more evidence is available, it makes sense to develop a plan of care that focuses on preventing symptoms. Successful management needs to be defined by the team that includes the resident or the resident's family. Although labeled as "self-care" behaviors, it seems logical that the AADE 7 behaviors can apply to "assisted-care" as well. Research, however, is lacking in this area of care. Ideas for individualized institutional diabetes care for residents using components from the AADE 7 can be found in Table 16.1.

As you read in Chapter 7, the meal plan should not be calorie restricted. Rather, carbohydrate intake should be as consistent as possible and, importantly, residents should not skip meals. Care staff should learn how to count and record carbohydrate intake. Residents should maintain a healthy level of hydration. Hyperglycemia exacerbates dehydration. Staff can keep a water glass full and accessible to the resident and give reminders to residents to take a drink during regular rounds. Chapter 9 noted that diabetes medications should be administered correctly and on time. Because insulin is considered a high-risk drug, medication nurses should receive annual updates. It is particularly important for staff to understand the relationship between timing of insulin delivery and mealtimes. Residents taking insulin or insulin secretagogues are at risk for hypoglycemia, and the risk intensifies when nutritional intake is compromised. The institution must have a protocol for hypoglycemia management that is communicated clearly and applied consistently. Both Chapter 5 and Chapter 11 suggest the development of a reasonable plan for monitoring. Well-defined blood glucose and A1C targets should be identified, and these targets should be communicated clearly to all staff. The schedule for blood glucose monitoring should be modified during periods of acute illness. Blood glucose values should be recorded in the resident's medical record and regularly reviewed by the attending staff. A regular schedule for contact with residents should be established and observed. Direct care staff must have clear-cut guidelines on what to report, when, and to whom.

None of this can be done in a vacuum. Team-based care is the norm in the LTC setting and frequent turnover of the front-line staff is not uncommon.[33] To put individualized plans of care into place, it is important to have ongoing training for all staff, good communication among all care team members, stable assignments that allow front-line caregivers to know the residents well, structured handoffs that outline the plan of care and identify potential areas for concern,

Table 16.1 Aspects to Incorporate into an Assisted Management Plan

AADE 7 self-care behaviors	Institutional/staff responsibility	Resident and family responsibility	Joint responsibility
Healthy eating	Eliminate calorie restricted meal plans (in favor of consistent carbohydrates) Transport to dining room on time Train staff to count carbohydrates for/with resident Document intake Weigh (weekly or monthly)	Select healthy foods Never skip meals Know sources of carbohydrate	Determine need for diabetes education and/or nutrition consultation
Being active	Transport to activities on time Be prepared to recognize and treat hypoglycemia	Participate in regular physical activities whenever possible Report symptoms of hypoglycemia as soon as they occur	Determine need for diabetes education and/or therapy consultation Plan best time for activities (to prevent or avoid hypoglycemia)
Taking medication	Annual staff training: diabetes medication Deliver diabetes medication on time	Take diabetes medication on time in nursing home and when off site Communicate problems to staff	Maintain accurate list of routine, PRN, and OTC medications Determine need for diabetes education and/or pharmacist consultation
Monitoring	Perform CBG on time Maintain schedule of routine monitoring for complications	Assist with CBG when able	Negotiate and identify specific glycemic goals and optimal testing frequency Determine need for diabetes education
Healthy coping	Avoid negative language (e.g., "cheating on your diet") Assess for depression regularly	Be aware of symptoms of hypoglycemia and hyperglycemia Report them to the staff as soon as the symptoms are noticed	Determine need for diabetes education

Problem solving	Provide regular staff training in job-specific principles of diabetes care	Communicate problems to staff (e.g., difficulty seeing plantar surfaces of feet, changes in appetite)	Determine need for diabetes education Determine need for assistive devices, or regimen changes
Reducing risks	Eliminate sliding-scale insulin Develop a routine of regular rounds on all residents with diabetes Develop hypoglycemia protocol and train all staff in how to use Develop mechanism to identify all residents at risk for hypoglycemia Have treatment for hypoglycemia, (e.g., glucose gel available in multiple locations) Remind resident to drink sufficient quantities of fluid daily Examine feet monthly	Take medication on time Do not skip meals Consume sufficient fluids Request blood glucose test when unwell	Determine fall risk Implement plan to reduce risk of falling Determine time frame for highest risk of hypoglycemia Determine need for diabetes education

Note: AADE = American Association of Diabetes Educators; CBG = capillary blood glucose; OTC = over the counter; PRN = as needed.

and a system of documentation that conveys the resident's status to all involved in the patient's care.

In the LTC setting, diabetes education must target multiple populations. All members of the staff must be comfortable with basic diabetes management strategies and familiar with the goals of the institution.[34–38] The resident with diabetes must be sufficiently knowledgeable about diabetes self-care to follow a reasonable plan of care and to know if and when to ask for help. Staff members must have position-specific knowledge and information on all aspects of care related to diabetes. Consultant diabetes educators, staff or consultant dietitians, and staff or consultant pharmacists are good resources for the administrative and the direct care staff. Chapters 2 and 3 make the point that a diabetes resource person or champion is an excellent way to guide the staff in moving toward an evidence-based approach to diabetes care in the nursing home.

CONCLUSION

In all areas of health care, it is incumbent on each member of the team to practice to the highest level of his or her training and education. To do so, each team member must stay current and perform his or her job function safely and effectively. In LTC, this is true for the medical director, the nursing administrator, the charge nurse, the certified nursing assistant, the consultant pharmacist, and the dietitian as well as all others involved in the care of our most vulnerable patients. Core knowledge about the best EBP is a fundamental component of safe and effective care at all levels of practice.

This book provides a compendium of information about management of diabetes in the LTC population. Each chapter focused on a geriatric-specific topic or a particular aspect of care. Each author identified an evidence-based approach to their assigned topic. As the chapters unfolded, it became increasingly clear that the extent of evidence supporting diabetes care and management in the older adult is limited. The result of this project is a source book of what currently is known about aspects of diabetes management most relevant to caregivers in an LTC setting. This is not the end of the story. As our population continues to age and the prevalence of diabetes continues to grow, ongoing research into the care and management of the older adult with diabetes will become ever more important.

REFERENCES

1. American Geriatrics Society. AGS *Guidelines for improving the care of the older adult with diabetes mellitus: 2013 update*. New York, NY, Author, 2013.
2. American Diabetes Association. Standards of medical care in diabetes—2013. *Diabetes Care* 2013;36(Suppl1):S11–S66.
3. American Medical Directors Association. *Guidelines for diabetes management in the long-term care setting*. Columbia, MD, Author, 2010.
4. Brown AF, Mangione CM, Saliba D, Sarkisian CA, California Healthcare Foundation/American Geriatrics Society Panel on Improving Care for Older Persons with Diabetes. Guidelines for improving the care of the

older person with diabetes mellitus. *Journal of the American Geriatric Society* 2003;51(5):S265–S280.

5. Sinclair AJ, Paolisso G, Castro M, Bourdel-Marchasson I, Gadsby R, Rodriguez Mañas L. European Diabetes Working Party for Older People 2011 clinical guidelines for type 2 diabetes mellitus. Executive summary. *Diabetes an Metabolism* 2011;37(Suppl3)(0):S27–S38.

6. U.S. Department of Veterans Affairs/Department of Defense. Clinical practice guidelines: Management of diabetes mellitus in primary care, 2010. Available at www.healthquality.va.gov/Diabetes_Mellitus.asp. Accessed 31 October 2013.

7. DiCenso A, Guyatt G, Ciliska D. *Evidence based nursing: A guide to clinical practice*. St. Louis, MO, Elsevier Mosby, 2005.

8. Montori VM, Guyatt GH. Progress in evidence-based medicine. *Journal of the American Medical Association* 2008;300(15):1814–1816.

9. Ebel MH, Siwek J, Weiss BD, Woole SH, Susman J, Ewigman B, Bowman M. Strength of recommendation taxonomy (SORT): A patient centered approach to grading evidence in the medical literature. *American Family Physician* 2004 Feb 1;69(3):548–556.

10. Guyatt GH, Oxman AD, Kunz R, Vist GE, Falck-Ytter Y, Schunemann HJ, Group GW. What is "quality of evidence" and why is it important to clinicians? [Review]. *British Medical Journal* 2008;336(7651):995–998.

11. Guyatt GH, Oxman AD, Vist GE, Kunz R, Falck-Ytter Y, Alonso-Coello P, Group GW. GRADE: An emerging consensus on rating quality of evidence and strength of recommendations. *British Medical Journal* 2008;336(7650):924–926.

12. Kirkman MS, Briscoe VJ, Clark N, Florez H, Haas LB, Halter JB, . . . Swift CS. Diabetes in older adults. *Diabetes Care* 2012;35(12):2650–2664.

13. Kirkman MS, Briscoe VJ, Clark N, Florez H, Haas LB, Halter JB, . . . Swift CS. Diabetes in older adults: A consensus report. *Journal of the American Geriatrics Society* 2012;60(12):2342–2356.

14. American Geriatrics Society Expert Panel on the Care of Older Adults with Multimorbidity. Guiding principles for the care of older adults with multimorbidity: An approach for clinicians. *Journal of the American Geriatrics Society* 2012;60(10):E1–E25.

15. American Medical Directors Association. *Guidelines for Diabetes Management in the Long-Term Care Setting: Clinical practice guideline*. Columbia, MD, AMDA, 2008, p. 1–42.

16. Yau CK, Eng C, Cenzer IS, John Boscardin W, Rice-Trumble K, Lee SJ. Glycosylated hemoglobin and functional decline in community-dwelling nursing home-eligible elderly adults with diabetes mellitus. *Journal of the American Geriatrics Society* 2012;60(7):1215–1221.

17. American Diabetes Association. A1C and eAG. Available at www.diabetes.org/living-with-diabetes/treatment-and-care/blood-glucose-control/a1c. Accessed 31 October 2013.

18. American DiabetesAssociation. Standards of medical care diabetes—2014. *Diabetes Care* 2014;37(Suppl1):S14–S80.

19. Garber A, Abrahamson M, Barzilay J, Blonde L, Bloomgarden Z, Bush M, . . . Davidson M. American Association of Clinical Endocrinologists'

comprehensive diabetes management algorithm 2013 consensus statement. *Endocrine Practice* 2013;19(0):1–48.

20. Davis S, Alonso MD. Hypoglycemia as a barrier to glycemic control. *Journal of Diabetes Complications* 2004;18(1):60–68.

21. Bremer JP, Jauch-Chara K, Hallschmid M, Schmid S, Schultes B. Hypoglycemia unawareness in older compared with middle-aged patients with type 2 diabetes. *Diabetes Care* 2009;32(8):1513–1517.

22. Briscoe VJ, Davis SN. Hypoglycemia in type 1 and type 2 diabetes: Physiology, pathophysiology, and management. *Clinical Diabetes* 2006;24(3):115–121.

23. Chelliah A, Burge MR. Hypoglycaemia in elderly patients with diabetes mellitus: causes and strategies for prevention. *Drugs and Aging* 2004;21(8):511–530.

24. The Diabetes Control and Complications Trial Research Group. The effect of intensive treatment of diabetes on the development and progression of long term complications in insulin-dependent diabetes mellitus. *New England Journal of Medicine* 1993;329:997–986.

25. U.K. Progressive Diabetes Study (UKPDS) Group. Intensive blood glucose control with sulfonylureas or insulin compared with conventional treatment and risk of complications in patients with type 2 diabetes (UKPDS 33). *Lancet* 1998;352(9131):837–853.

26. Albers JW, Herman WH, Pop-Busui R, Feldman EL, Martin CL, Cleary PA, . . . Complications Research Group. Effect of prior intensive insulin treatment during the Diabetes Control and Complications Trial (DCCT) on peripheral neuropathy in type 1 diabetes during the Epidemiology of Diabetes Interventions and Complications (EDIC) Study. [Research Support, N.I.H., Extramural Research Support, Non-U.S. Gov't]. Diabetes Care 2010;33(5):1090–1096.

27. The Diabetes Control and Complications Trial/Epidemiology of Diabetes Interventions and Complications Research Group (EDIC). Retinopathy and nephropathy in patients with type 1 diabetes four years after a trial of intensive therapy. *New England Journal of Medicine* 2000;342(6):381–389.

28. White NH, Sun W, Cleary PA, Tamborlane WV, Danis RP, Hainsworth DP, DCCT-EDIC Research Group. Effect of prior intensive therapy in type 1 diabetes on 10-year progression of retinopathy in the DCCT/EDIC: Comparison of adults and adolescents. [Research Support, N.I.H., Extramural]. *Diabetes* 2010;59(5):1244–1253.

29. Bodenheimer T, Wagner EH, Grumbach K. Improving primary care for patients with chronic illness. *Journal of the American Medical Association* 2002;288(14):1775–1779.

30. Piatt GA, Orchard TJ, Emerson S, Simmons D, Songer TJ, Brooks MM, . . . Zgibor JC. Translating the chronic care model into the community. *Diabetes Care* 2006;29(4):811–817.

31. Siminerio LM, Piatt G, Zgibor JC. Implementing the chronic care model for improvements in diabetes care and education in a rural primary care practice. *Diabetes Educator* 2005;31(2):225–234.

32. Peeples M, Tomky D, Mulcahy K, Peyrot M, Siminerio L, on behalf of AADE Outcomes Project AADE/UMPC Diabetes Education Outcomes Project. AADE7™ Self-care behaviors: Evolution of the American Association of

Diabetes Educators' diabetes education outcomes project. *Diabetes Educator* 2008;34(3):445–449.

33. Harrington C, Swan JH. Nursing home staffing, turnover, and case mix. [Research Support, Non-U.S. Gov't]. *Medical Care Research and Review* 2003;60(3):366–392; discussion 393–369.

34. Allsworth JE, Toppa R, Palin NC, Lapane KL. For the patient. Many nursing home patients do not receive diabetes medicine. [Comparative study patient education handout]. *Ethnicity and Disease* 2005;15(2):351.

35. Douek IF, Bowman C, Croxson S. A survey of diabetes management in nursing homes: the need for whole systems of care. *Practical Diabetes International* 2001;18(5):152–154.

36. Feldman SM, Rosen R, DeStasio J. Status of diabetes management in the nursing home setting in 2008: A retrospective chart review and epidemiology study of diabetic nursing home residents and nursing home initiatives in diabetes management. *Journal of the American Medical Directors Association* 2009;10(5):354–360.

37. Maas ML, Specht JP, Buckwalter KC, Gittler J, Bechen K. Nursing home staffing and training recommendations for promoting older adults' quality of care and life: Part 1. Deficits in the quality of care due to understaffing and undertraining. [Research Support, Non-U.S. Gov't Review]. *Research in Gerontological Nursing* 2008;1(2):123–133.

38. Maas ML, Specht JP, Buckwalter KC, Gittler J, Bechen K. Nursing home staffing and training recommendations for promoting older adults' quality of care and life: Part 2. Increasing nurse staffing and training. [Research Support, Non-U.S. Gov't Review]. *Research in Gerontological Nursing* 2008;1(2):134–152.

Index